Recent Results in Cancer Research 108

Recent Results in Cancer Research

Volume 98: Perioperative Chemotherapy
Edited by U. Metzger, F. Largiadèr, H.-J. Senn
1985. 48 figures, 45 tables. XII, 157. ISBN 3-540-15124-9

Volume 99: Peptide Hormones in Lung Cancer
Edited by K. Havemann, G. Sorenson, C. Gropp
1985. 100 figures, 63 tables. XII, 248. ISBN 3-540-15504-X

Volume 100: Therapeutic Strategies in Primary and Metastatic Liver Cancer
Edited by Ch. Herfarth, P. Schlag, P. Hohenberger
1986. 163 figures, 104 tables. ISBN 3-540-16011-6

Volume 101: Locoregional High-Frequency Hyperthermia and Temperature Measurement
Edited by G. Bruggmoser, W. Hinkelbein, R. Engelhardt, M. Wannenmacher
1986. 96 figures, 8 tables. IX, 143. ISBN 3-540-15501-5

Volume 102: Epidemiology of Malignant Melanoma
Edited by R. P. Gallagher
1986. 15 figures, 70 tables. IX, 169. ISBN 3-540-16020-5

Volume 103: Preoperative (Neoadjuvant) Chemotherapy
Edited by J. Ragaz, P. R. Band, J. H. Goldie
1986. 58 figures, 49 tables. IX, 162. ISBN 3-540-16129-5

Volume 104: Hyperthermia and the Therapy of Malignant Tumors
Edited by C. Streffer
1987. 52 figures, 63 tables. IX, 207. ISBN 3-540-17250-5

Volume 105: Breast Cancer
Edited by S. Brünner and B. Langfeldt
1987. 59 figures, 43 tables. IX, 132. ISBN 3-540-17301-3

Volume 106: Minimal Neoplasia
Edited by E. Grundmann and L. Beck
1988. 82 figures, 61 tables. IX, 194. ISBN 3-540-18455-4

Volume 107: Application of Hyperthermia in the Treatment of Cancer
Edited by R. D. Issels and W. Wilmanns
1988. 118 figures, 56 tables. XII, 277. ISBN 3-540-18486-4

H.-J. Senn A. Glaus L. Schmid (Eds.)

Supportive Care in Cancer Patients

With 60 Figures and 97 Tables

Springer-Verlag
Berlin Heidelberg New York
London Paris Tokyo

Professor Dr. Hans-Jörg Senn
Oberschwester Agnes Glaus
Dr. Luzius Schmid

Medizinische Klinik C, Kantonsspital St. Gallen
9007 St. Gallen, Switzerland

ISBN-13:978-3-642-82934-5 e-ISBN-13:978-3-642-82932-1
DOI: 10.1007/978-3-642-82932-1

Library of Congress Cataloging-in-Publication Data
Supportive care in cancer patients/H.-J. Senn, A. Glaus, L. Schmid (eds.).
p. cm. - (Recent results in cancer research; 108) Includes index.
ISBN-13:978-3-642-82934-5 (U.S.)
1. Cancer-Palliative treatment. 2. Cancer-Patients-Rehabilitation. 3. Cancer pain-Treatment. 4. Cancer-Complications and sequelae-Treatment. I. Senn, Hansjörg. II. Glaus, A. III. Schmid, L. IV. Series.
[DNLM: 1. Neoplasms-therapy. W1 RE106P v. 108 / QZ 266 S9588]
RC261.R35 vol. 108 [RC271.P33] 616.99'4 s-dc 19 [616.994'4]
DNLM/DLC 88-4496

Softcover reprint of the hardcover 1st edition 1988

2125/3140-543210

Preface

The symposium on supportive care in cancer patients, which took place in St. Gallen, Switzerland, on February 18–21, 1987, welcomed renowned experts in the field and more than 600 participants from 25 countries with the aim of stimulating discussion on how to improve our professional skills and personal attitudes toward cancer patients in all stages of their disease. Why did we organize such a symposium on supportive care in cancer patients? Recent decades have witnessed remarkable success in cancer treatment, and we have learned how to cure a finite number of neoplastic diseases. Some malignant tumors that previously entailed high fatality rates, such as leukemias, lymphomas, and testicular cancers, can now be cured, even when at an advanced stage. Yet it seems to many that our struggle to improve results and to fight death from cancer has also imposed greater toxicity on patients. Conventional scientifically based oncology has only recently made adequate efforts to improve the subjective quality of life of cancer patients, for example through prophylaxis against emesis, nausea, and scalp hypothermia, pain control and the development of psychosocial support structures. The search for less toxic and yet equally effective treatment measures has not been one of our primary goals in the past.

Supportive care has always been part of nurses' professional aim, even though many have not known how best to offer it. The title and scope of this symposium was apparently still less attractive to physicians. This is reflected by the fact that two-thirds of the participants were nurses and other health care professionals, and barely one-third physicians. But we can at least state that those physicians who took part really understand what supportive care means and therefore are surely the very best in their profession!

The contribution of nonphysicians in the area of supportive care should not be underestimated. Participants at this conference shared their experiences from different perspectives and with different styles. They described not only what they do, but also what they are. I am glad that along with sessions for nurses and sessions for physicians we also offered joint sessions where nurses were able to learn from doctors and doctors from nurses.

Such thoughts lead to the question: "Who is the most important supporter for cancer patients?" This conference brought together nurses, physicians, social workers, psychologists, and fortunately also some clergymen. Different experts in supportive care from various fields consider themselves or at least their professional colleagues to be the true provider of support to the patient. Is the most important person the one who fights bleeding and infection? The one who tries to manage treatment side effects? The one who most successfully fights cancer pain? The one who best provides terminal care? Or the one who skillfully offers psychosocial support? In preparing this conference we realized that supportive care in cancer patients is a very extensive and holistic affair. Every one of the mentioned topics is a part of it. Full support can only be successful if it is comprehensive in its basic approach and if it starts at the time of prevention and proceeds through diagnosis, treatment, and terminal care. Supportive care will, however, involve different goals and aspects in different stages of the disease, from diagnosis to life or to death.

Today, at least in Europe, we also have to face sociomedical attitudes in our society which attack "conventional" medicine, and especially oncology, as being an inhuman, science-oriented system. There is a demand for "human, nontoxic, soft, alternative" medicine. If we truly learn to be more supportive - without compromising treatment effectiveness - our practice will correspond more closely to such desires. Patients will feel the effect of our efforts not only in their battle against cancer but also on their whole personality. Supportive care also includes the support of the care givers. Many of the topics raised at this conference touched on ourselves and hopefully also provided personal and professional support.

St. Gallen, March 1988

H. J. Senn
A. Glaus
L. Schmid

Contents

*List of Contributors**

* The address of the principal author is given on the first page of each contribution.

[1] Page on which contribution begins.

Management of Cancer Pain

Differential Diagnosis of Pain in Cancer Patients

R. H. Adler and C. Hürny

Medizinische Abteilung, C. G. Lory Haus, Inselspital, Universität Bern,
3010 Bern, Switzerland

Defintion of the Problem

Pain in cancer inpatients is due to the underlying disease in 78%, is caused by or associated with cancer therapy in 19%, and is due to other medical conditions in 3%. The corresponding figures for outpatients are 65%, 25%, and 10% [1,2]. Although the pain is of somatic origin in most cases, it is nevertheless important to establish an exact diagnosis of the pain in the individual patient because this will determine the therapeutic approach. Coping with the cancer diagnosis is a difficult task for the patient. Therefore it is no surprise that psychic decompensation may occur, leading to a contribution of psychological factors to organically determined pain or to psychogenic pain.

A further problem is the question of whether the pain which initially leads the patients to a physican is of somatic origin (perhaps due to a hidden malignancy or a metastasis) or ist "only" psychogenic. Which physician does not know patients in whom pain was assumed to be psychogenic in origin because of a lack of organic findings but later proved to be of malignant somatic origin?

Table 1 shows possible diagnostic categories of pain in cancer patients.

Table 1. Diagnostic categories of pain in cancer patients

1. Pain due to tumour infiltration/compression
2. Pain associated with cancer treatment
a) Surgery
b) Chemotherapy
c) Radiation therapy
3. Pain of organic origin other than cancer
4. Pain of organic origin enhanced by psychosocial factors
5. Psychogenic pain
a) Conversion
b) Psychophysiological (fight-flight)

Recent Results in Cancer Research, Vol. 108

Table 2. The seven dimensions of the symptom pain

1. Bodily location: Where is the symptom located?
2. Quality: What is it like?
3. Quantitiy: How intense is it?
4. Chronology: When did the symptom begin and what course has it followed?
5. Setting: Under what circumstances does it take place?
6. Aggravating and alleviating factors: What makes it worse or better?
7. Associated manifestations: What other symptoms or phenomena are associated with it?

Establishment of the Diagnosis

The exact diagnosis is made by means of a thorough anamnesis with an appropriate technique which allows the physician to obtain biological, psychological, and social data at once and to understand the meaning of these data in the biographical context of the individual patient. During the interview, the physician follows the patient's associations and only asks more specific questions when he needs more precise information; that is, information not given spontaneously by the patient in response to open-ended questions. Practical advice regarding application of this interview technique is available both in English (Morgan and Engel [3]) and in German (Adler and Hemmeler [4]).

The part of the interview dealing with the present illness needs special attention. Each symptom - including pain - has seven dimensions. The symptom "pain" must be analyzed wih respect to its "localization," "quality," "quantitiy," "time," "accompanying symptoms," "aggravating/alleviating factors," and "the circumstances" in which it appears, is present, or disappears (Table 2).

The comprehension of these dimensions is of vital importance, and essential in determining whether we deal with somatic pain - where psychogenic factors play an important role - or with psychogenic pain.

A reliable diagnosis is certainly not established by exclusion of a somatic disorder. As mentioned above, not being able to find a somatic explanation does not prove that the pain is psychogenic.

Differential Diagnostics

Organic Pain of Neoplastic Origin

Organic pain of neoplastic origin is typically described by the patient in matter-of-fact, simple language and without use of any medical terms. The pain is well localized, its irradiation is well defined, and it conforms to anatomical structures. Its presence and worsening are not influenced by the presence of family or friends. The accompanying symptoms are limited in number. The interviewer is able to listen carefully, with composure and is not confused, irritated, impatient, or bored.

Organic pain is dependent - with respect to intensity and quality - on the patient's voluntary motor activity. This is an important phenomenon that requires special attention.

Clinical examples: A 70-year-old retired worker on a steamboat had received a total right hip prosthesis 1 year prior to evaluation. Six months later he fell on that hip and subsequently began to complain of hip pain, at first perodically, later constantly. Several X-rays taken over a period of 4 months showed an intact prosthesis. The pain, however, became so severe that the patient had to be hospitalized for 3 months and was seen in consultation by a neurologist, a rheumatologist, an orthopedic surgeon, and finally by a neurosurgeon who diagnosed a pain syndrome most likely to be of a psychogenic nature. During the interview the patient complained of constant severe pain. When asked whether he had observed a movement which would regularly increase or diminish his pain, he described how his pain had suddenly disappeared when he was seated in the car for the 40-mile ride to this hospital with his right thigh slightly externally rotated and then abruptly came back while passing trough a village 10 miles from the hospital after he changed the position of his right leg. Review of the X-rays revealed an intact prosthesis, but the comparison between the bone structures surrounding the prosthesis and the left pelvic area suggested a slightly more pronounced radiolucency on the right side. A needle biopsy revealed metastic carcinoma which was confirmed 2 months later at autopsy.

A 32-year-olt Sports teacher had suffered continuously from pain in the right foot for the past 4 years. Diagnostic tests, including X-rays and an electroneurogram to exclude a tarsal tunnel syndrome, were normal. Finally the patient entered psychotherapy where he made great progress, but without any pain reduction. After the 4 years, the orthopedic surgeon who works with us in the pain clinic was told by the patient that he had originally felt the pain only when walking on his right heel and not when walking on the ball of his foot. Later, walking on the ball of the foot became painful as well. When lying down, the pain always disappeared in the beginning. The physician intensified the diagnostic tests; electroneurography of the lateral side of the foot showed denervation potentials, computerized tomography of the foot showed infiltration of the aponeurosis, and operation yielded a malignant synovioma.

The explanation of this phenomenon, the dependence of organic pain on voluntary motor activity, has already been discussed elsewhere [7].

Symptoms which turn out to be of a somatic nature are usually characterized by a change in their intensity when the patient changes his body position, and by the ability of the patient to describe this to his physician, providing the latter gives him the opportunity to do so by means of openended questions. Pains of a psychogenic nature lack this relationship; they follow other laws [5, 6, 8]. Patients with psychogenic pains sometimes also describe pains which change when there is a change in motoric behavior, but the correlation is vague, highly variable, and inconsistent upon repeated description. Patients can even suffer from organic pain upon which a psychogenic pain is superposed, e.g., angina and pseudo-angina pectoris. The former is correlated with characteristic motoric behaviors, e.g., exertion, while the latter's dependence on activity is vague and inconsistent.

These observations raise the question of how one can recognize whether a perception is derived from within the psychic apparatus of the patient or from his body or its environment. Freud states in *The Metapsychological Supplement to the Theory of Dreams* and in *Instincts and Their Vicissitudes* [9, 10] that an organism interprets a perception as an external and as a real one if that organism can make it disappear by means of motoric action, while the organism must interpret a perception as originating internally if it cannot be altered by such an action. This statement can be clarified by means of analogies: If we perceive something which seems to us to be unbelievable, we close our eyes (make the perception disappear by motoric action) and take a second look in order to make sure it is real. A patient in an intensive care unit who is motorically restrained may lose his ability to differentiate perceptions originating in his environment from those originating intrapsychically; eventually he begins to hallucinate. When dreaming we can experience a perception as real, e.g., falling or running while we are actually not moving. When we consider that one of the characteristics of dreaming is the blocked motoric activity (which contributes to our inability to judge the perceptions as originating intrapsychically), we understand why one of the outstanding features of pain of organic origin must be its correaltion with the motoric behavior of the patient. We should also begin to suspect that the substrates of dream formation and of psychogenic symptoms might be similar (which they actually are) [9, 10].

On the other hand one should bear in mind that overly cautious and scant administration of analgesics to patients with pain due to cancer leads to many differential diagnostic considerations that would not be necessary if the dosis were accurate.

Organic Pain of Nonmalignant Origin

The characteristics of organic pain of nonmalignant origin are the same as those described for organic pain of neoplastic origin.

Clinical example: A 66-year-old female federal officer who retired 4 years ago was admitted to the pain clinic because of chronic backaches. In March 1984, after lifting the bed mattress, the pain suddenly appeared, and since then lumbar pains which spread into the left dorsal aspect of the thigh have persisted. The X-rays showed a compression fracture of the second lumbar vertebral body, in April 1984 impressions of the cortex of the 12th thoracic and 1st lumbar vertebrae, in July 1984 an additional fish vertebra deformation of the 5th lumbar vertebra, and finally in November 1984 a fracture of the right pubic bone. Since 1962 the patient had been suffering from repeated urinary tract infections and from a slight chronic renal insufficiency due to bilateral chronic interstitial nephritis. In April 1983 she underwent a partial resection of an ovarian carcinoma metastatic to the peritoneum. Since then the patient has been treated with 5-fluorouracil and Cytoxan. At the moment she is in complete remission. No tumor manifestations can be found using noninvasive diagnostic methods. The laboratory findings are normal except for a slightly increased alkaline phosphatase and restricted kidney function.

Bone biopsy shows simply osteopenia and no signs of osteomalacia or tumour infiltration. Treatment with calcium, vitamin D and sodium fluoride yielded a normalization of the alkaline phosphatase; no new fractures appeared and the backaches diminished. The reason for the pain is an involutional osteoporosis. The ovarian carcinoma was not responsible for the backaches.

Differential diagnosis between pain of neoplastic origin and, as in this case, pain of nonneoplastic origin is often difficult but is of major importance as it affects treatment.

Organic Pain to Which Psychogenic Factors Contribute

Psychogenic factors can also increase organic pain due to cancer. Insecurity, anxiety, and social isolation may be contributing factors. Adequate disclosure of information about diagnosis, prognosis, and treatment plans, a solid working alliance with the physician, and mutual trust diminish it.

Clinical example: A 56-year-old housewife who underwent surgery for breast cancer 7 years previously was treated with combined chemotherapy for 8 months after she developed generalized bone metastases. The strong pains in the pelvic region showed only slight regression, although the initially osteolytic metastases were sclerosing progressively.

It occured to the physician that the patient opened each report of the medical findings when returning from the X-ray examinations. She did so although the doctor always explained the new results to her fully. Asked why she repeatedly did this, she showed shame and reluctantly confessed that she cannot trust doctors. Only much later did the physician learn the following: the gynecologist who had operated on her previously had told her that if no metastases appeared in the subsequent 5 years she could consider herself cured. Five years and several months following the mastectomy, back pains appeared and bone metastases were discovered. The forecast of the operating physician proved wrong and led to deep insecurity in the patient. Continuous fear aggravated the pains caused by tumour infiltration. The clarification of the problem alleviated the pains markedly.

Pain of Psychophysiological Origin

Pains which also have to be considered are muscle tension pains in the head, jaw, shoulders, neck and thorax as accompanying signs of the "fligh-fight" state. The patients show fright and/or rage and the somatic correlates such as perspiration, palpitation of the heart, and tremor.

Clinical example: A 36-year-old secretary was sent for diagnostic clarification of thoracic pains 2 years after curative treatment of Hodgkin's disease stage IIB. Since the completion of her treatment the patient had felt pressure-like pains - independent of strain and movement - in the right anterior thorax. Simultaneously with the thoracic pains, she experienced paresthesia in the face and in the left arm. She was breathing with sighs, appeared discouraged and agitated, developed insomnia, felt tired even in the morning, had trouble concentrating, and lost her joy in living. As treatment was completed, her partner moved out, the patient began working part-time as a secretary, and with the responsibility for her two young children she felt constantly overburdened and exhausted.

In the case of this secretary with reactive depression, the thoracic pains have to be considered as a symptom of chronic hyperventilation, which is confirmed by a low PCO_2 and otherwise normal arterial blood gases.

Psychogenic Pain Due to Conversion

If an individual gets into a conflictual situation with which for psychic reasons he cannot cope, he might repress parts of the conflict and feelings that arose through the conflict and instead suffer from somatic symptoms. He expresses that part of the conflict which is not in harmony with his conscience and the tendency suppressing the conflict through body language. The suppressive tendency originates in the ethical and moral background of the patient's personality. The resulting symptom thus neutralizes the conflict. For those who are not familiar with the psychodynamics of conversion, analogies can help one to understand the process. Physical reactions in dreams - such as an escape or a fall - are intrapsychic events which are experienced physically. In the game called "charades" the performer expresses a notion physically and the spectator must guess which notion is expressed

Table 3. Conversion pain. (Adler and Hemmeler 1986)

Confirmatory criteria:
Intrapsychic conflict anteceding pain onset
"Choice" of the symptom pain in relation to conflict
Localization of the symptom pain in relation to conflict
Neutralization of the conflict (belle-indifférence)
- Primary gain
- Secondary gain
Additional nonspecific criteria:
Dramatic but vague symptom description
Symptoms not corresponding to anatomical and physiological conditions
Multiple disturbances, work-ups, and operations without clear-cut indication in the past
Egocentricity, lability, eccentricity, vanity, demanding dependency
Unstable relationships
Substance abuse
Suicide attempts

by the physical action; the performer corresponds to the patient, the spectator to the physician. The difference between conversion and charades is the following: the patient does not know which notion is expressed through body language - since the notion is unconscious - whereas the performer is conscious of the notion he expresses.

The conversion partially expresses a wish - usually of an aggressive nature - in the form of pain but at the same time punishes the individual for it, protects him from the conflict becoming conscious, and establishes novel possibilities of relationship to his surroundings.

The diagnosis "conversion" is only valid if (see Table 3):

1. The main characteristics of the conflict can be tracked from the patient's statements
2. The conflict is connected with the beginning of the symptoms.
3. The choice of the symptom "pain" can be explained as well as the choice of the pain localization
4. The secondary gain from the symptom can be established

Clinical example: One year after mastectomy of the right breast (carcinoma stage $T_2N_0M_0$) a 42-year-old waitress was sent to the oncology clinic for further treatment because of bone metastases. Four months before, lumbar pains had appeared, irradiating into the left leg. Bone scintigraphy suggested the possible presence of metastases in the lumbar vertebrae and in the sacrum. The laboratory findings were normal. Based on radiological evidence of osteolytic metastases, radiomenolysis and pain irradiation were carried out without success. During the examination in the clinic the patient complained of constant pains in the back and left leg. No aggravating or alleviating factors could be detected. The patient was not able to describe the exact localization. She complained about the symptoms in a dramatic way. While speaking about her intense pains, she remained affectively uninvolved and smiled in a strange manner ("belle-indifférence").

During the following consultations the physician learned that the patient brought her disabled husband to physical therapy on the day her pain began. The husband, an alcoholic, was unable to work because of chronic back pain after several laminectomies, and had to be cared for by the patient.

The vague pain description, the belle-indifférence, and the preceding conflict (unconscious, forbidden rage against the sick husband) which is both expressed and neutralized by the back pains allow the diagnosis of "conversion." A new evaluation of the X-rays identified the suspected osteolytic lesions in the lumbar vertebrae as actually being superimposed intestinal gas.

The above-mentioned confirming criteria are identical with those in DSM III, with the exception that the definition in DSM III does not demand explanations for the choice of symptoms and localization. If the listed criteria are strictly applied, the diagnosis will be reliable [5, 6, 8] and there is no reason to fear that an organic disease could be missed.

Individuals who are predisposed to develop conversion symptoms often describe their complaints in a colorful, dramatic, unspecified way. The complaints do not fit into anatomical or physiological concepts. In the patient's past many disturbances, diagnostic procedures, and interventions are found; however, their indications are not clear. Patients are often self-centered, psychologically unstable, vain, demanding and dependent, have superficial relationships and sexual problems, and tend toward drug abuse, suicide attempts, and depressive moods. The observed emotional state during the description of the pain does not correlate with the content of the patient's descriptions (belle-indifférence). The language is mostly pseudointelligent, bombastic, and full of medical terms. While listening to the patient, the interviewer feels confused, bored, irritated, and frustrated (countertransference) [11].

All these criteria are not confirmatory however. There are individuals with less pathological personality traits who might suddenly develop conversion symptoms under stress, whereas others with the above-mentioned characteristics might get an organic disease.

Summary

The differential diagnosis of pain in cancer patients and in patients in whom cancer is suspected can be best attained using a technique of anamnesis that

1. Follows the associations of the patient
2. Accepts biological, psychological, and social factors without prejudice
3. Comprehends the symptom "pain" in its seven dimensions

The list of possible pains includes pain of neoplastic origin, pain due to cancer therapy, somatic pain of nonneoplastic origin, cancer pain increased by psychic factors, and psychogenic pain. The last category includes pain due to conversion and pain as an accompanying sign of the "flight-fight" reaction.

References

1. Foley KM (1979) The management of pain of malignant origin. In: Tyler HR, Dawson DM (eds) Current neurology, vol 2. Houghton-Mifflin, Boston, pp 279-302
2. Kanner RK, Foley KM (1980) Patterns of narcotic drug use in a cancer pain clinic. Ann NY Acad Sci 362: 161-172
3. Morgan WA Jr, Engel GL (1968) The clinical approach to the Patient. Saunders, Philadelphia
4. Adler R, Hemmeler W (1986) Praxis und Theorie der Anamnese. Der Zugang zu den biologischen, psychischen und sozialen Aspekten des Kranken. Fischer, Stuttgart
5. Drossman DA (1982) Patients with psychogenic abdominal pain: six year's observation in the medical setting. Am J Psychiatry 193: 1549-1557
6. Sauvant JD, Hürny C, Hemmeler W, Adler RH (1986) The reliability in time of the diagnosis of psychogenic pain: a five year follow-up study. Submitted for publication.
7. Adler RH (1981) The differentiation of organic and psychogenic pain. Pain 10: 249-252
8. Engel GL (1970) Conversion symptoms. In: MacBryde CM (ed) Signs und symptoms. Applied physiology and clinical interpretation, 5th edn. Lippincott, Philadelphia, pp 650-668
9. Freud S (1957) The metapsychological supplement to the theory of dreams, SE XIV, Hogarth, London, pp 217-237
10. Freud S (1957) Instincts and their vicissitudes, SE XIV. Hogarth, London, pp 109-140
11. Adler R (1987) Psychosomatische, diagnostische und therapeutische Überlegungen zum Gesichtsschmerz. In: Bergener M, Herzmann C (eds) Das Schmerz-Syndrom - eine interdisziplinäre Aufgabe. VCH, Weinheim, pp 169-177

Optimal Pharmacological Control of Chronic Cancer Pain

R. G. Twycross

Sir Michael Sobell House, The Churchill Hospital, Old Road, Headington,
Oxford OX3 7LJ, Great Britain

From a pharmacological point of view, pain in cancer falls into three categories:

1. Opioid non-responsive pains
2. Opioid responsive pains - but do *not* use opioids
3. Opioid responsive pains - do use opioids

The term "opioid responsive pain" is used as shorthand to describe pains that respond increasingly well to increasingly powerful analgesics. In other words, if pains is moderately severe, it responds to codeine; if very severe, to morphine.

Sometimes, there is overlap between the three categories. Metastatic bone and nerve compression pains, for example, are best considered partially responsive to opioids. The purpose of the classification is, however, to remind doctors that opioids are of limited value for certain pains, and that sometimes they are of no value at all (Table 1).

Table 1. Types of pain and implications for treatment [12]

Type of pain	Treatment	
Somatic (nociceptive)		
Muscle spasm	Physical therapy Diazepam Non-opioid analgesics	
Tissue distortion	Analgesics	
Nerve compression	Analgesics Corticosteroids Nerve blocks	
Deafferentation (nerve destruction)	Antidepressants Anticonvulsants	
	Opioids Corticosteroids Nerve blocks Cordotomy	If peripheral nerve lesion occasionally useful; if spinal cord lesion of no benefit

Recent Results in Cancer Research, Vol. 108

Opioid Non-responsive Pains

Muscle Pain

Muscle spasm pain secondary to underlying bone pain and/or skeletal deformity is common in cancer patients. So are myofascial trigger point (TP) related pains [7]. Treatment consists of explanation, physical therapies (local heat and massage), diazepam and relaxation therapy, and injection of TPs with local anaesthetic and a corticoid (e.g. bupivacaine and depot methylprednisolone). However severe, *morphine is not indicated for muscle spasm and TP pains.*

Bone Pain

Pain caused by bone metastases is ofen only partially opioid responsive. Best results are usually obtained wih a combination of aspirin, or an alternative non-steroidal anti-inflammatory drug (NSAID), and morphine. Many osseous metastases produce a prostaglandin (PG) which causes osteolysis [2]. The PG also lowers the "peripheral pain threshold" by sensitizing the nerve endings [1]. Aspirin and other NSAIDs inhibit the synthesis of PGs and thereby alleviate pain. Radiotherapy should, of course, be used if feasible. This often totally relieves the pain and makes the continued use of analgesics unnecessary.

Nerve Compression Pain

Neuralgic pain is often not controlled by morphine alone. In this circumstance, a corticoid should be prescribed (e.g. dexamethasone 4 mg daily b.i.d.). A marked improvement is often seen within 48 h. If the nerve compression relates to an identifiable bone metastasis or soft tissue mass, radiotherapy should be considered. For patients who do not respond adequately to the combined use of morphine and dexamethasone, a neurolytic or neuro-ablative procedure may have to be considered.

Other Corticoid Responsive Pains

A corticoid should be considered as a "co-analgesic" whenever there is a large tumour mass within a relatively confined space, e.g. nerve and spinal cord compression, certain head and neck cancers, and headache caused by raised intracranial pressure. A tumour is often surrounded by an area of inflammation; and pressure on neighbouring veins and lymphatics may lead to further local or regional swelling. Corticoids reduce the inflammation and thereby reduce the total tumour mass (Fig. 1).

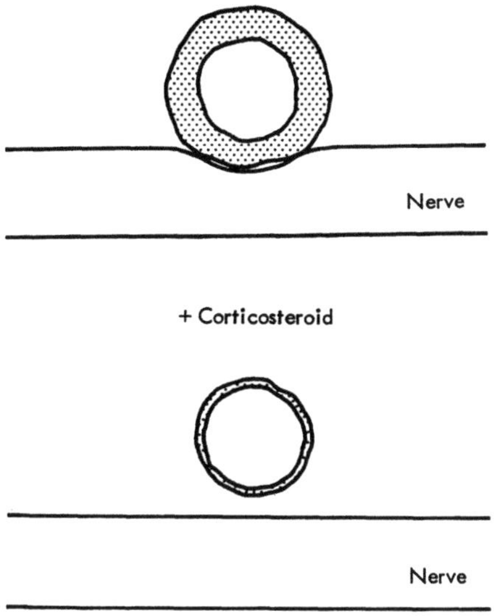

Fig. 1. Presumed mechanism of action of corticoids in relief of nerve compression pain. Total tumour mass = neoplasm + surrounding hyperaemic oedematous tissue. General anti-inflammatory effect of corticoid reduces total tumour mass, resulting in reduction of pain [9]

Deafferentation Pain

Deafferentation pain is associated with nerve destruction. In cancer, it usually results from infiltration of a nerve by the malignancy. The pain is superficial and burning in character, and dermatomal in distribution. There is often associated allodynia (i.e. light touch exacerbates the pain). Stabbing pain may also be a feature. *Deafferentation pain does not respond to opioids.* It is, however, much helped by an antidepressant [5].

Amitriptyline is generally too toxic for debilitated elderly patients. Dothiepin is a useful alternative. A 25 mg capusle is given at bedtime as an initial test dose. This is increased to 50 mg the next night and to 75 mg a few days later. Sometimes a higher dose is needed. For patients intolerant of dothiepin, mianserin is used, starting with 10-30 mg at bedtime, and increasing step by step to 60-120 mg. If stabbing is the main problem or persists despite the prescription of an antidepressant, sodium valproate (an anticonvulsant) is prescribed. In the elderly and the very debilitated, the initial dose is 200 mg bedtime; in stronger patients, 500 mg.

Opioid Responsive Pains - But Do Not Use Opioids

Functional Bowel Pains

Although functional bowel pains can be relieved with opioids, this is clearly not the best approach. Colic associated with constipation should be treated by treating the constipation. Irritable bowel syndrome occurs in about 10% of cancer patients (as in the general population) and calls for appropriate measures.

Intestinal colic associated with obstruction responds to opioids. Sometimes, however, an antispasmodic is preferable. Mild recurrent colic often responds to agents such as mebeverine 135–270 mg q.i.d., propantheline 15 mg b.-t.i.d. and hyoscine *butylbromide* 10–20 mg p.o./i.m. q.i.d. Unpredictable, occasional severe colic is perhaps better treated with sublingual hoyscine *hydrobromide* 0.3 mg as required.

Squashed Stomach Syndrome

In squashed stomach syndrome, epigastric pain is caused by relative gastric distension. This often occurs in patients with a grossly enlarged liver, even when the stomach is completely normal. It is important to recognize the postprandial discomfort for what it is, because explanation to the patient is crucial in management. The aim of treatment is to prevent distension. This requires a combination of dietary and pharmacological measures (Table 2). Some patients, particularly those with an endo-oesophageal tube, also experience retrosternal pain caused by reflux oesophagitis.

Table 2. Squashed stomach syndrome

Symptoms	Treatment
Early satiation Epigastric fullness Epigastric discomfort/pain Flatulence Hiccup Nausea Vomiting (especially postprandial) Heartburn	Explanation Dietary advice Antiflatulent (e.g. Asilone 10 ml after meals and at bedtime) Metoclopramide (after meals and at bedtime or 4 hourly if also receiving morphine) Cyclizine 50 mg 8 hourly is occasionally also necessary

Opioid Responsive Pains – Do Use Opioids

Three important concepts govern the use of analgesics in the management of opioid responsive pains, namely:

1. "By the mouth"
2. "By the clock"
3. "By the ladder"

"By the Mouth"

Morphine and other strong opiods are effective by mouth. Because of reduced bioavailbility, the doses are some two to three times larger than when given by injection. If there is intractable vomiting as well as pain, parenteral medication will, of course, be necessary. It is, however, usually possible to convert to the oral route once the vomiting has been controlled.

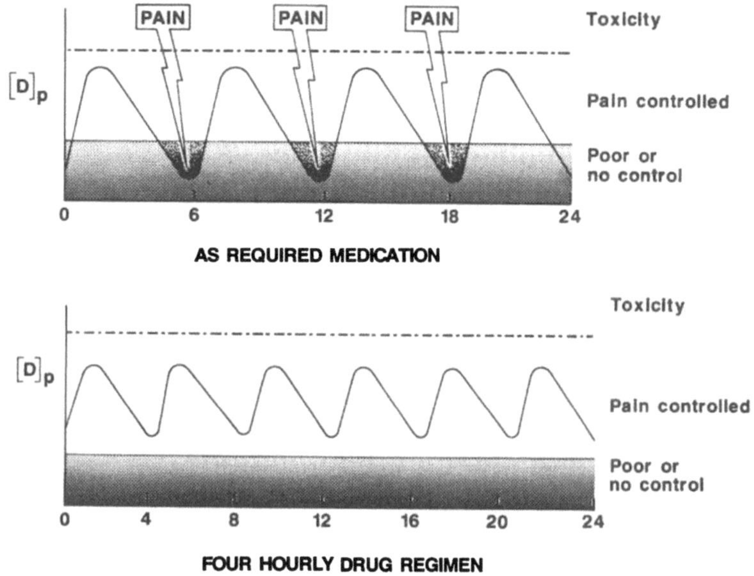

Fig. 2. The results of "as required" compared with regular 4-hourly morphine sulphate. $[D]_p$, plasma concentration of drug [9]

"By the Clock"

"As required" medication has no place in the treatment of persistent pain (Fig. 2). *Continuous pain requires regular prophylactic therapy.* This means that the next dose is given before the effect of the previous one has worn off and, therefore, before the patient may think it necessary.

For codeine and morphine a 4-hourly regimen is optimal. If a strong analgesic other than morphine is used, the doctor must be familiar with its pharmacology. For example, pethidine - effective for an average of only 2-3 h - is commonly given every 4 or 6 h, leaving the patient in pain for as many as 3 out of every 6 h. On the other hand, levorphanol is usually satisfactory when given every 6 h; and buprenorphine and methadone every 8 h. In the case of methadone, with a plasma half-life of over 2 days when taken regularly by mouth, there is a danger of increasing side-effects as a result of cumulation.

"By the Ladder"

The three standard analgesics are aspirin, codeine and morphine (Fig. 3). Other analgesics should be considered alternatives of fashion or convenience. It is necessary, however, to be familiar with one or two alternatives for patient intolerant of the standard drugs. Aspirin has two alternatives; paracetamol (which has no anti-inflammatory effect) and NSAIDs. The author uses dextropropoxyphene in preference to codeine. It is less constipating and, in Great Britain, the compound tab-

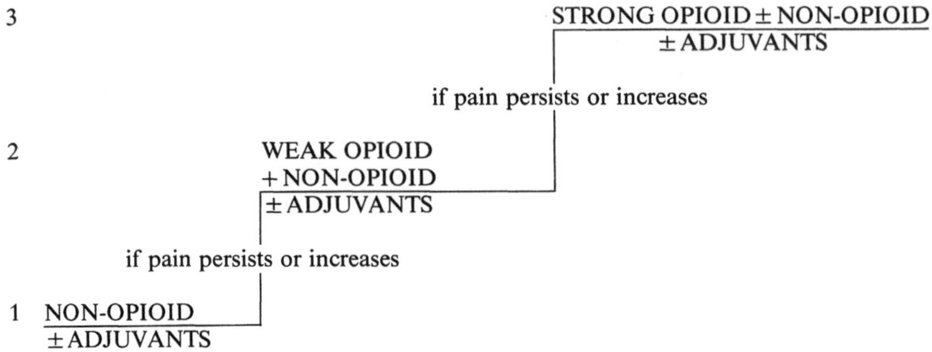

Fig. 3. The analgesic ladder for cancer pain management

let with paracetamol (co-proxamol) has a greater "codeine-equivalent" content than other weak opioid compound tablets.

With opioid responsive pains, the aim is to titrate the dose of the analgesic against the pain, gradually increasing the dose until the patient is pain-free. The effective analgesic dose varies considerably from patient to patient. The right dose of morphine, for example, is that which gives adequate relief for 4 h without unacceptabel side-effects. "Maximum" or "recommended" doses, derived mainly from postoperative parenteral single dose studies, are not applicable in cancer. The following should be noted:

1. Oral morphine is prescribed when non-opioids and weak opioids fail to control the pain despite regular use at an appropriate dose level. The use of oral morphine is determined by analgesic need, not by the doctor's estimate of life expectancy - which is often wrong.
2. Oral morphine can be given either as an aqueous solution of morphine sulphate or as slow-release tablets (MST-Continus). Most patients changing form a weak opioid commence on *60 mg a day*, i.e. aqueous morphine sulphate 10 mg every 4 h or MST-Continus 30 mg every 12 h.
3. The top of ladder is not reached simply by prescribing oral morphine, as doses from as little as 5 mg to more than 1 g every 4 h may be given. The majority of patients never need more than 100 mg, and many considerably less.
4. A double dose of aqueous morphine at bedtime usually circumvents the need for a dose in the middle of the night.
5. When a twice daily regimen is preferable, MST-Continus is used. This is available in Britain and several other countries in 10, 30, 60 and 100 mg sizes [4].
6. Avoid short-acting preparations like pentazocine (weak opioid), pethidine/meperidine (intermediate), and dextromoramide (strong opioid).
7. Do not prescribe an opioid agonist-antagonist (e.g. pentazocine, buprenorphine) with an opioid agonist (i.e. codeine, morphine).

Adjuvant Medication

Psychotropic Drugs

Discomfort is worse at night when the patient is alone with his pain and his fears. The cumulative effect of may sleepless, pain-filled nights is a substantial lowering of the patient‘s pain threshould with a corresponding increase in pain intensity. Temazepam is a useful hypnotic and may be given in doeses ranging from 10 mg to 60 mg. If a patient is very anxious, an anxiolytic should be prescribed instead (e.g. diazepam 5-20 mg nocte). If a patient remains depressed after two or more weeks of improved pain relief and psychological support, an antidepressant should be considered.

Analgesic Side-effects

Constipation

A laxative is almost always necessary for patients receiving an opioid. The author uses a colonic stimulant in conjunction with a feacal softener [10]. Possibly because of a greater small bowel component to the constipation, some patients need lactulose 20-40 ml two or three times a day instead. Rectal measures (suppositories and enemas) may also be necessary.

Nausea and Vomiting

At Sobell House, 60% of patients receiving morphine require an anti-emetic. Haloperidol 1-2 mg at bedtime is the author’s anti-emetic of choice. In about 10% of patients receiving morphine, this is ineffectual. In these, the morphine retards gastric emptying. Thus, if a patient does not respond to haloperidol and the pattern of vomiting is suggestive of gastric stasis, a gastrokinetic anti-emetic (metoclopramide or domperidone 10 mg up to every 4 h) should be substituted. In patients with raised intracranial pressure or with intestianl obstruction, cyclizine is the drug of choice [10].

Drowsiness

In the majority of patients, drowsiness is an initial side-effect which clears after a few days on the same dose.

Respiratory Depression

Pain is the physiological antagonist to the central depressant effects of morphine (Hanks, personal communication). Thus, respiratory depression is not a problem when using morphine or other strong opioid regularly by mouth to relieve pain in cancer. The fact that a double dose of morphine at bedtime causes no excess night-time mortality indicates that there is a reasonable safety margin [6].

On the other hand, if the pain is treated successfully by neurolytic or neuroablative techniques, life-threatening respiratory depression can occur if the dose of morphine is not reduced considerably [3]. *A reduction to 25% is recommended.* If the nerve block is totally successful, the morphine can be tailed off completely over the next 1-2 weeks. If only partly successful, the dose may need to be increased again to 50%-60% (or more) of the original dose.

Expectations

One hundred and fifty-six patients were treated in accordance with the "three-step" analgesic ladder [8]. Of these patients, 87% had complete relief, 9% had "acceptable relief" and 4% had partial relief. In a second survey of more than 1200 patients, the analgesic ladder proved efficacious in 71% of cases [11]. In the remainder, neurolytic procedures were also used.

Relief is obtained within 2-3 days in some patients, but in others (particularly those whose pain is made worse by movement and in the very anxious and depressed) it may take 3-4 weeks of in-patient treatment to achieve satisfactory control. Even so, it should be possible to achieve significant improvement within 1-2 days in all patients. Although the ultimate aim is complete freedom from pain, there will be less disappointment but more success if in practice the aim is "graded relief". As some pains respond more readily than others, improvement must be assessed in relation to each pain.

The initial target should be a pain-free, sleep-full night. Many patients have not slept well for weeks and are exhausted and demoralized. To sleep through the night pain-free and wake refreshed is a boost to their morale (and that of the doctor). The next target is relief during the day when sitting in bed or a chair. Finally, one aims at freedom from pain on movement. This ultimate goal is not always possible.

Acknowledgements. Table 1 and Figure 3 are reproduced by permission of the World Health Organization. An expanded version of this paper entitled "The Management of Pain in Cancer" will appear in Nimmo W.S. and Smith G (eds) *Anaesthesia*. Blackwell Scientific, London and Oxford, 1988.

References

1. Ferreira SH (1972) Prostaglandins, aspirin-like drugs and analgesia. Nature 240: 200-203
2. Galasko CSB (1981) The development of skeletal metastases. In: Weiss L, Gilbert AH (eds) Bone metastasis, Hall, Boston, pp 83-113
3. Hanks GW, Twycross RG, Lloyd JW (1981) Unexpected complication of successful nerve block. Anaesthesia 36: 37-39

4. Hanks GW, Twycross RG, Bliss JM (1987) Controlled-release morphine tablets: a double-blind trial in patients with advanced cancer. Anaesthesia 42: 840-844
5. Raftery H (1979) The management of postherpetic pain using sodium valproate and amitriptyline. Ir Med J 72: 399-401
6. Regnard CFB, Badger C (1987) Opioids, sleep and the time of death. Palliative Med 1: 107-110
7. Sola AE (1981) Myofascial trigger point therapy. Resident Staff Physician 27: 38-45
8. Takeda F (1986) Field testing in Japan of WHO guidelines for relief of cancer pain. The Pain Clinic 1: 83-89
9. Twycross RG, Lack SA (1983) Symptom control in far-advanced cancer: pain relief. Pitman, London
10. Twycross RG, Lack SA (1986) Control of alimentary symptoms in far-advanced cancer. Churchill Livingstone, Edinburgh
11. Ventafridda V, Tamburini M, Caraceni A, De Conno F, Naldi F (1987) A validation study of the WHO method for cancer pain relief. Cancer 59: 851-856
12. World Health Organization (1986) Cancer pain relief. World Health Organization, Geneva

Epidural Opiates and Nerve Blocks

M. Zenz

Klinik für Anästhesiologie, Intensiv- und Schmerztherapie, „Bergmannsheil Bochum“
Ruhr-Universität, Gilsingstraße 14, 4630 Bochum, FRG

The pharmacological treatment of pain in cancer patients with oral nonnarcotics and narcotics is the mainstay of therapy. In more than 90% of our own patients, pain is controlled by oral administration of peripheral acting analgesics and opioids or the combination of both. In a very small number of patients there is an indication for invasive measures.

Ladder of Pain Therapy

The first step in the ladder of pain therapy is always the introduction of causal measures in controlling pain. Typical examples are radiation, chemotherapy, or surgery for the tumour or the metastases. Only when these methods are not possible or are exhausted is there an indication for chronic pharmacological treatment or invasive methods like nerve blocks (Fig. 1).

Regional Blocks

Nerve blocks are one of the first steps in palliative pain therapy. They can be performed on the combined peripheral nerves, on the sympathetic nerve trunks, or on the CNS (epidural, intrathecal, intracerebroventricular). The substances used for different indications are local anaesthetics, opioids, neurolytic agents, corticosteroids, and alpha-agonists (Table 1).

Local Anaesthetics

Not all of the theoretically indicated and possible regional blocks are actually indicated in the patient with cancer pain. The block of nerve plexus or peripheral nerves with local anaesthetics is very seldom indicated, because the effect only lasts some hours and the block has to be performed again and again. Diagnostic blocks with local anaesthetics might be indicated in certain cases.

Recent Results in Cancer Research, Vol. 108

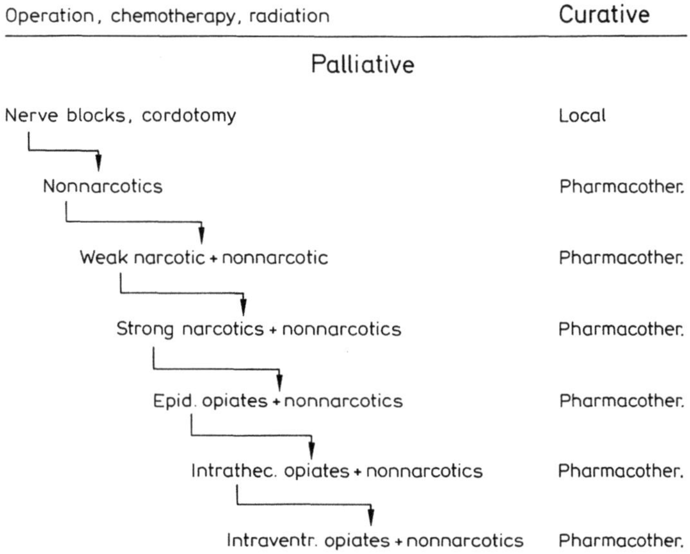

Fig. 1. Analgesic ladder in cancer pain

Table 1. The different drugs used in regional blocks

Substances / Site	Nerve plexus	Peripheral nerve	Sympathetic nerve	CNS		
				Epidural	Intrathecal	Intraventricular
Local anaesthetics	+	+	+	+	+	Ø
Neurolytic agents	Ø	(+)	+	+	+	Ø
Corticosterioids	–	–	–	+	–	–
Opioids	(+)	(+)	(+)	+	+	+
Alpha-agonits	–	–	–	+	+	–

+, indicated; –, not indicated; (+), possible; Ø, contraindicated

The local anaesthetic block at the epidural or intrathecal space is also only indicated for diagnosis, e.g., before a planned neurolytic block. In some cases a continuous epidural local anaesthetic block might be valuable, namely when pain is due to decreased peripheral blood supply. The arterial flow is increased by several hundred percent following an epidural block [25], but the method is certainly limited by the side-effects of sympathetic block of the lower extremities, e.g., hypotension, and the concomitant motor block, which is not suitable in outpatient treatment.

Local anesthetics in cancer pain are mostly used to block a carcinomatous neuritis by injecting on sympathetic ganglia. A carcinomatous neuritis is identical to reflex sympathetic dystrophy [7] and is characterized by burning pain, hyperpathia, and sudomotor malfunction. The distribution of pain is related to the sympathetic innervation and does not follow the dermatome of a peripheral nerve. Sympathetic block can be performed at the stellate ganglion, the thoracic and lumbar sympathetic trunks, the celiac plexus, the trigeminal ganglion, and the pterygopalatine ganglion. When a typical sympathetic block is not possible, e.g., in cases in which the tumour is in the direct neighborhood of the sympathetic nerve, the block can also be performed via a combined peripheral nerve trunk. For example an alternative to stellate ganglion block is the supraclavicular plexus block or the axillary plexus block.

The local anaesthetic to be used is preferentially one of the long-acting amide-type local anaesthetics, optimally bupivacaine 0.125%-0.5%. Etidocaine is not suitable, because the sympathetic block is inconstant and limited with this substance.

Neurolytic Blocks

When a local anaesthetic block (diagnostic block) has shown efficacy in controlling pain, neurolytic agents can be injected to induce a longer lasting effect. Neurolytic substances are contraindicated for nerve plexus blocks because motor function is impaired. Neurolytic blocks with alcohol or phenol can be performed at the level of a peripheral somatic nerve, e.g., the intercostal nerve. This might be indicated when a single pain is diagnosed in one single nerve. On the other hand, neurolytics like alcohol often (~20%) induce an alcohol neuritis as a consequence of therapy, which is frequently far more severe than the previous pain. As a consequence we no longer perform neurolytic blocks in peripheral nerves.

In sympathetic nerve trunks neurolytic blocks can be performed without any danger of neuritis or motor block. One of the most established methods is celiac plexus block in intractable pain limited to intra-abdominal organs, e.g., pain caused by pancreatic or stomach tumours. After a diagnostic block with local anaesthetics, 30-50 ml of 50% alcohol is injected. The favorite technique today is ultrasonic controlled fine-needle puncture from the ventral side. This technique is less dangerous and less complicated than all other techniques. The effect lasts from several weeks to 6 months [12]. Most side-effects and complications (one exception is hypotension) can be excluded by the ultrasonic technique.

Neurolytic sympathetic block is not possible at the level of the stellate ganglion because there are essential nerves directly adjacent to the sympathetic nerve (n. phrenicus, n. recurrens). Block of the sympathetic ganglion at the thoracic level is in the author's opinion too dangerous compared with the alternatives.

Subarachnoid neurolytic blocks are performed when intractable pain has a strong limited distribution. For example the "saddle pain" in rectal cancer can easily be treated by an intrathecal block. One may use 98% alcohol (1-1.5 ml), which is hypobaric to CSF, with the patient lying in a position in which the sacral area is the highest point. Alternatively, 5%-7% phenol in glycerine (0.4-0.8 ml) can be used with the patient sitting. The specific weight of phenol in glycerine is higher than that of CSF and the drug therefore concentrates at the lowest point of the CSF.

The effectiveness of subarachnoid neurolytic blocks is limited to 60%-80% [16, 18]. The duration of effect is also limited: pain relief is obtained for a period of 2 weeks to 3 months [16, 18].

Side-effects include motor paralysis and bladder and bowel dysfunction and depend on the site of injection, the volume, the injection speed, and the position of the patient.

Corticosteroids

Corticosteroids are often given orally in patients with nerve compression pain [17]. In the same way, corticosteroids can be administered topically, preferentially into the epidural space. Four to eight milligrams of dexamethasone are given together with the local anaesthetic. The effect is not long lasting, so that the procedure has to be repeated. This treatment is indicated only in cases in which a local anaesthetic block is performed. In all other cases oral administration is to be preferred (Table 1).

Opioids

Somatic and Sympathetic Nerves

Very few authors have reported the effect of opioids given topically on peripheral nerves [11, 15]. These authors report long-lasting pain relief in different pain situations. However, no controlled studies have been performed to confirm the results. Surprisingly, even in cases of sympathetic block long-lasting pain relief is described following topical opioid injection.

Spinal Opioids

In the German-speaking countries cancer pain therapy with opioids really began with the introduction of spinal opioids, followed some years later by the routine use of oral narcotics. Fear of side-effects and complications have favored use of various weak narcotics almost unknown in English-speaking countries, e.g., tilidine and tramadol. Since epidural opioids were introduced into therapeutic practise there has been increasing interest in strong narcotics, even for oral administration. In this respect the German-speaking countries are certainly some decades behind the United States and the United Kingdom. Another aspect is the unique discussion of *Sterbehilfe* - a word without a parallel in English. The ratio of German publications on oral and on spinal opioids in cancer pain is 1:10, although the ratio of indication is the inverse of this.

It is often not realized that the first anecdotal report on spinal opioids in humans was provided by Wang as early as 1977. In 1979 the unique success of the method started all over the world [1, 19]. Its theoretical background was the demonstration of opioid receptors in the spinal cord in the substantia gelatinosa of the dorsal horn [14, 21]. Injecting into the close neighborhood of these receptors, e.g., epidurally or intrathecally, leads to long-lasting hypalgesia. It starts after 30-40 min and lasts for about 12 h. Motor and sympathetic functions are not affected, but all typical opioid side-effects may occur. The most dangerous is respiratory depression. Other side-effects include nausea, vomiting, urinary retention, itching, sedation, and constipation. However, most side-effects are less frequent in spinal than in oral application.

Choice of the Opioid

Morphine has mostly been used for epidural opioid analgesia in cancer pain. However, the physicochemical properties of morphine are not ideal for this purpose. The low liposolubility and pronounced hydrophilic properties of this drug make it more likely to induce side-effects. The reason is that morphine diffuses slowly across the lipophilic neuronal barriers and remains active in the CSF for a long time. This makes diffusion to the respiratory center in the brain more possible than with lipophilic drugs. The lipophilic drugs diffuse very quickly into the spinal cord and back to the vascular system; in this way their transport with the CSF to the vital centers in the brain is rendered less likely. Buprenophine, sufentanil, alfentanil, and fentanyl are lipophilic drugs that are theoretically more appropriate for spinal application.

Route of Administration

The more logical way to administer opioids to the spinal opiate receptors is the intrathecal route, because by this route the opioid does not have to pass the dura mater before entering the CSF. However, other problems may occur in comparison to the epidural route. CSF may pass along the catheter, producing a continuous leakage. The danger of infection is increased by injecting directly into the CSF. The danger of respiratory depression might be greater because the active drug concentration within the CSF might be higher, even if the dose is reduced. The advantage of the intrathecal route is the possibility of obtaining excellent results with minimal doses, in this way making possible the use of small pumps with a limited volume for chronic application.

A new route is the direct intracerebroventricular injection of the opioid. Surprisingly, the side-effects reported up to now have been of minor severity. Because the method is the most invasive, it has to be reserved for special indications (Table 2).

Epidural Opiates

Most experience exists with the epidural application of opiates for cancer pain therapy [3, 13, 24]. Afer the initial enthusiastic reports it is essential not to overtreat every patient with epidural opiates but to ensure the method is properly indicated, because most pain situations can be treated by oral opiates. Epidural opiates are indicated when oral opiates are going to be ineffective even at high doses. Another indication is the existence of severe side-effects with oral opiates, e.g., nausea and

Table 2. Indications for epidural, intrathecal, and intraventricular opiates

Epidural opiates
Severe pain
Opiates effective
Oral opiates ineffective
Oral opiates - severe side-effects
Causal therapy impossible
Intrathecal opiates
Severe pain
Opiates effective
Epidural opiates tested
Epidural opiates - high doses
Epidural opiates - pump problems
Intraventricular opiates
Severe pain
Opiates effective
Epidural/intrathecal opiates tested
Epidural/intrathecal opiates - high doses
Epidural/intrathecal opiates - pump problems

vomiting or severe constipation. In contrast to our own opinion of some years ago, there is no indication for the epidural route before the oral route has been tried extensively.

The technique is simple and can be performed on an outpatient basis. An epidural catheter is inserted in the usual way via a Tuohy needle as near as possible to the main segment of pain. The position of the catheter can be established by X-ray or by injection of a local anaesthetic. After that an opioid is injected dissolved in saline solution, e.g., morphine 5 mg in 10 cc saline or 0.3 mg buprenorphine in the same volume. When pain relief has been obtained the patient can be sent home with exact instructions for the injections and the catheter care.

Usually the injections can be performed by the patient himself or his relatives. Continuous contact with the patient has to be guaranteed. In cases where this is not possible, a hospital stay might be indicated.

The dose of opioid has to be adjusted to the pain level. Doses might vary from 2 mg to 100 mg morphine (Zenz et al. 1985). The duration of action may also vary, from 6 to 24 h. The best way is to start with a short hospital stay to adjust doses and the time interval of injection.

Correct catheter care is very important in making long treatment periods possible without the need for catheter removal due to infection. We advise patients to take a whole body bath with povidone-iodine soap every second day. On the same occasion the cover is changed, together with the bacterial filter. The puncture site is covered by povidone-iodine unguent. The catheter has to be fixed by a suture for longer treatment periods [23]. This simple method of catheter fixation has some advantages: the catheter is better protected against removal or dislodgement, and compared to tunneling the simple suture fixation makes catheter change very easy and the invasive procedure minimal for the patient.

Tunneling. After a test period of some days the catheter can be tunneled (Carl 1986). This can be performed under local anaesthesia. Tunneling a catheter possibly makes catheter care easier and reduces the risk of infections and removal, although these have been reported [3]. The tunneled catheter can be used for bolus injections or connection to an external pump.

Pumps. When the prognosis of the patient is better, a pump implantation is an alternative that minimizes the need for care, supervision, and patient cooperation. However, this is not possible in every case, and the conditions for a pump implantation must be borne in mind. The effectiveness of epidural opiates has to be tested in advance. One must test that low volumes are sufficient to control pain, because the volume of the pumps is limited. One must also test that the dose of opiate needed does not exceed a certain limit set by the industrial concentration of opiate per milliliter. For example, the highest concentration of morphine is 20 mg/ml; when a pump delivers 4 ml/day the highest morphine dose will be 80 mg/day, and in some cases this is not sufficient to control the pain [24].

Two different pump systems can be chosen. The completely implantable pump (e.g., Infusaid) is limited in volume and rate: the Infusaid pump can contain 50 ml and deliver 4 ml/day [5, 6, 13]. External pumps are an alternative to completely implantable systems and can be connected to a percutaneous or tunneled catheter. All kinds of pumps exist, syringe infusors, reservoir infusors, and self-powered portable infusors. Prices vary according to the technical standard. The least expensive is the Travenol self-powered infusor, while the most expensive are programmable systems, which very seldom seem indicated for cancer pain therapy. A precondition for the therapy with pumps is testing of the possible adjustment of the pump characteristics to match the patients pain.

Side-effects. The theoretically most severe side-effect, respiratory depression, has never been reported in cancer pain treatment when exclusively epidural opiates have been given and no technical mistakes made. I would exclude respiratory depression when oral opiates have been given in the preceding period and when a cautious dose adjustment is performed. Nausea and vomiting may occur, but as in oral treatment they often disappear after 2–3 weeks of treatment. Constipation is seldom seen with spinal opioids compared to systemic application. Urinary retention and pruritus are rare side-effects.

All side-effects can be treated by intravenous application of naloxone. However, the cardiovascular side-effects of this opioid antagonist (hypertension, tachycardia, increased O_2 consumption) have to be borne in mind. In most cases it is better to treat the side-effects with symptomatic measures. We regularly give a laxative. When nausea is reported we give an antiemetic. There is no effective symptomatic treatment against pruritus or urinary retention.

Intrathecal Opioids

When the epidural doses of opioids increase there can be an indication for changing the catheter to the intrathecal space. Doses decrease by a factor of 10. A lower volume of the opioid is required – making a pump implantation more possible.

Analgesia is more constant and longer lasting. However, side-effects are more severe and more frequent. Postspinal headache is possible, and if infection occurs, the consequences are more serious. In the author's opinion intrathecal opiates should not be the first step, but the next step after epidural opiates (Fig. 1; Table 2).

The technical modalities are similar to the epidural route [5]. Greater attention is to be given to the catheter care because of the greater danger of infection.

Intracerebroventricular Opioids

As the next (last) step in therapy the intraventricular injection of opioids may be chosen. The indication for this most invasive method must be checked very carefully. Failure of epidural or intrathecal treatment might be an indication, when there is a guarantee that opiates act at all (Fig. 3). Pain in the head and neck area is another indication. In most cases the technique is performed by a neurosurgeon. [2, 8, 9, 10] have presented large series showing the great effectiveness of this method. Very small doses of opiates (0.5 mg morphine/day) are sufficient to control the pain. It has to be realized that 0.5 mg morphine intraventricularly corresponds to 500 mg morphine intravenously. In one of our own patients the final dose of opiate was 9.5 mg intraventricular morphine, which corresponds to 9500 mg intravenous morphine (Table 3).

Table 3. Morphine equivalents in chronic pain therapy

Oral	30 mg
Intravenous	10 mg
Epidural	2–5 mg
Intrathecal	0.2–0.5 mg
Intraventricular	0.01 mg

Surprisingly, side-effects following this direct injection of opiates into the fourth ventricle have been rare up to now. In three cases of overdose respiratory depression was observed. Euphoria and somnolence are frequently seen. Constipation is rare.

Alpha-agonists

Alpha-adrenergic agents have a direct antinociceptive action [22]. In cancer pain drugs like clonidine have only been used in combination with opioids. [4, 6] has reported the combination of clonidine with opioids by the intrathecal route. We give clonidine when opiate doses exceed a certain level or when opiate doses suddenly increase. Another indication is the prevention of withdrawal symptoms. It is also possible to administer clonidine orally (3 × 75–150 μg) to increase the effect of the epidural opiate, but we have the impression that this effect ceases after some weeks. There have been no controlled studies on the effect of alpha-agonists in cancer pain (Table 1).

Conclusion

Nearly all patients with cancer pain can be treated adequately using a stepwise approach. Nerve blocks are only indicated in certain situations, because most patients suffer from multiple pains. Oral opiates control pain in some 90% of patients. In the remaining 10% all kinds of spinal opioids are indicated, starting with a simple percutaneous epidural catheter and bolus injections. For patients with a better prognosis a pump implantation can be a good decision. At the moment the intrathecal catheter and the intraventricular route seem indicated only rarely.

The drug of choice for spinal application is a lipophilic one. But the lipophilic drugs have limitations. Buprenorphine has a ceiling effect, fentanyl is too short acting, and sufentanil has not been introduced in all countries.

Spinal opioid analgesia has made pain therapy in cancer patients more effective and easy. There remain only very few patients not controlled by these methods. However, it has to be stated that all the technical approaches cannot substitute for the human relationship between patient and doctor. Pain is not a symptom alone; it has to be treated holistically, and spinal opiates are only one aspect of the care.

References

1. Bahar M, Magora F, Olshwang D, Davidson JT (1979) Epidural morphine in treatment of pain. Lancet 1 (8115): 527–9
2. Blond S, Meynadier J, Chrubasik J, Dupard TH et al. (1985) Intrathekale und intraventrikuläre Morphin-Analgesie bei Karzinompatienten: Langzeit-Erfahrungen. Pain 4: 129
3. Carl P, Crawford ME, Ravlo O, Bach V (1986) Longterm treatment with epidural opioids. A retrospective study comprising 150 patients treated with morphine chloride and buprenorphine chloride. Anaesthesia 41 (1): 32
4. Coombs DW, Saunders RL, Savage S, Jensen L, Murphy C (1985) Chronic intrathecal clonidine and narcotic tolerance. Can Anaesth Soc J 32 (3): 63
5. Coombs DW, Maurer LH, Saunders RL, Gaylor M (1984) Outcomes and complications of continuous intraspinal narcotic analgesia for cancer pain control. J Clin Oncol 2 (12): 1414–20
6. Coombs DW, Saunders RL, Fratkin JD, Jensen LE, Murphy CA (1986) Continuous intrathecal hydromorphone and clonidine for intractable cancer pain. J Neurosurg 64 (6): 890
7. Gerbershagen H (1979) Blocks with local anaesthetics in the treatment of cancer pain. In: Bonica JJ, Ventafridda V (eds) Advances in pain research and therapy, vol 2. Raven, New York, p 311
8. Leavens ME, Hill CS JR, Cech DA, Weyland JB, Weston JS (1982) Intrathecal and intraventricular morphine for pain in cancer patients: initial study. J Neurosurg 56 (2): 241–5
9. Lenzi A, Galli G, Gandolfini M, Marini G (1985) Intraventricular morphine in paraneoplastic painful syndrome of the cervicofacial region: experience in thirty-eight cases. Neurosurgery 17 (1): 6–11

10. Lobato RD, Madrid JL, Fatela LV, Rivas JJ, Reig E, Lamas E (1983) Intraventricular morphine for control of pain in terminal cancer patients. J Neurosurg 59: 627-33
11. Mays K, North WC, Schnapp M (1981) Stellate ganglion blocks with morphine in sympathetic type pain. J Neurol Neurosurg Psychiatry 44: 189-90
12. Moore DC (1979) Role of nerve block with neurolytic solutions for pelvic visceral cancer pain. In: Bonica JJ, Ventafridda V (eds) Advances in pain research and therapy, vol 2, Raven, New York, p 593
13. Müller H, Aigner K, Zierski J (1985) Behandlung von Tumorschmerzen mit Pumpsystemen zur rückenmarksnahen Opiatapplikation. Dtsch Ärztebl 82 (35): 2475-84
14. Pert CB, Snyder SH (1973) Opiate receptor: demonstration in nervous tissue. Science 179: 1011
15. Sprotte G (1984) Einsatz von Regionalanaesthesie beim Risikopatienten. In: Koßmann, Seeling (eds) Stellenwert der Regionalanaesthesie beim Risikopatienten. Keitz und Fischer, Eschwege, p 17
16. Swerdlow M (1979) Subarachnoid and extradural neurolytic blocks. In: Bonica JJ, Ventafridda V (eds) Advances in pain research and therapy, vol 2. Raven, New York, p 325
17. Twycross R, Lack S (1983) Symptom control in far advanced cancer: pain relief. Pitman, London
18. Ventafridda V, Martino G (1976) Clinical evaluation of subarachnoid neurolytic blocks in intractable cancer pain. In: Bonica JJ, Albe-Fressard D (eds) Advances in pain research and therapy, vol 2. Raven, New York, p 689
19. Wang JK (1977) Analgesic effect of intrathecally administered morphine. Reg Anaesth 2 (1): 3-4
20. Wang JK, Nauss LA, Thomas JE (1979) Pain relief by intrathecally applied morphine in man. Anaesthesiology 50: 149-51
21. Yaksh TL, Rudy TA (1976) Analgesia mediated by a direct spinal action of narcotics. Science 192: 1357-8
22. Yaksh TL, Reddy SV (1981) Studies in the primate on the analgetic effects associated with intrathecal actions of opiates, alpha-adrenergic agonists and baclofen. Anaesthesiology 54 (6): 451-67
23. Zenz M, Piepenbrock S, Hüsch M, Schappler-Scheele B, Neuhaus R (1981 A) Erfahrungen mit länger liegenden Periduralkathetern - peridurale Morphin-Analgesie bei Karzinompatienten. Reg Anaesth 4: 26-28
24. Zenz M, Piepenbrock S, Tryba M (1985) Epidural opiates: long-term experiences in cancer pain. Klin Wochenschr 63 (5): 225-9
25. Zenz M, van den Berg B, van den Berg E (1981 B) Plethysmographische Untersuchungen zur Sympathikusblockade nach Periduralanaesthesie und periduraler Morphin-Analgesie. Anaesthesist 30 (10): 70-3

Electrostimulation and Neurosurgical Measures in Cancer Pain

J. Siegfried

AMI Klinik im Park, Seestraße 220, 8002 Zürich, Switzerland

In 1975 Gildenberg [1] published the results of a survey of the procedures used to combat pain by 1998 neurosurgeons in the United States and Canada. Approximately 2000 percutaneous cordotomies, 135 thalamotomies, 20 mesencephalotomies, 40 cingulotomies, and 24 implantations of stimulating electrodes were performed annually. It is difficult to speculate on to day's figures, but thalamotomies, mesencephalotomies, and cingulotomies are probably almost no longer performed. Percutaneous cordotomies are considered even more rarely following the tremendous development of stimulating techniques and the epidural/intrathecal or ventricular application of morphine or morphine-like substances. If 10 years ago neurosurgical techniques had already been markedly improved by the use of percutaneous techniques like cervical cordotomies and sterotactic thalamotomies or mesencephalotomies (without general anaesthesia, without loss of blood, with minmal stress for the patient, and with short hospitalization), in the last few years new advances in the field of pain physiology have modified our neurosurgical therapeutic spectrum still further. In the choice of operation it is of decisive importance to distinguish between neurogenic (deafferentation) pain and somatogenic pain. Neurogenic pain is taken to mean pain (mainly a burning sensation) in an area of disturbed sensitivity, e. g. pain due to invasion of nerve roots by the cancer or to radiation or surgical damage of nervous structures. Somatogenic pain occurs because of irritation of pain receptors, e.g., bone pain in bone metastases.

In accordance with this clinical classification of pain, two neurosurgical methods are considered:

1. Interruption of the tracts conducting pain between the periphery and the cerebral intergration centers or intrathecal (intraventricular) administration of morphine-like substances trough an implanted drug delivery system in cases of somatogenic pain.
2. Intermittent electrical stimulation of a tract or of a center aimed at producing inhibition of the pain information through an implanted electrical neurostimulation system (neuropacemaker) in cases of neurogenic pain. It is generally accepted today that morphine does not really control deafferentation pain.

Recent Results in Cancer Research, Vol. 108

Somatogenic Pain

Destructive Techniques

Destructive techniques for the treatment of pain have traditionally centered on the sectioning of pain fibers, either at the roots, dorsal horn, of spinothalamic tract level. The advances in technology have simplified the surgery and decreased the attendant risk; however, the goal remains unchanged. The ablative approach to pain control characteristically has a high early succes rate. Unfortunately, early success yields to a progressive decline in pain relief. More importantly, in these ablative techniques, dysesthetic pain may subsequently occur and may actually be worse than the presenting pain.

In a similar paper [11], we considered destructive techniques a very attractive approach in the treatment of somatogenic pain in advanced cancer and mentioned in detail neurotomies, sympathectomies, rhizotomies, cordotomy, myelotomy, medullary tractotomy, mesencephalotomy, thalamotomy, and hypophysectomy. Three years later we retain only percutaneous cervical cordotomy as a last resort, and use it under even more restrictive conditions.

The first open cordotomy for pain was reported in [12]. In [6] described his technique for a percutaneous method. In [8] suggested a radiofrequency lesion, which has become the standard technique. The surgical goal is the sectioning of the lateral spinothalamic tract, which results in loss of contralateral analgesia and loss of temperature sensation with preservation of touch and position sensation.

With the advent of neurostimulation techniques as well as subarachnoidal administration of opiates by implantable systems, the indications for percutaneous cervical cordotomy have decreased. Presently we feel that the only indication for this procedure should be poorly controlled, severe, chronic pain which is of malignant origin and unilateral. If the patient has bilateral pain, an open thoracic bilateral cordotomy at T2-3 is perferable to bilateral cervical cordotomy in that it avoids postoperative respiratory insufficiency, although not bladder dysfunction. The risk of respiratory embarrassment is high following a bilateral high cervical cordotomy, even when the procedure is performed in two stages. Percutaneous C1-2 bilateral cordotomy may result in reductions of vital capacity, forced expiratory volume, maximal breathing capacity, and maximal midtidal thoracic pressure [3]. Moreover, involuntary respiration is suppressed with preservation of voluntary respiratory activity, resulting in sleep-induced apnea. Postoperative death following bilateral cordotomy is frequently caused by nocturnal apnea [2]. Respiratory dysfunction is usually reversible but may require ventilation monitoring as well as assistance for up to 3 weeks. Extremely poor pulmonary function is a relative contraindication to unilateral percutaneous high cervical cordotomy. Pulmonary function test should be performed if the patient's pulmonary status is poor. The patient and his family should be aware that preexisting neurological deficits, such as paresis or bladder, bowel, and sexual dysfunction, may be increased postoperatively. Although the increase is usually transient, it may be permanent.

Intrathecal Opiates

In the early 1970s, opiate receptors were identified in the brain and spinal cord [7]. In the spinal cord, the greatest concentration of opiate receptors is in rexed laminae 1 and 2. Subsequent animal experimentation using chronic spinal subarachnoid catheters in rats demonstrated that intrathecal morphine produces a dose-dependent increase in the nociceptive threshold. Experimental evidence demonstrated that morphine reduces ascending nociceptive activity by a direct effect at the level of the substantia gelatinosa. In the late 1970s epidural and intrathecal opiates were used extensively in the treatment of acute postoperative pain following procedures involving the thorax, abdomen, and lower extremities. Relatively small doses of morphine (0.5-3.0 mg) provided complete and prolonged (12-48 h) analgesia below the level of injection without any change in non-nociceptive perception. The clinical application quickly included use of implanted reservoirs and infusion pumps. Complications have included pruritus (15%), urinary retention (15%-20%), nausea and vomiting (infrequently), and respiratory depression (which seems unlikely with the use of hyperbaric solutions when the patient maintains a sitting or half-sitting position for 4-6 h after application). The complications are transient and rapidly subside.

Neurosurgeons have quickly applied the method in the treatment of chronic cancer pain in the pelvic region or in the lower extremities by implanting a catheter in the lumbar or thoracic subarachnoid space and connecting this catheter with subcutaneous drug reservoir placed in the abdominal region. An alternative method is the subcutaneously implanted pump, which avoids repetitive punctures but which is still very expensive. When chronic cancer pain is located in the cervical, the throat, or the facial regions, the application of opiates in microdosage will be performed through an implanted delivery system connected with a ventricular catheter.

One problem still open is the development of tachyphylaxis and tolerance. The rapidity with which tolerance develops fluctuates greatly in patients who receive intrathecal opiates. However, with the advent of morphine agonists and opiate analogues that can be used following the development of tolerance to morphine, the indications for the technique may be broader in the future. At present, this technique offers the best treatment for midline or bilateral somatogenic pain secondary to malignancy. If pain is of deafferentation origin, morphine application will be of almost no help.

Neurogenic Pain

Neurogenic pain which is due to damage to nervous structures and is accompanied by a neurological sensory deficit or hyperactivity (e.g., anesthesia dolorosa or hyperpathia) is the most distressing pain and the most difficult to treat. With the introduction of neurostimulation techniques, it became possible for the first time to relieve this kind of pain, and these techniques were subsequently applied for other types of pain.

If the postulation of the gate-control theory of pain [5] was the major incentive for the development of the neurostimulation technique, many other theories were suggested. However, even in the absence of a definite, convincing pain-inhibiting mechanism, clinical data have proved that neurostimulation can produce analgesia.

The first surgical experiment to relieve pain by electrical stimulation was performed on a peripheral nerve by Sweet [13]; this closely followed the publication of the gate-control theory of pain, which postulated that activation of large myelinated nerve fibers might block the transmission of pain impulses in the spinal cord. The largest accumulation of afferent fibers is found in the dorsal columns of the spinal cord, which suggests that neurostimulation could also be carried out at this level. [9] was the first to perform such a stimulation of the dorsal columns. Later on, [4] chose the specific sensory thalamic nuclei as a target. The introduction of neurostimulation with so-called non-destructive or non-ablative techniques opened up a new direction in the neurosurgical treatment of pain; today these techniques are the most attractive method in the treatment of chronic persistent pain of benign origin, and the only one in the treatment of neurogenic pain in patients with benign or malignant disease. On can now say that perturbed neural function may be modified by crude electrical signals and that destructive means of pain relief may some day be come obsolete [10].

The surgery required for spinal cord or thalamic stimulation causes minimal somatic pain and can be performed using a local anaesthetic. In the awake patient the electrode can be placed in the optimal position for pain relief, and postoperatively the parameters of stimulation may be adjusted to optimize pain relief. Most importantly, if the procedure is unsuccessful, the electrode can be removed, and there has been no destruction of neural function.

For dorsal cord stimualtion, an electrode is introduced percutaneously into the dorsal epidural space of the vertebral canal cephalad to the site of the pain for monopolar stimulation. If the patient obtains satisfactory pain relief with repetitive stimulation over a few days, the electrode is connected to a programmable neuropacemaker placed in a subcutaneous pocket, usually in the right abdominal region. For deafferentation pain, this technique is appropriate when the nerve lesion is peripheral or postganglionic. When the neural lesion is central (preganglionic) or when the neurogenic pain is located in the face, the stimulation will be performed at the thalamic level. The monopolar electrode is then introduced stereotactically in the sensory thalamic nucleus somatotopically corresponding to the location of pain. The connection to a subcutaneously implanted neuropacemaker under the clavicula is performed in the second stage, when the intermittent stimulation elicits statisfactory pain relief. Excellent results can be obtained in 80% of the cases of neurogenic pain when cancer is invading nerve roots or plexus or when radiotherapy has elicited an anaesthesia or hypesthesia dolorosa.

Summary

Neurosurgery for cancer pain may always be considered when the pain no longer responds to conservative treatment methods or only at the cost of undesirable side-effects. Almost all these operations that can be considered for the cancer patient can be performed percutaneously, without general anaesthesia, without loss of blood, and with short hospitalization.

Chronic pain has to be differentiated according to whether it is somatogenic or neurogenic. For somatogenic pain (pain without any neurological deficit), intrathecal or intraventricular administration of morphine-like substances through an implanted drug delivery system is the most attractive method. The classical neurosurgical interruption of a tract conducting pain between the periphery and the cerebral integration centers is an almost obsolete method, and percutaneous cordotomy can only be discussed when the pain is strictly unilateral and the prognosis of the disease relatively favorable. For neurogenic pain (pain with sensory disturbances) the only method which can be helpful is electrical stimulation with an implanted neuropacemaker connected to an electrode in the dorsal columns of the cord or in the sensory thalamic nucleus (depending on the location of the pain), since morphine has at best only a poor analgesic effect on deafferentation pain.

References

1. Gildenberg PL (1975) Survery of stereotactic and functional neurosurgery in the United States and Canada. Appl Neurophysiol 38: 31-37
2. Krieger AJ, Rosomoff HL (1974) Sleep induced apnea: 1. A respiratory and anatomic dysfunction syndrome following bilateral percutaneous cordotomy. J Neurosurg 39: 168-180
3. Kupermann AS, Krieger AJ, Rosomoff HL (1971) Respiratory function after cervical cordotomy. Chest 59: 128-132
4. Mazars G, Merienne L, Cioloca C (1973) Stimulations thalamiques intemittentes antalgiques. Rev Neurol (Paris) 128: 273-279
5. Melzack R, Wall PD (1965) Pain mechanisms: a new theory. Science 150: 971-979
6. Mullan S, Harper PV, Hekmatpanah J, Torres H, Dobben G (1963) Percutaneous interruption of spinal pain tracts by means of a Strontium-90 needle. J Neurosurg 20: 931-939
7. Pert CB, Snyder SH (1973) Opiate receptor: demonstration in nervous system. Science 179: 1011-1013
8. Rosomoff HL (1971) Communication at the 39th meeting of American Association of Neurological Surgeons, Houston, Texas
9. Shealy CN, Mortimer JT, Reswick J (1967) Electrical inhibition of pain by stimulation of the dorsal column: preliminary clinical reports. Anaesth Analg 46: 489-491
10. Siegfried J, Hood T (1983) Current status of functional neurosurgery. Adv Technical Standards Neurosurg 10: 19-79
11. Siegfried J, Kühner A, Sturm V (1984) Neurosurgical treatment of cancer pain. Rec Results Cancer Pain 89:148-156
12. Spiller WG, Martin E (1912) The treatment of persistent pain of organic origin in the lower part of the body by division of the anterolateral column of the spinal cord. JAMA 58: 1489-1490
13. Sweet WH, Wepsic JG (1968) Treatment of chronic pain by stimulation of fiber of primay afferent neuron. Trans Am Neurol Ass 93: 103-105

Treatment of Pain in the Cancer Patient: The Role of the Nurse

B. Dicks

114 Kingsley Road, Maidstone, Kent ME15 7UP, Great Britain

Nurses often say that because prescribing drugs is a medical responsibility the role of the nurse in the treatment of pain in the cancer patient is limited. However, it can be asserted (a) that pharmacological management alone does not constitute the sum total of pain control and (b) that effective pharmacological management is not only a matter of good prescribing. The intention of this chapter is to illustrate the necessity of a broad concept of pain management and to highlight in particular the role of the nurse in the treatment of cancer pain.

There would be common agreement among nurses that one of the main goals of oncology nursing in general is to assist a person to live as full a life as possible with his disease. However, this is not easily accomplished, particularly as the disease progresses and restrictions increase. In this paper, therefore, I shall try and identify some of the problems which we may encounter when assisting the patient in pain to live as full a life as possible. I intend to consider these problems under three main headings:

1. Society's view of cancer pain
2. Loss of control
3. Iatrogenic problems

Society's View of Cancer Pain

Patients are influenced by society's view of cancer and pain. A cancer diagnosis is still often seen as not only a sentence of death, but as a very nasty, painful end. That cancer is held to be synonymous with pain is revealed by this woman's reluctance to accept her diagnosis: "There was no lump, and I thought you'd get a lump or something. And I pressed it ... and no pain. I always understood you had dreadful pain. I thought if it was cancer, I should have felt it ... Then it spread to the bones and I *did* start to get some pain, so I thought well ... maybe I *have* got it" [1].

Professionals too can hold a distorted view of cancer pain. It is often quoted that pain is a major symptom in up to 85% of cancer patients [2]. It is, however,

Recent Results in Cancer Research, Vol. 108

important to remind ourselves that hospice data are likely to overestimate the incidence of pain in cancer as unrelieved pain is a main reason for referral [2].

The pessimism with which many people view cancer probably stems in part from the widespread misconception that cancer is a single disease. Individuals who contract particularly painful forms of cancer with a high mortality are therefore taken to represent all cancer patients.

It is generally recognised that pain is a dual phenomenon; a simple clinical model portrays it as having a cognitive component (the actual physical perception of pain) and an affective component (the emotional reaction to that perception). As the affective component is said to preadominate in chronic pain, preconceived ideas concerning the inevitability and degree of pain can result in an increase in anxiety which in turn can lead to an increase in the perceived intensity of pain [3]. It is therefore essential that nurses recognise that the control of pain requires comprehensive management which considers *all* sources of distress, whether physical, psychological, spiritual, social or cultural.

Loss of Control

"Scientific medicine tends to make some patients feel like a feather in the wind" [1]. This comment made by a medical oncologist highlights the tendency that orthodox treatment often has, of leaving patients feeling that they have been reduced to a vehicle for their disease, a collection of symptoms that only the experts can alleviate. Of course, to some extent cancer treatment in general and pain management in particular inevitably necessitate some loss of control over one's life. In fact coming into hospital for whatever reason involves to some extent the relinquishment of personal autonomy, the sacrificing of autonomy in the short term for a long-term gain often being essential. However, nurses caring for patients in pain need to be aware of the importance of minimising loss of control as it can be extremely frustrating and stressful for a patient, damage his self-esteem, increase his anxiety and actually heighten his sense of pain [4].

How, then, can we minimise loss of control? One of the main ways of assisting patients in this respect is to facilitate the mobilisation of resources to cope with their disease. A longitudinal study carried out by Poletti et al. which looked at factors affecting coping mechanisms in cancer patients identified several important factors [5]. Below I refer to two which are particularly relevant to this discussion:

1. Mobilisation of resources requires information. Information concerning the cause of pain, the reason why a particular analgesic or co-analgesic has been selected, the formulation of goals for pain management and the identification of methods of intervention all need to be discussed with the patient. A study was carried out at the Royal Marsden Hospital which involved designing a pain assessment chart for use with chronic cancer pain. It was intended that the chart incorporate the patient's perception of his or her pain so it was designed for completion by the patient alone or with assistance from his primary nurse. Amongst other things, the results of this study indicated that the involvement of many patients in their pain management helped to increase their confidence in it.

2. Mobilisation of resources requires retaining a maximum of power over the environment and over oneself. I think it is true to say that on the whole nurses and doctors expect patient compliance. One only has to look at some of the numerous studies on nurse-patient communication or just attach oneself to an average ward round to have this opinion reinforced. We are all aware that in recent years there has been something of a backlash against orthodox treatment methods. I am sure that this is not simply because surgery, radiotherapy or chemotherapy may have distressing side-effects but also because medicine tends to remove power from an individual or, to use the oncologist's words referred to earlier, "can make some patients feel like a feather in the wind". I am not, of course, saying that orthodox treatment is inappropriate, but rather that it should be given within a holistic framework. By holistic I do not merely mean the incorporation of a complementary method of pain relief. A holistic approach may involve the utilisation of such techniques but the techniques themselves are not synonymous with holism. Holism is about seeing people as a whole, the person, not the disease or the symptoms, being the focus of the treatment or care. It is about allowing the individual to take as much responsibility as he wants to for himself and his health. Much of the scepticism surrounding the incorporation of some non-pharmacological interventions relates to a lack (in some instances) of proven efficacy. Although I believe that it is the responsibility of the nurse to contribute to the evaluation of such techniques, I do not believe that we should allow a lack of proven efficacy to stop us from utilising interventions which at best can give back to the patient a degree of control and at the least provide him with a means of diversion which can be used to place pain at the periphery of awareness [6].

Iatrogenic Problems

Although the past 20 years have seen a revolution in the area of pain management there is still a lot of evidence to indicate that the nature of cancer pain is still misunderstood. Here I shall discuss two examples of this under the umbrella term "iatrogenic problems".

Let us consider the placebo effect in relation to phamacological methods of pain control. It is increasingly recognised that a considerable proportion of the behavioural effect of drugs is not achieved by way of their assumed specific site of action. For example, double-blind clinical trials of antidepressants and related drugs (drugs which are often used as co-analgesics in the management of cancer pain) generally show at least a 30% improvement in patients (rated on various types of mood scales) after treatment with placebo [1]. This of course does not mean that pharmacological management of pain is inappropriate; rather it emphasises the fact that the efficacy of a drug is not just dependent upon its biochemical action but has a lot to do with contact with the prescribing doctor and nurse. I believe that nurses involved in caring for patients in pain can have an enormous placebo effect which can result in significant analgesic sparing effects.

Ignorance concerning the use of opioids can be justifiably classified as an iatrogenic problem too. Hesitation to use morphine when a weak opioid is ineffective is usually based on unfounded fears concerning addiction and respiratory depression. Neither respiratory depression nor addiction occur in patients receiving long-term opioids for cancer pain [7]. We have a responsibility to dispel these often deeply ingrained myths about morphine as misconceptions held by doctors and nurses can result in a lot of unnecessary suffering. However, because the principal side-effects of morphine are inevitable drowsiness, universal constipation and possible nausea and vomiting, colleagues need to be educated concerning the management of these symptoms and patients and relatives require careful explanation and reassurance.

Conclusion

The importance of the provision of adequate information was emphasised earlier in this chapter. It is very important that we recognise that alongside the need for information exists the need for hope. Hope is a vital factor where the mobilisation of coping mechanisms is concerned. Interestingly, a small study carried out by Morris et al. [8] in the 1970s on the relationship between mental attitudes and prognosis in breast cancer recorded some significant findings in this respect. In this study patients' responses to their illness were divided into four categories: denial, fighting spirit, stoic acceptance, and helplessness and hopelessness. It was noted both at 5- and at 10-year intervals after diagnosis that recurrence-free survivals were significantly more common among patients in the "denial" and "fighting spirit" categories than among patients in the "stoic acceptance" and "helpless/hopeless" categories. It is significant that patients defined as rejecting evidence about their cancer and not wanting information should do as well in terms of survival as those defined as planning to conquer cancer by marshalling all their resources and wanting to know everything about their illness. This apparent paradox should remind us of the importance of paying attention to the fundamental principle of pain management, which is that we tailor make our care to the individual needs of each patient. This can only be achieved, however, when the recipient of our care is the centre of our focus. Control must shift from professional to patient if effective pain management is to be achieved and the patient enabled to live the remainder of his life as fully as possible.

References

1. Open University (1985) Experiencing and explaining disease. Oxford University Press, Oxford
2. Twycross RG, Lack SA (1983) Symptom control in far advanced cancer; pain relief. Pitman, London
3. Gartside G (1986) Alternative methods of pain relief. Nursing 3 (11): 405–407
4. Turton P (1985) When the team doesn't work. Nursing Times 81 (12): 23
5. Poletti R (1985) Clinical oncology and cancer nursing. Pergamon, London
6. McCaffery M (1979) Nursing the patient in pain. Harper and Row, New York
7. Hanks GW, Hoskin PJ (1986) Pain control in advanced cancer; pharmacological methods. J R Coll Physicians Lond 20 (4): 276–281
8. Morris T (1983) Practising what is preached. National society for Cancer Relief, London

Management of Bleeding and Infection

Coagulation Disorders Associated with Neoplastic Disease

R. H. Steingart

Division of Hematology/Oncology, Baystate Medical Center, Springfield, MA 01199, USA

Hemorrhagic, thrombotic, and embolic complications occur frequently in cancer patients. Diverse hemostatic alterations, including impaired plasma coagulation, platelet abnormalities, and vascular disorders, account for these defects.

Hypercoagulability and Thrombosis

The association between malignancy and thrombosis has been recognized since 1865, when Trousseau described the syndrome of recurrent migratory thrombophlebitis in a series of patients with gastric carcinoma [1]. Since then, a number of clinical and postmortem studies have appeared describing arterial and venous thrombosis, migratory thrombophlebitis, pulmonary embolism, and nonbacterial thrombotic endocarditis in patients with neoplasms [2]. The overall incidence of thrombosis in patients with malignancies is between 5% and 15% [3]. Thromboembolic events rank second only to infections as causes of death in patients with solid tumors. Although patients with mucin-secreting tumors of the gastrointestinal tract have long been known to be prone to thromboembolic complications, other tumor types are also associated with an increased risk of thromboembolic disease. Pancreatic carcinoma has historically been associated with the greatest risk of thrombosis, which is reported to occur in as many as 50% of patients. However, since the prevalence of lung cancer far exceeds that of pacreatic cancer, the presence of thrombosis is most likely to be associated with tumors of the lung than of the upper gastrointestinal tract. The other more common tumors associated with thrombosis include gastric, colon, prostate, ovarian, breast, and renal in descending order.

Episodes of thrombosis, particularly superficial thrombophlebitis, may actually antedate by months or even years the clinical diagnosis of cancer in many patients [4]. However, the indications for conducting an extensive search for an occult malignancy in patients with deep vein thrombophlebitis or pulmonary embolism are vague.

Nonbacterial thrombotic endocarditis has been described primarily with adenocarcinoma of the lung, pancreas, and colon. The aortic valve is the most fre-

Recent Results in Cancer Research, Vol. 108

quently involved, followed by the mitral valve. The spleen is the most commonly infarcted viscus. However, end organs associated with greatest morbidity and mortality include cerebral vessels, coronary arteries, and the renal bed.

The increased incidence of thromboembolic disease has led several investigators to examine various aspects of the coagulation system in patients with cancer. Subclinical coagulopathy is frequent in patients with malignancy. Abnormalities of routine tests of blood coagulation have been reported to occur in as many as 98% of patients with cancer [5]. The most common clotting abnormalities in cancer patients are elevated concentrations of fibrin split products (FSPS), prolonged thrombin times, thrombocytosis, and hyperfibrinogenemia. Other common abnormalities include decreased antithrombin III levels (AT III) and elevation of plasma coagulation factors, including factors V, VIII, IX, and XI. These abnormalities have been said to be consistent with the presence of "overcompensated intravascular coagulation with secondary fibrinolysis." It is theorized that low-grade intravascular coagulation with accelerated clotting factor utilization is accompanied by increased synthetic rates for fibrinogen, clotting factors, and platelets, resulting in actual increases in their levels in the circulation and a relative hypercoagulable state.

The mechanism by which malignant tissue initiates disseminated intravascular coagulation (DIC) is poorly understood. Three basic mechanisms for the activation of blood coagulation in patients with neoplastic disorders have recently been described: (1) the activation of platelets by tumor cells, (2) the production of procoagulants by monocytes and macrophages, stimulated by the tumor, and (3) the production of procoagulants directly by tumor cells [6]. The tissue procoagulants derived from extracts of human breast, colon, kidney, and lung cancer can directly initiate coagulation by activation of factor X to Xa [6]. This differs from the conventional method of activation by thromboplastic substances via factor XII or factor VII.

The treatment of thromboembolic complications in patients with cancer is difficult. It does appear that succes in controlling the coagulopathy ultimately requires successful control of the tumor. When laboratory abnormalities are found in the absence of clinical complications, treatment of the coagulopathy is generally not indicated. One exception is when subclinical DIC complicates acute promyelocytic leukemia (to be discussed later). The use of anticoagulants (warfarin, heparin) and antiplatelet drugs (salicylates, dipyridamole) has been associated with some correction of altered coagulation factors and clinical improvement. In spite of this, cancer patients are notoriously resistant to anticoagulation therapy and rethrombosis is common [4].

Hemorrhage

Disseminated intravascular coagulation is present in many patients with cancer and manifests varying clinical patterns, the most extreme form being acute DIC and fulminant catastrophic hemorrhage. The occurrence of overt DIC, characterized by consumption of platelets and clotting factors with resultant bleeding complications, is less common with solid tumors than is "chronic" DIC manifested by thrombosis. Although acute DIC has been reported in association with almost all types of solid tumor, it is most commonly observed with carcinoma of the lung, gallbladder, stomach, colon, breast, ovary, and melanoma [2, 3]. It is especially common in both local and metastatic carcinoma of the prostate. The incidence in different series ranges from 6% to 40%. The neoplastic disorder most frequently associated with fulminant DIC is acute promyelocytic leukemia.

Hemorrhagic complications in affected patients with solid tumors may range from minor mucocutaneous bleeding to extensive gastrointestinal, genitourinary, pulmonary, or intracerebral hemorrhage. Patients with acute dcompensated DIC will commonly manifest thrombocytopenia, hypofibrinogenemia, prolonged thrombin, prothrombin, and partial thromboplastin times, and elevated levels of circulating FSPs. Antithrombin III as well as other clotting factors levels are usually reduced due to consumption. Less commonly, the peripheral blood smear will show evidence of microangiopathic red cell fragmentation.

Unlike the "chronic" hypercoagulable form of this entity, in "acute" DIC clotting factors are consumed in excess of production. The mechanisms by which tumors can cause any form of DIC have been discussed. The reason some tumors tend to favor clot formation and others clot lysis is not clear. However, in the case of prostatic carcinoma, the neoplastic tissue contains procoagulant-like materials which can trigger both the extrinsic coagulation system as well as the fibrinolytic system. Acute promyelocytic leukemia is frequently associated with DIC. In many instances, subclinical DIC is converted to fulminant DIC with the initiation of cytotoxic chemotherapy. This ist attributed to the release of a thromboplastin-like material localized to the nuclear membrane and granules within the cells [7]. Endotoxin derived primarily from gram-negative organisms also can cause acute DIC in the neutropenic cancer patient.

Therapy in the acute DIC of neoplastic disease should be initially directed at treatment of the underlying malignancy or infection itself. Until antitneoplastic therapy is initiated, control of bleeding is often unsuccessful. The first line of therapy for active bleeding often consists of treatment with replacement products such as platelets and clotting factors. A major controversy exists concerning heparin usage. Although anticoagulant therapy has a more clear benefit with respect to chronic as opposed to acute DIC, no randomized trials of heparin therapy in the DIC of malignancy have been conducted.

Heparin should be used cautiously in the setting of severe renal or hapatic failure, when extensive vascular damage is present, or when very severe thrombocytopenia and hypofibrinogenemia are found. Despite the controversy regarding the use of heparin, in patients with acute promyelocytic leukemia there appears to be a decreased incidence of fatal hemorrhage and therefore an increased incidence of remission induction in the prophylactically heparin-treated group [8].

Primary Fibrin(ogen)olysis

Primary fibrin(ogen)olysis is a hemostatic disorder in which there is either local or systemic activation of the fibrinolytic pathway resulting in plasmin degradation of fibrinogen, fibrin, factor V, and factor VIII. Hypofibrinogenemia, very high circulating levels of FSP, low plasminogen levels, and relatively normal levels of platelets are usually present.

Although primary hyperfibrinolysis occurs in malignancy, DIC with secondary fibrinolysis is a much more common cause of hemorrhage. The more common tumors that are capable of spontaneous fibrinolytic activity include prostatic carcinoma and sarcomas [9]. In addition, Davidson et al. described a patient with metastatic large cell carcinoma of the lung whose tumor produced plasminogen activators that caused bleeding at the site of a surgical incision [10].

Distinction from a coexisiting DIC syndrome may be difficult but must be made before treatment with an inhibitor of plasminogen activation such as ε-aminocaproic acid is considered. These drugs can cause severe thrombotic complications in the setting of DIC.

Other Coagulation Defects

Patients with neoplastic disease may develop bleeding from other coagulation factor abnormalities. These are less common and are usually associated with less serious hemorrhage than when DIC develops. Hepatic dysfunction, due to neoplastic parenchymal damage or to obstruction of the biliary system, may produce a variety of coagulation defects. Reduced synthesis and poor absorption of vitamin K may lead to deficiencies in particular of the vitamin K dependent factors (II, VII, IX, and X). Vitamin K supplementation is usually ineffective and hemorrhage must be controlled with fresh frozen plasma.

Isolated deficiencies of individual coagulation factors are rare, and for the most part the etiology of the acquired deficiency state is unknown. Most have only mild decreases in factors and are therefore clinically asymptomatic.

The vast majority of acquired circulating anticoagulants are antibodies either neutralizing a specific blood coagulation factor or interfering in some fashion with factor function. Inhibitors may occur with a wide variety of tumors. They are usually more significant clinically in paraproteinemias than in solid tumors. Table 1 outlines these isolated deficiencies and inhibitors.

Table 1. Selective impairment of plasma coagulation in cancer

Pathological inhibitors
Paraproteins in plasma cell dyscrasias
Lupus-like: Hodgkin's disease, non-Hodgkin's lymphoma, myelofibrosis, carcinoma
Factor XI inhibitors: carcinomas of the colon, prostate
Factor VII inhibitor: bronchogenic carcinoma
Isolated factor deficiencies
XIII: chronic myelocytic leukemia (CML), metastatic liver disease
XII: CML
XI: malignant melanoma
X: multiple myeloma with amyloidosis
VIIR: RC and/or VIIIR:Ag: macroglobulinemia, chronic lymphocytic leukemia, Wilms' tumor
V: CML
Abnormal fibrinogen: hepatocellular carcinoma

Thrombocytopenia

Thrombocytopenia is the most common cause of bleeding in patients with both solid tumors and hematological malignancies. Decreased production of platelets can result from systemic chemotherapy, radiotherapy, or direct invasion of the marrow with tumor. Ineffective thrombopoiesis, characterized by dysplastic or megaloblastic marrow hypercellularity and peripheral cytopenia, is usually caused by sepsis, B_{12} or folate deficiency, or primary myelodysplastic syndromes. Correction of the underlying infection or nutritional deficiency may result in improved counts. Platelet counts of less than 10000 mm^{-3} are often associated with spontaneous hemorrhage and therefore most advise support with platelet concentrates.

Thrombocytopenia due to increased peripheral destruction most commonly indicates the presence of DIC, hypersplenism, or an autoimmune phenomenon. A syndrome resembling idiopathic thrombocytopenic purpura (ITP) is most often associated with lymphoproliferative malignancies. Case reports of patients with non-smal cell and small cell lung cancer, as well as adenocarcinomas of the rectum, colon, ovary, and gallbladder, have shown associations with ITP-like syndromes [11]. These may develop prior to, concident with, or following the diagnosis of cancer.

Thrombocytosis

Thrombocytosis occurs in up to 30%-40% of cancer patients. It is more often associated with carcinomas but has been described in both Hodgkin's and non-Hodgkin's lymphomas. The etiology may be due to increased thrombopoietic activity. The platelet count is usually modest, ranging from 400000 mm^{-3} to 800000 mm^{-3}. Clinical bledding or thrombosis from this isolated problem is rare, and specific treatment is not necessary. Treatment of thrombocytosis is ordinary required only in the myeloproliferative disorders when the platelet count exceeds 1000000 mm^{-3} and there is clinical evidence of thrombosis or hemorrhage.

Qualitative Platelet Disorders

Abnormal platelet function is common in both solid tumors and hematologic malignancies. In solid tumors, the most common cause of defective platelet function is the presence of FSPs resulting from DIC or fibrinolysis.

Hemorrhagic manifestations frequently occur in the dysproteinemias, where abnormalities of platelet function much more commonly account for clinical bleeding than do thrombocytopenia or factor deficiencies. The actual incidence of hemorrhage in malignant paraprotein disorders varies depending upon the particular disease.

About 15% of patients with IgG myeloma and over 38% with IgA myeloma experience bleeding. Patients with Waldenström's macroglobulinemia have a greater than 60% incidence of hemorrhage [12]. Impaired in vitro platelet function is attributed to coating of the platelet canalicular system with paraprotein. Treatment of hemorrhage is directed towards decreasing the paraprotein by either chemotherapy or, more acutely, with plasmapheresis. Other causes of acquired qualitative platelet defects in patients with cancer include uremia, liver disease, and the use of certain antibiotics.

Vascular Disorders

Neoplastic diseases of the endothelium may result in purpuric and hemorrhagic lesions. Chief among these is Kaposi's sarcoma. Once primarily a disease of older Italian and Jewish men, this disease has become increasingly more common and noticeable due to its association with acquired immune deficiency syndrome (AIDS). Amyloid, in association with both plasma cell dyscrasias and other tumors, may be deposited in the area between the endothelium and the basement membrane, thereby infiltrating the subendothelium in both the microcirculation and the macrocirculation. The infiltrated vessel has decreased tensile strength and constriction abilities. Extravasation, including purpura, may occur. Purpura may be one of the presenting signs in as many as 16% of all patients with amyloidosis [13, 14]. The distribution of the lesion has a peculiar predilection for the face.

In malignant dysproteinemic states, such as multiple myeloma and Waldenström's macroglobulinemia, purpuric lesions may result from associated cryoglobulinemia or cryofibrinogenemia.

Purpura may be seen in patients who have received glucocorticoids for extended periods. This type of purpura is typically superficial and limited to the forearms. Glucocorticoids decrease collagen synthesis and may result in reduction of structural support for the microcirculation.

Effects of Chemotherapy on Hemostasis

Chemotherapy may alter hemostasis by a variety of mechanisms. The most common and significant of these have been previously discussed and include the thrombocytopenia associated with bone marrow suppressive cytotoxic drugs and

Table 2. Antineoplastic agents which may alter hemostasis

Agent	Mechanism
L-Asparaginase	Hypofibrinogenemia Depression IX, XI
Mithramycin	Platelet dysfunction Depression II, V, VII, X
Doxorubicin Daunorubicin	Primary fibrinolysis
Ara-C	Platelet dysfunction
L-Phenylalanine mustard	Platelet dysfunction

the enhancement of DIC by drug-induced destruction of some malignant neoplasms. Antineoplastic agents which may interfere with hemostasis are listed in Table 2.

References

1. Trousseau A (1865) Phlegmasia alba dolens. Clinique medicale de l'Hotel-dieu de Paris, London. New Sydenham Society 3: 94
2. Sack GH, Levin J, Bell W (1977) Trousseau's syndrome and other manifestations of chronic disseminated coagulopathy in patients with neoplasms. Clinical, pathologic and therapeutic features. Medicine (Baltimore) 56: 1-37
3. Bick RL (1978) Alterations of hemostasis with malignancy. Semin Thromb Hemost 5: 1-26
4. Schafer AI (1985) The hypercoagulable states. Ann Intern Med 102: 814-828
5. Sun NC, McAfee WM, Gibert JM et al. (1979) Hemostatic abnormalities in malignancy, a prospective study of one hundred and eight patients. Am J Clin Pathol 71: 10-16
6. Rickles FR, Edwards RL (1983) Activation of blood coagulation in cancer: Trousseau's syndrome revisited. Blood 62: 14-31
7. Gralnick HR, Sultan C (1975) Acute promyelocytic leukemia: haemorrhagic manifestation and morphologic criteria. Br J Haematol 29: 373-376
8. Drapkin RI, Gee TS, Dowling MD et al. (1978) Prophylactic heparin therapy in acute promyelocytic leukemia. Cancer 41: 2482-2490
9. Goldsmith GH Jr (1984) Hemostatic disorders associated with neoplasia. Ratnoff OD, Forbes CD (eds) Disorders of hemostasis. Grune and Stratton, Orlando, pp 351-363
10. Davidson JR, McNicol GP, Frank GC (1969) Plasminogen-activator producing tumor. Br Med J [Clin Res] 1: 88-91
11. Bellone JD, Kunicki TH, Aster RH (1983) Immune thrombocytopenia associated with carcinoma. Ann Intern Med 99: 470-472
12. Perkins HA, Mackenzie MR, Fudenberg HH (1970) Hemostatic defects in dysproteinemias. Blood 35: 695-707
13. Kitchens CS (1984) The purpuric disorders. Semin Thromb Hemost 10: 173-189
14. Kyle RA, Bayrd ED (1975) Amyloidosis. Review of 236 cases. Medicine (Baltimore) 54: 271-299

Hematological Support in Patients Undergoing Allogenetic Bone Marrow Transplantation

B. Osterwalder, A. Gratwohl, P. Reusser, A. Tichelli, and B. Speck

Abteilung für Onkologie, Medizinische Klinik C, Kantonsspital,
9007 St. Gallen, Switzerland

Bone marrow transplantation (BMT) is not possible without the substitution of blood cell components [1]. Cytostatic conditioning and total body irradiation (TBI) as the usual preparative regimen for BMT induces severe bone marrow aplasia lasting at least 2-4 weeks until marrow function takes place, as well as profound humoral and cellular immunosuppression. Under these circumstances transfusion of blood cells can be associated with several hazards. Clinical consequences of HLA-sensitization due to leukocyte contamination in random donor blood products include febrile transfusion reactions, random donor platelet transfusion refractoriness, and poor granulocyte increments after granulocyte transfusions. Because of possible sensitization for non-MHC-antigens, transfusions from close relatives should be strictly avoided prior to transplantation. Use of single random donors for platelet substitution [2] and leukocyte depletion of red blood cell (RBC) and platelet (PLT) concentrates [1] are important in patients when BMT is attempted. For patients with severe aplastic anemia, blood transfusion therapy should be restricted as much as possible since the survival of untransfused patients is significantly better [3]. In the post-transplantation period there is hardly a risk of alloimmunization owing to the profound immunosuppression. Major risks after BMT, however, include transmission of viral disease (Epstein-Barr virus, cytomegalovirus, and recently HIV), since these viruses can be latently present in the circulating leukocytes [4, 5, 6, 7]. Viral reactivation occurs as a consequence of the severe immunodeficiency state. These risks increase greatly when granulocyte transfusions are administered. Selection of seronegative blood donors, use of frozen RBC units, leukocyte depletion of RBC and PLT concentrates, and use of the marrow donor for PLT substitution are effective in reducing some of these hazards.

The present report reviewed the requirements for RBC and PLT transfusions in 42 patients with aplastic anemia and hematological malignancies undergoing allogeneic bone marrow transplantation during a 2-year study with anti-CMV-hyperimmunoglobulin prophylaxis. In addition an attempt was made to identify factors associated with an increased need for transfusions.

Recent Results in Cancer Research, Vol. 108

Patients and Methods

Between 1 January 1984 and 31 December 1985, 44 patients were admitted to our hospital for allogeneic BMT (43 HLA-A, -B, -C, and DR-identical, MLC-negative; one DR-mismatch). Two patients were excluded, one for nonmedical reasons and one due to septic death on day 5 post-BMT. The remaining 42 patients (22 females, 20 males, median age 26.5 years, range 5-44 years) had the following underlying disease: 13 acute lymphocytic leukemia (ALL), 13 acute myelocytic leukemia (AML), 13 chronic myelogenous leukemia (CML), and 3 severe aplastic anemia (SAA). Leukemic patients were conditioned with cyclophosphamide (60 mg/kg body wt. and day × 2) and TBI (1000 cGy midline dose, fractionated in nine patients). Patients with SAA received cyclophosphamide (50 mg/kg body wt. × 4). Cyclosporin A (plus additional high-dose methylprednisolone in 12 patients) was given for prevention of graft-versus-host disease (GvHD) according to the standard Basel protocol [8]. All patients were nursed in sterile laminar air flow units with an intensive PEPA program [9]. Frozen deglycerolized RBC concentrates (Regional Blood Transfusion Center of Basel, Dr. H. P. Burri) were administered in order to keep the patient's hemoglobin above 100 g/liter. PLT concentrates were collected mainly from the marrow donor, in a few cases from other family members, and rarely from HLA-typed unrelated donors, using the cell separator Fenwall CS-3000, in order to keep the patient's platelet counts above 20×10^9/liter [10]. All blood products were irradiated in vitro with 1500 cGy in order to inactivate lymphoid cells that might initiate or enhance GvHD [11]. For CMV prophylaxis the anti-CMV-hyperimmunoglobulin CYTOTECT (Biotest, Frankfurt, FRG) was used as described [12].

Graft-versus-host disease was graded according to Thomas et al. [13]. A major ABO incompatibility was defined as the presence of antibodies against donor-type RBC (e.g., A→O). A minor ABO mismatch was present when the donor had antibodies against recipient-type RBC (e.g., O→A) [14].

All transfusions of RBC, PLT, and granulocyte concentrates (in one patient) were recorded during the study time within the laminar air flow unit pre- and post-BMT, until death or transfusion independency.

Student's *t*-test was used for comparison of the different transfusion subgroups.

Results

All patients needed transfusions after marrow grafting. The transfusion requirements for the whole patient group and for some subgroups according to factors which can influence the need for blood products are shown in Table 1. Overall a median of eight RBC concentrates (mean 9.6 ± 7.2, range 1-32) and four PLT concentrates (mean 4.6 ± 3.2, range 1-11) per patient were administered postgrafting according to our criteria. Figures 1 and 2 illustrate the need for RBCs and PLTs in relation to the time post-BMT. RBC transfusion need started after a median of 8.5 days (mean 9.2 ± 5.6, range 1-31 days), which is significantly later ($P < 0.0005$) than for PLT transfusions (median 6 days, mean 6.1 ± 1.9, range 1-10).

Table 1. Overall transfusion requirements in 42 patients after allogeneic bone marrow transplantation, and factors influencing transfusion requirements

Factors	No. of patients	Red cell transfusions			Platelet transfusions		
		Med.	Mean ± SD	Range	Med.	Mean ± SD	Range
Overall							
Pre-BMT	23/7	3	3.1 ± 1.9	1- 8	3	2.7 ± 1.2	1- 4
Post-BMT	42	8	9.6 ± 7.2	1-32	4	4.6 ± 3.2	1-11
Diagnosis							
ALL	13	11	9.9 ± 6.3	1-20	3	4.6 ± 3.5	1-11
AML	13	7	8.4 ± 6.1	1-23	5	5.1 ± 2.6	2-11
CML	13	10	10.1 ± 8.9	1-32	4	4.9 ± 3.7	1-11
SAA	3		8, 22, 2			2, 1, 2	
Age							
5-20 years	15	8	8.8 ± 6.2[a]	1-22	2.5	3.9 ± 2.8[c]	1- 9
21-30 years	14	5.5	6.6 ± 5.6[b]	1-22	4	4.6 ± 3.1	1-11
31-44 years	13	11	13.6 ± 8.3[a, b]	2-32	5	5.6 ± 3.8[c]	1-11
ABO compatibility							
Minor/no barrier	34	7	8.9 ± 6.5[d]	1-23	3.5	4.5 ± 3.1	1-11
Major barrier	8	9	12.5 ± 9.6[d]	3-32	5.5	5.4 ± 3.7	1-11
Graft-versus-host disease:							
Grades 0-I	11	6	5.0 ± 3.1[e]	1-11	4	4.0 ± 2.3	1- 8
Grades II-IV	31	11	11.2 ± 7.5[e]	2-32	4	4.9 ± 3.5	1-11

[a] $P<0.05$
[b] $P<0.01$
[c] $P<0.1$, >0.05
[d] $P=0.1$
[e] $P<0.01$

Red blood cell transfusion dependency post-BMT lasted a median of 27.5 days (mean 35.5 ± 25.3, range 1-98), which again is significantly longer ($P<0.005$) than the PLT transfusion dependency (median 11.5 days, mean 20.3 ± 24,4, range 1-90). Thus the need for platelets is greatest in the first 2 weeks after BMT, which reflects the usually good engraftment of megakaryopoiesis [15].

The *underlying disease* did not influence the transfusion need for RBCs and PLTs. Higher numbers of nucleated *bone marrow cells* ($\times 10^8$/kg body wt.) infused at day 0 into the patient also did not reduce transfusion demands (data not shown). In addition, no correlation was found with *engraftment* (day post-BMT with leukocytes $>1 \times 10^9$/liter) (data not shown). The need for transfusions, however, increased with *age* (above 30 years). This is statistically significant for RBCs, but only of borderline significance for PLTs.

Eight patients had a *major ABO barrier* to the donor. Seven of these patients received a median of four (mean 3.3 ± 1.7, range 1-5) RBC concentrates during the conditioning phase in the context of an immunoadsorption procedure for in vivo removal of residual antibodies [14]. Eight patients had a minor ABO incom-

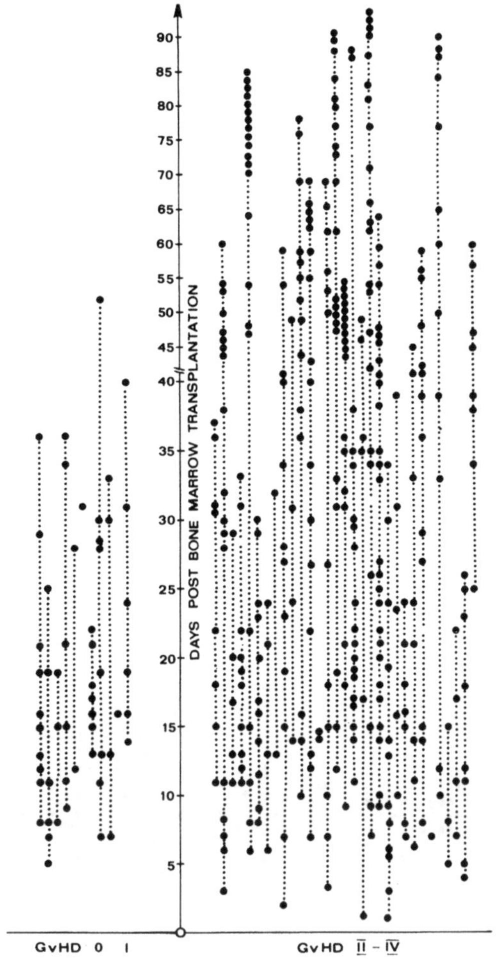

Fig. 1. Requirements for RBC transfusions in 11 patients with GvHD grades 0-I and in 32 patients with GvHD grades II-IV in relation to the time after allogeneic bone marrow transplantation. Each *dot* (●) represents one single unit of RBC; each *dotted line* (●····●) represents one patient's transfusion course

patibility to the donor and therefore had plasma centrifuged from the donor marrow. Postgrafting there is an increased demand for RBC transfusion ($P=0.1$), mainly due to ABO incompatible RBC transfusions for in vivo adsorption of isohemagglutinins against the marrow donor's RBCs. PLT requirements were not altered.

Severe GvHD (grades II-IV) was associated with a statistically significant increase in RBC requirements but not in PLT need. This difference is still present when patients with a major ABO barrier are excluded from this comparison (mean 5.0 ± 3.4, range 1-11 in patients with GvHD 0-I versus mean 10.3 ± 6.8, range 1-23 in patients with GvHD II-IV, $P<0.025$). The mean age did not differ significantly in these two groups (GvHD 0-I: 22.6 ± 6.1, range 13-32; GvHD II-IV: 25.4 ± 11.1, range 5-44 years, $P<0.25$), indicating that the increase in RBC requirements is due to severe GvHD. As could be expected, patients with GvHD grades II-IV required RBC transfusion for a significantly longer period post-BMT

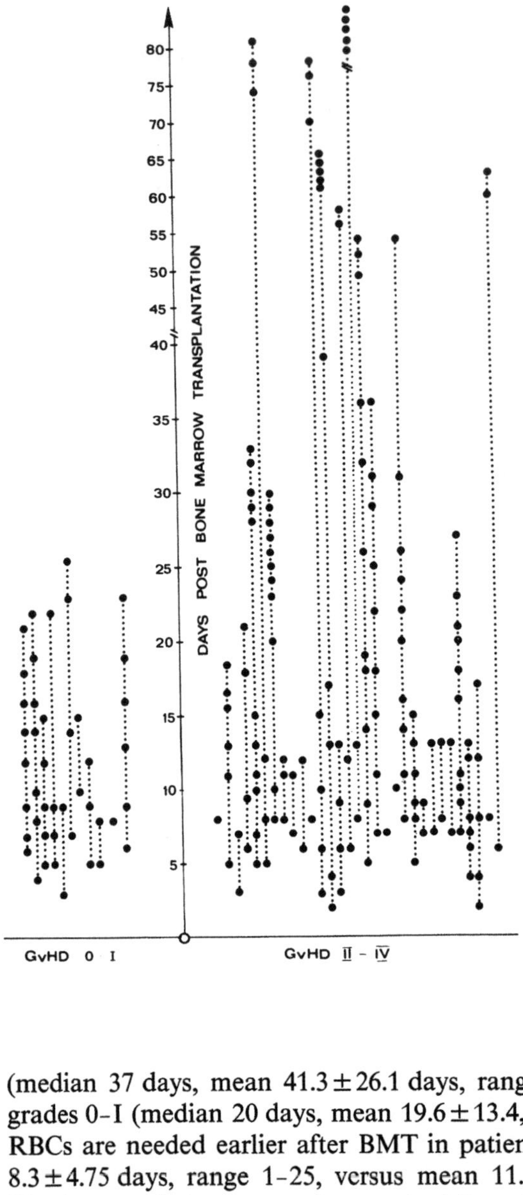

Fig. 2. Requirements for PLT transfusions in 11 patients with GvHD grades 0-I and in 32 patients with GvHD grades II-IV in relation to the time after allogeneic bone marrow transplantation. Each *dot* (●) represents one single unit of PLT; each *dotted line* (●·····●) represents on patient's transfusion course

(median 37 days, mean 41.3±26.1 days, range 1-98) than patients with GvHD grades 0-I (median 20 days, mean 19.6±13.4, range 1-45) ($P<0.01$). In addition RBCs are needed earlier after BMT in patients with GvHD grades II-IV (mean 8.3±4.75 days, range 1-25, versus mean 11.8±7.2 days, range 5-31, $P<0.05$). Platelet transfusions were also required for a longer period after BMT in patients with GvHD grades II-IV (median 11.5 days, mean 24.4±27.5, range 1-90) than in patients with GvHD grades 0-I (median 10 days, mean 9.9±6.9, range 1-19) ($P>0.05$ <0.1). PLTs needs to be started in both groups at day 6 post-BMT (Figs. 1, 2).

Overall 24 patients are alive (February 1987), two of them with relapse of leukemia and three with chronic GvHD. Seven patients died of GvHD, three of leukemic relapse, two of CMV-associated interstitial pneumonia, three of idiopathic interstitial pneumonia, and one each of veno-occlusive disease, bone marrow aplasia, and cerebral hemorrhage. At autopsy CMV-associated interstitial pneumonia was also found in the patient with cerebral hemorrhage and the patient with veno-occlusive disease. This latter CMV-seronegative patient with a CMV-negative marrow donor had inadvertently received PLT concentrates from a CMV-seropositive relative in the period before death. Thus CMV might have been transferred by transfusion.

Discussion

Our transfusion policy in BMT included the use of irradiated frozen deglycerolized RBC concentrates in an attempt to minimize transmission of viral disease (especially cytomegalovirus), as well as the use of irradiated PLT concentrates, collected by the cell separator mainly from the marrow donor. Hemoglobin had to be maintained above 100 g/liter and platelet counts above 20 $\times$ 10^9/liter. Although all patients required transfusions after allogeneic BMT, the numbers of units needed are in general smaller than in patients with leukemia undergoing conventional intensive chemotherapy or in patients with severe aplastic anemia following antilymphocyte globulin therapy [16].

On average, eight RBC and four PLT transfusions were necessary in the 42 patients following BMT. Requirements for RBCs started a median of 8.5 days post-BMT and lasted a median of 27.5 days, whereas requirements for PLTs already began at day 6 and lasted only a median of 11.5 days. Among the variables evaluted statistically for their effect on transfusion requirements, only age above 30 years and the development of grade II-IV GvHD were associated with a significant increase in RBC transfusions. There was a tendency for a higher RBC transfusion need when the transplant was across a major ABO barrier. PLT transfusion needs were not significantly influenced by these variables, although we noted a tendency for higher PLT transfusion requirements in older patients.

In a study of 82 patients with severe aplastic anemia the group from Seattle analyzed transfusion requirements using a multivariate statistical analysis of 22 variables [17]. On average, 8 RBC units (1-82) and 44 PLT units (6-468) were necessary postgrafting. Requirements for RBCs and PLTs increased significantly with increasing age and when the patient had isohemagglutinins against the marrow donor's RBCs. Their transfusion strategy was different to ours. Normal packed RBCs were transfused. Patients received pooled random platelets until platelet refractoriness, after which single donor pheresis products were used.

The fact that we used single donor platelet products with high yields of platelets [10] from the beginning might explain the lower number of PLT transfusions necessary in our study. In addition we mainly studied leukemic patients. However, as far as it is possible to draw conclusions from the small number of patients with SAA, we saw no difference in the need for transfusions in relation to the underlying disease.

In the Seattle patient group AB0 blood group incompatibility between marrow donor and recipient was a significant factor in increased RBC need [17]. Our patient group might be too small to reach the level of significance. However, the persistence of isohemagglutinins postgrafting always led to repeated in vivo adsorption of the antibodies by donor-type RBCs, whereas recipient-type RBCs were administered for maintenance of the hemoglobin [14].

Most important with regard to the transfusion need in our patients was the development of severe GvHD. Not only did it increase the number of RBC transfusions necessary, but these patients also required transfusions significantly earlier after BMT and for a significantly longer period (Fig. 1). This is well understandable from the much more complicated clinical course postgrafting, primarily in the second month post-BMT, with the occurrence of hemolytic syndromes and gastrointestinal hemorrhage. The influence on PLT transfusions was much less prominent. Wulff et al. [17] observed no increased risk for the development of acute GvHD in patients receiving larger amounts of blood products. Although our patients with severe GvHD required RBC transfusions earlier after BMT, our data suggest that the increase in numbers and in time of transfusion dependency in these patients is mainly due to the complications of GvHD in the second and third months after BMT.

Due to the profound immunosuppression after BMT, alloimmunization can hardly play a role. Patients in the Seattle study who were refractory to random-donor platelets at the time of BMT had no increase in transfusion requirements [17]. Our patients with CML, who had received few or no transfusions before BMT, required comparable numbers of transfusions to patients with acute leukemia, who all received a considerable number of transfusions during conventional chemotherapy. Of our three patients with SAA, two were untransfused and one had received three units of blood before BMT. It is well known that patients with aplastic anemia who are untransfused do significantly better after BMT [3]. Therefore special attention is necessary prior to BMT to prevent immunization for MHC antigens and also non-MHC-antigens, e.g., those present within the family. Family members are thus available for substitution only after BMT. There are also good reasons for preventing alloimmunization during chemotherapy in leukemic patients awaiting BMT [2]. Careful depletion of DR (class II)-expressing leukocytes and leukocyte fragments in all blood products should be an essential part of the transfusion policy from diagnosis onward.

Of more importance after BMT is the possibility of transmitting viral diseases by the marrow or by leukocyte contamination. This is illustrated in our patient who died of veno-occlusive disease, where at autopsy CMV-associated interstitial pneumonia was also found despite the fact that patient and donor were both seronegative. Obviously one single seropositive transfusion might transmit the virus. The CMV hyperimmunoglobulin could not prevent the development of CMV pneumonia. New problems arise with HIV, as reflected by several reports [4, 5, 6, 7]. For granulocyte transfusions which are, fortunately, rarely necessary in BMT, selection of donors poses special problems. Although GvHD is a rare complication of RBC and PLT transfusions, it can easily be prevented by gamma irradiation of concentrates prior to transfusion. This should be an integral part of the transfusion strategy in BMT [11].

In conclusion, an optimal transfusion strategy should commence from the time of diagnosis in leukemic as well as in aplastic patients awaiting BMT. Careful selection of donors and blood products, effective leukocyte depletion, and strict criteria for RBC, PLT, and granulocyte transfusions might all reduce the risks resulting from alloimmunization and transmission of viral disease. An optimal transfusion policy can contribute to successful bone marrow transplantation.

Summary

Bone marrow transplantation is impossible without effective support with blood components during the period of pancytopenia before graft function appears. We analyzed 39 patients with leukemia and three patients with severe aplastic anemia with regard to the pre- and postgrafting requirements for RBC and PLT transfusions. Overall a median of eight RBC and four PLT concentrates were necessary in all 42 patients after allogeneic BMT (ranges, 1-32 RBC and 1-11 PLT units). Requirements were identical irrespective of the underlying disease (ALL, AML, CML, SAA). Transfusion need for RBC and PLT concentrates increased in patients over 30 years old and with a major red blood group AB0 barrier between marrow donor and recipient. The presence of grade II-IV GvHD increased RBC requirements significantly, but not PLT requirements. In addition these patients were dependent on RBC transfusions for significantly longer periods. Only one patient required therapeutic granulocyte transfusions. In a CMV-negative patient with a CMV-negative marrow donor, who died of veno-occlusive disease, cytomegalovirus was transmitted inadvertently by a seropositive PLT concentrate in his final course. Our transfusion strategy included frozen deglycerolized RBC concentrates and single donor PLT concentrates, collected mainly from the marrow donor by a cell separator. All blood products were irradiated in vitro with 1500 cGy before transfusion. An optimal transfusion policy starting before BMT can contribute to successful bone marrow transplantation.

References

1. Brand A, Claas FHJ, Falkenburg JHF et al. (1984) Blood component therapy in bone marrow transplantation. Semin Hematol 21: 141-155
2. Gmür J, von Felten A, Osterwalder B et al. (1983) Delayed alloimmunization using random single donor platelet transfusions: a prospective study in thrombocytopenic patients with acute leukemia. Blood 62: 473-479
3. Storb R, Thomas ED, Buckner DC et al. (1980) Marrow transplantation in thirty "untransfused" patients with severe aplastic anemia. Ann Intern Med 92: 30-36
4. Bierling P, Cordonnier C, Duedari N et al. (1985) LAV/HTLV III in allogeneic bone marrow transplantation. Ann Intern Med 104: 131-132
5. Vilmer E, Devergie A, Gluckman E (1986) Lymphadenopathy AIDS virus (LAV) infection after bone marrow transplantation. Bone Marrow Transplant 1 [Suppl 1]: 37
6. Rombos Y, Apperley JF, Rice SJ et al. (1986) Seroconversion for HTLV-III antibody status after BMT for CGL. Bone Marrow Transplant 1 [Suppl 1]: 38
7. Novakovitch G, Maranchini D, Bagarry D et al. (1986) LAV/HTLV III infection after bone marrow transplantation. Bone Marrow Transplant 1 [Suppl 1]: 39
8. Speck B, Gratwohl A, Osterwalder B et al. (1985) Experience with 100 allogeneic marrow grafts using cyclosporin-A (CyA) for prophylaxis against GvHD. Exp Hematol 13 [Suppl 17]: 126
9. Osterwalder B, Szucs T, Gratwohl A et al. (1983) Infectious problems in bone marrow recipients on a protected-environment-prophylactic-antibiotic program (PEPA). Pro-

ceedings of the 13th international congress of chemotherapy, Vienna 1983 (part 71/8-12)
10. Osterwalder B, Gratwohl A, Levak A et al. (1986) Analysis of results of three different methods for the isolation of platelet and granulocyte concentrates-practical and economic considerations. Plasma Ther Transfus Technol 7: 61-66
11. Leitman SF, Holland PV (1985) Irradiation of blood products. Indications and guidelines. Transfusion 25: 293-303
12. Osterwalder B, Reusser P, Gratama JW et al. (1986) Prophylactic application of an anti-cytomegalovirus hyperimmunoglobulin in allogeneic bone marrow transplantation. Bone Marrow Transplant 1 [Suppl 1]: 47-48
13. Thomas ED, Storb R, Clift RA et al. (1975) Bone marrow transplantation. N Engl J Med 292: 832-843, 895-902
14. Osterwalder B, Gratwohl A, Nissen C et al. (1986) Immunoadsorption for removal of anti-A and anti-B blood group antibodies in AB0-incompatible bone marrow transplantation. Blut 53: 379-390
15. Osterwalder B, Haberthür C, Gratwohl A et al. Can beta-lactam antibiotics in vivo prolong cytostatic-induced bone marrow aplasia? A study in 115 patients undergoing allogeneic bone marrow transplantation. To be published
16. Osterwalder B, Gratwohl A, Tichelli A et al. Long-term transfusion support in patients with severe aplastic anemia undergoing antilymphocyte globulin therapy (manuscript in preparation).
17. Wulff JC, Santner TJ, Storb R et al. (1983) Transfusion requirements after HLA-identical marrow transplantation in 82 patients with aplastic anemia. Vox Sang 44: 366-374

Empirical Antimicrobial Therapy for Febrile Granulocytopenic Cancer Patients: Lessons from Four EORTC Trials

J. Klastersky

Service de Médicine et Laboratoire d'Investigation Clinique H.J. Tagnon,
Institut Jules Bordet, Centre des Tumeurs de l'Université Libre de Bruxelles,
1 Rue Héger-Bordet, 1000 Bruxelles, Belgium

In the 1960s, treatment of infectious complications in cancer patients became a major issue since sepsis was recognized as a major complication of chemotherapy and/or neoplastic disease and a leading cause of death. A major step forward was the recognition that granulocytopenia was the most important factor predisposing cancer patients to frequent and severe sepsis. Improvements in the results of antimicrobial therapy under these conditions are probably to be attributed to the early treatment of granulocytopenic cancer patients (GCPs) with combinations of broad spectrum antibiotics - a so-called empirical therapy - as soon as they become febrile, even if the clinical source and the microbiological nature of the presumed infection are unknown at that time. The value of this approach, which conflicts with the basic rules of antimicrobial therapy requiring the demonstration of a site and of a pathogen prior to commencement of the therapy, has never been confirmed in a controlled trial. However, its immediately observable benefits led to its general acceptance.

Our group (EORTC Antimicrobial Therapy Cooperative Group) has contributed to this approach by setting the standards for definition of infection in GCPs, and criteria of antimicrobial response. Both have been adopted widely and are still the "golden standards" used by most investigators involved in this area of research [4].

Febrile episodes in GCPs are caused by bacterial sepsis (i.e., bacteremia) in about 20% of the patients; gram-negative bacillary bacteremia (GNBB) accounts for two-thirds of these episodes and gram-positive infections for the rest. *Candida* fungemia is relatively rare as an initial cause of fever in GCPs: it is found in approximately 5% of the patients. It is possible, however, that undocumented fungal infections cause fever in some patients in whom no bacterial sepsis can be demonstrated (clinically documented and possible infections). This is probably relatively rare since febrile episodes that are not documented microbiologically usually respond readily to antimicrobial empirical therapy.

Over the years there has been a slight decrease in the incidence of GNBB in GCPs and a corresponding increase in bacteremic infections caused by gram-positive bacteria (Table 1). These observations fully justify the special concern of our group, and of others, to continue to cover GNBB mainly with empirical antimicrobial regimens.

Recent Results in Cancer Research, Vol. 108

Table 1. Bacteremic isolates in three consecutive trials conducted by the EORTC Antimicrobial Therapy Cooperative Group

Microorganisms	Trial I (1978)		Trial II (1980)		Trial III (1982)		Trial IV (1986)	
E. coli	46	68%	33	64%	30	57%	63	57%
P. aeruginosa	18		18		15		34	
Klebsiella sp.	26		14		6		9	
Other gram-negative	13		9		6		23	
S. aureus	28	28%	10	32%	10	37%	25	40%
S. epidermidis	5		9		15		18	
S. pneumoniae	5		6		5		6	
Other Gram-positive	4		12		7		41[a]	
Candida sp.	7	5%	4	4%	5	5%	6	3%
Total	152		115		99		225	

[a] 21 *Streptococcus viridans.*

Another observation made in trial I [4], which is of general significance, is the role of the "spontaneous" changes in the neutrophil count for the response to antimicrobial therapy. Both the initial granulocyte count and the subsequent changes in the level of granulocytopenia during the administration of antimicrobial agents are of prognostic significance for the clinical response to therapy. A low initial granulocyte count and/or a further decline in the number of circulating granulocytes is a major determinant of poor prognosis of a treated infection. It is important, therefore, that any clinical trial of empirical therapy in GCPs involves a sufficient number of severely granulocytopenic patients whose granulocyte counts do not "spontaneously" increase during antimicrobial therapy.

In addition, it has been demonstrated that a higher antibacterial activity of the serum (which is predictive of the outcome of bacteremia in GCPs and in other conditions) is necessary in severely neutropenic patients as compared to those with less severe granulocytopenia. As shown in a recent study from our center [9], the outcome in patients with more than 1000 granulocytes per cubic millimeter is uniformly good when the serum bactericidal activity of the serum is 1:8 or greater; on the other hand, in severely granulocytopenic patients, a higher level (at least 1:16) is required to safely predict a favorable outcome.

Finally, the first EORTC trial clearly indicated that the risk of further infection (i.e., superinfection) increases with the duration of granulocytopenia. The duration of antimicrobial therapy was also found to influence the frequency of further infection in patients whose granulocyte count increased; however, it was unclear to what degree the duration of severe granulocytopenia influences the length of antimicrobial therapy.

It can be concluded at this point that the level and the dynamics of the granulocyte count play a major role in the incidence and the response to antimicrobial therapy in GCPs and influence the frequency of further infection. Severely neutropenic patients whose granulocytopenia remains stable or deteriorates represent the group in which the assessment of antimicrobial therapy is most meaningful.

Any study that does not include sufficient numbers of such patients is necessarily biased owing to the uniformly good results observed in other categories. These considerations support the plea for large cooperative trials to compare and evaluate antimicrobial therapy in GCPs.

The first EORTC trial [4] was a relatively simple comparison between three antimicrobial regimens: carbenicillin + cephalothin, cephalothin + gentamicin, and carbenicillin + gentamicin, the prototype of empirical antimicrobial therapy in GCPs. All three regimens were actually used at that time as empirical therapy in GCPs. It was clearly shown that carbenicillin + gentamicin had the best therapeutic ratio; it was clearly superior to carbenicillin + cephalothin, mainly because strains resistant to both carbenicillin and cephalothin were quite common. Most of the bacteremic patients infected with these strains and receiving carbenicillin + cephalothin died early during the course of therapy; this explains why that regimen resulted in only a 39% response rate while carbenicillin + gentamicin was effective in 62%. Chephalothin + gentamicin was also effective in 62% but was associated with an unacceptable incidence of serious nephrotoxicity.

These observations raised a series of basic questions, among which was the role of aminoglycosides in the control of sepsis in GCPs. It was known at the time that aminoglycosides were disappointing as the sole treatment of GNBB in GCPs; however, on the basis of in vitro studies, these antibiotics appeared the most active and led to a minimal rate of emergence of resistant strains. As a matter of fact, there is evidence that aminoglycosides are helpful as salvage therapy in patients who do not respond to double β-lactam antibiotic combinations; these latter combinations have been associated, in our studies and in other investigations, with a high failure rate owing to the frequency of doubly resistant pathogens. Thus from the point of view of antimicrobial sensitivity it appears that the inclusion of aminoglycosides in empirical antimicrobial therapy regimens makes sense.

There are other considerations that militate in favor of the inclusion of aminoglycosides in empirical regimens to be used in GCPs. They appear to prevent the emergence of resistance to the β-lactams that occasionnally takes place during therapy. This conclusion is based on extensive in vitro and animal work and was confirmed by [3] in a carefully conducted clinical trial in which the emergence of resistant isolates during therapy as well as the numbers of treatment failures, superinfections, or both was found to be siginficantly decreased with the use of carbenicillin + gentamicin as compared to that of piperacillin alone. Moreover, the combinations of β-lactams plus an aminoglycoside are regularly synergistic in vitro; a phenomenon whose significance has been shown in several clinical trials [6]. Especially in severely neutropenic patients, synergistic combinations appear to be more effective clinically than nonsynergistic ones.

Potential occurrence of nephro- and ototoxicity is a frequently advocated reason for deleting the aminoglycosides from the empirical antimicrobial regimens to be used in GCPs. Our first EORTC trial [4] confirmed that cephalothin + gentamicin was indeed associated with an unacceptable rate of nephrotoxicity; however, this was not the case for carbenicillin + gentamicin. Furthermore, subsequent studies (trial II) failed to confirm an increased nephrotoxicity of regimens consisting of cephalosporins and aminoglycosides, as will be discussed later. It should be recognized, however, that aminoglycosides can be synergistically nephrotoxic with several drugs (cyclosporin, cisplatin) that are frequently used in cancer patients and that they may aggravate other conditions predisposing to impairment of renal function.

Trial II [11] was a logical attempt to improve the clinical response by combining all the antibiotics used in our preceding trial. The precise question posed was whether the addition of a cephalosporin (cefazolin) would improve the response rate in CGPs as compared to a combination of an antipseudomonal β-lactam (ticarcillin) plus an aminoglycoside (amikacin). Cefazolin was substituted for cephalothin and was administered at a much lower dosage owing to the fear that nephrotoxicity would be caused by the combination with the aminoglycoside. Amikacin was used instead of gentamicin because in several centers participating in the trial, the rate of resistance to gentamicin was reported to be about 20%, while that to amikacin was lower than 1%. The study also investigated the possible benefit that accrues from early empirical granulocyte transfusions; patients with available donors of granulocytes were randomly allocated to receive or not to receive multiple transfusions, starting not later than 24 h after the onset of the febrile episode. All these patients were treated with carbenicillin + amikacin, without cefazolin. Moreover, the study allowed the oral administration of nonabsorbable antibiotics as prophylaxis against sepsis as long as the attitude was uniform for all patients from one single center; this permitted retrospective evaluation of the effect of chemoprophylaxis with orally administered nonabsorbable antibiotics on the frequency of severe infection.

The clinical results were good with carbenicillin + amikacin whether cefazolin was added or not: 64%. Interestingly enough, the response rate in *Klebsiella* sp. infections was lower (33%) with the triple drug regimen than with carbenicillin + amikacin (63%). Nephrotoxicity of our triple drug combination, which, as mentioned above, might have been feared owing to combination of a cephalosporin with an aminoglycoside, was not verified in trial II; with both regimens, the frequency of renal function impairment was 6%, a relatively low figure; and it was mild and reversible in most patients.

Trial II also established that the empirical use of granulocyte transfusions in combination with a broad spectrum regimen such as carbenicillin + amikacin was not useful for the management of GCPs [2].

Moreover it provided us with an opportunity to test the hypothesis that orally administered nonabsorbable antibiotics might be helpful in preventing severe sepsis in GCPs. Although our observations were retrospective, they suggested that the patients who had received chemoprophylaxis presented a significantly lower incidence of microbiologically documented infections than those who had not.

Trial III compared three different antibiotic regimens: ticarcillin + amikacin, serving as the control therapy, azlocillin + amikacin, and cefotaxime + amikacin [4]. In addition, a question regarding the optimal duration of empirical therapy in responding patients and another about the possible usefulness of empirical therapy with amphotericin B in nonresponding patients were added to the evaluation of the antimicrobial therapy. Our investigation of the optimal duration of empirical therapy in responding patients remained inconclusive because of the similarity of the duration of neutropenia between the two study groups: the median duration was 11 days in the patients randomized to receive antibiotics until granulocytopenia subsided. No difference in outcome could be observed between the two groups. Some investigators have suggested that the therapy in responding GCPs should be extended until the granulocytopenia subsides. Others have not found any benefit from prolonged therapy in responding patients and have stressed its risk in predisposing to further infection.

In the portion of trial III involved with evaluation of antimicrobial therapy, our goal was to compare with a standard therapy (ticarcillin + amikacin) two newer β-lactams in combination with amikacin: azlocillin (an antipseudomonal ureidopenicillin) and cefotaxime (a broad spectrum, so-called third generation cephalosporin). These choices were made on the basis of experimental studies in neutropenic mice which suggested a synergistic activity for these combinations but not for azlocillin + cefotaxime, which was thus not included in the clinical trial [12]. Azlocillin + amikacin was found to be a more effective therapy (66% response rate) than cefotaxime + amikacin (37%) and ticarcillin + amikacin (47%); the differences were particularly striking for *E. coli* (82%, 50%, and 47%). The results of trial III were especially disappointing as far as cefotaxime + amikacin was concerned. The relative inefficacy of cefotaxime against *P. aeruginosa* might in part account for these poor results (0/5 responses in *P. aeruginosa* bacteremia). However, the results with cefotaxime + amikacin were also disappointing in bacteremias due to *E. coli* (50%); this might have been related to the relatively low dosage of cefotaxime used in our study (1.7 g every 6 h).

Azlocillin + amikacin and ticarcillin + amikacin were equally effective in the treatment of GNBB caused by the organisms that were sensitive in vitro to azlocillin or ticarcillin; the response rate was 70% and 74% respectively. However, in our study, ten GNBBs were cause by ticarcillin-resistant strains in the group of patients receiving ticarcillin + amikacin and only one patient responded. Among the patients who received azlocillin + amikacin, six GNBBs were caused by azlocillin-resistant strains, among which three responded. Thus the overall response rate was 20/30 (66%) for GNBB treated with azlocillin + amikacin and 15/29 (50%) for GNBB treated with ticarcillin + amikacin, a statistically significant difference. As already mentioned, the mortality rates in these two groups were not significantly different, suggesting that amikacin, to which all strains were sensitive, played a role in the outcome.

EORTC trial IV was directed to the specific question of whether a cephalosporin (ceftazidime) might be as effective for empirical therapy in GCPs as a combination of ceftazidime + amikacin. Because our group felt that the role of synergism was important in the management of these patients, especially those with GNBB, we decided to compare ceftazidime + a short course of amikacin (3 days) with ceftazidime + a full course of amikacin (at least 9 days) [1].

In patients with GNBB a full course of amikacin, combined with ceftazidime, was associated with an 80% response rate while the shorter course of amikacin + ceftazidime resulted in only a 48% response rate ($P = 0.006$). Mortality resulting from infection was 9% and 19% respectively. These results suggest that the combination of ceftazidime + amikacin, the latter being given as a full course, might be more advantageous. The full course of amikacin in combination with ceftazidime was not associated with an excess of nephrotoxicity (6%) as compared to the regimen including only a short course of amikacin (9%). The advantage of a full course of amikacin in combination with ceftazidime was particularly obvious in patients with sepsis caused by *P. aeruginosa* and in patients with severe and persistent granulocytopenia. The precise reasons for the advantage of the β-lactam plus aminoglycoside combination remain speculative; it may be suspected that these results support the role of synergism.

Other investigators have reported different results: [8] reported favorable results in GCPs with ceftazidime alone; however, their study was performed in less severely neutropenic patients and in a pediatric group with solid tumors rather than acute leukemia. In addition, their protocol allowed for very early change of the antibiotics in the event of suspected failure. They concluded that ceftazidime alone was as effective as a triple drug regimen (carbenicillin + cephalothin + gentamicin) in the total population of febrile GCPs studied; however, they indicated that in GNBB these conclusions should be applied only cautiously and that emergence of resistance of the β-lactam antibiotic was to be carefully monitored.

Trial IV confirmed a series of observations made by us and others, which represent the fundamental principles of antimicrobial therapy in GCPs; namely differences in antibiotic efficacy could only be detected in patients with microbiologically demonstrated infection. In clinically documented episodes and in "possible" infections, the outcome is uniformly good whatever the antibiotic regimen. Trial IV also confirmed the importance of the dynamics of granulocytopenia in GCPs undergoing empirical therapy for febrile episodes. Both response and mortality were related to it.

In trial IV we continued to evaluate the role of empirically administered amphotericin B (Fungizone) in patients with no proven bacterial infection who remained febrile after a course of empirical antimicrobial therapy. Previous studies had suggested the empirical use of amphotericin B to be useful in these patients, many of whom presumably might have fungal infections. We indeed found that the patients who received amphotericin B empirically had better control of fever and lower incidences of microbiologically demonstrated fungal infections and of deaths caused by fungal infections [7].

Some other interesting conclusions can be drawn from the overall comparison of our four trials. It was found that the response rate of GNBB in GCPs receiving various empirical antimicrobial regimens has remained quite constant during the last decade: 68% in trial I, 61% in trial II, 57% in trial III, and 62% in trial IV (Table 2). These results varied to some extent, as already discussed, with the different antimicrobial regimens that were used. Mortality from GNBB also remained stable over the period considered here and was in the range of 20%–25%. No relationship was found between the response rate and the mortality; differences in response between regimens did not translate into differences in mortality. These observations suggest that empirical therapy was capable of "buying time", perhaps because of the role of aminoglycosides that were included in most of our trials, and permitted changes of antimicrobial therapy once the pathogen and its sensitivities were known and/or if the response was clinically suboptimal. In addition, other investigations have indicated that death from GNBB in GCPs usually occurs early during the course of the infection and that it is often associated with septic shock, uncontrolled neoplastic disease, and/or inadequate therapy as indicated by

Table 2. Response rates to empirical therapy of gram-positive (G+) and gram-negative (G−) bacteremia in patients with granulocytopenia

		Overall response	Deaths
Trial I	Carbenicillin + cephalothin	G+: 43/54 (80%)	3/28 (11%)
	Cephalothin + gentamicin	G−: 50/73 (68%)	18/73 (25%)
	Carbenicillin + gentamicin		
Trial II	Ticarcillin + amikacin	G+: 13/19 (68%)	
	Ticarcillin + cefazolin + amikacin	G−: 45/74 (61%)	
Trial III	Ticarcillin + amikacin	G+: 17/39 (44%)	9/39 (23%)
	Azlocillin + amikacin	G−: 32/56 (57%)	12/56 (21%)
	Cefotaxime + amikacin		
Trial IV	Azlocillin + amikacin		
	Ceftazidime + short amikacin	G+: 20/47 (42%)	2/47 (4%)
	Ceftazidime + long amikacin	G−: 35/56 (62%)	13/56 (23%)

EORTC trial I: 1978; trial II: 1980; trial III: 1982; trial IV: 1985

the lack of sensitivity of the offending pathogens to the antibiotics prescribed empirically [10].

Over the years, gram-positive bacteremias have become more prevalent, as discussed previously, and the response rate of these infections to the empirical antibiotic regimens - aimed chiefly at the control of GNBB - has progressively decreased. It was 80% in trial I and only 42% in trial IV. This evolution is probably related to the increasing numbers of pathogens which are intrinsically resistant to the drugs used in empirical regimens and to the role of focal infections related to intravenous catheters. The mortality due to these infections was found to be surprisingly low (4% in trial IV). These observations suggest that the control of gram-positive infections in GCPs might be achieved by attention to the local factors that cause them rather than by extending the antimicrobial spectrum.

EORTC trial V poses a very specific question: whether the addition of vancomycin to ceftazidime + amikacin improves the response rate and possibly eliminates the mortality resulting from gram-positive bacteremia. Since the mortality due to these infections is quite low, it is possible that the benefits of a drug as expensive and toxic as vancomycin are insufficient to justify its use. No data are as yet available regarding this study.

References

1. Calandra T, and the EORTC Antimicrobial Therapy Cooperative Group (1986) Amikacin short (AS) or full (AF) course plus ceftazidime (C) versus amikacin (A) plus azlocillin (AZ) for gram-negative rod bacteremia (GNB) in granulocytopenic cancer patients (GCP). Proc 26th ICAAC, New Orleans
2. EORTC International Antimicrobial Therapy Project Group (1983) Early granulocyte transfusions in high risk febrile neutropenic patients. Schweiz Med Wochenschr [Suppl 14] 113: 46-48
3. Gribble MJ, Chow AW, Naiman SC, Smith JA, Bowie WR, Sacks SL, Grossman L, Buskard N, Growe GH, Plenderleith LH (1983) Prospective randomized trial of piperacillin

monotherapy versus caboxypenicillin-aminoglycoside combination regimens in the empirical treatment of serious bacterial infections. Antimicrob Agents Chemother 24: 388-393

4. Klastersky J, Gaya H, Glauser MP, Schimpff SC, Tattersall MHN, Zinner SH, and the EORTC Antimicrobial Therapy Project Group (1978) Three antibiotic regimens in the treatment of infection in febrile granulocytopenic patients with cancer. J Infect Dis 137: 14-29
5. Klastersky J, Glauser MP, Schimpff SC, Zinner SH, Gaya H, and the European Organization for Research of Treatment of Cancer Antimicrobial Therapy Project Group (1986) Prospective randomized comparison of three antibiotic regimens for empirical therapy or suspected bacteremic infection in febrile granulocytopenic patients. Antimicrob Agents Chemother 29: 52-57
6. Klastersky J, Zinner SH (1982) Synergistic combinations of antibiotics in gram-negative bacillary infections. Rev Infect Dis 4: 294-301
7. Meunier F, and the EORTC Antimicrobial Therapy Cooperative Group (1986) Empiric therapy with Fungizone (FUNG) in febrile neutropenic patients (FNP). Proc 26th ICAAC, New Orleans
8. Pizzo PA, Hathorn JW, Hiemenz J, Browne M, Commers J, Cotton D, Gress J, Longo D, Marshall D, McKnight J, Rubin M, Skelton J, Thaler M, Wesley R (1986) A randomized trial comparing ceftazdime alone with combination antibiotic therapy in cancer patients with fever and neutropenia. N Engl J Med 315: 552-558
9. Sculier JP, Klastersky J (1984) Significance of serum bactericidal activity in gram-negative bacillary bacteremia in patients with and without granulocytopenia. Am J Med 76: 429-435
10. Sculier JP, Weerts D, Klastersky J (1984) Causes of death in febrile granulocytopenic cancer patients receiving empiric antibiotic therapy. Eur J Cancer Clin Oncol 20: 55-60
11. Zinner SH, Gaya H, Glauser MP, Klastersky J, Schimpff SC, Tattersall MHN, and the EORTC Antimicrobial Therapy Project Group (1983) Combination of amikacin and carbenicillin with or without cefazolin as empirical treatment of febrile neutropenic patients. J Clin Oncol 1: 597-603
12. Zinner SH, Klastersky J, Gaya H, Bernard C, Ryff JC, and the EORTC International Antimicrobial Therapy Project Group (1981) In vitro and in vivo studies of three antibiotic combinations against gram-negative bacteria and *Staphylococcus aureus*. Antimicrob Agents Chemother 20: 463-469

Managing Fungal and Viral Infection in the Immunocompromised Host

U. Jehn*

Medizinische Klinik III, Klinikum Großhadern, Ludwig-Maximilians-Universität, Marchioninistraße 15, 8000 München 70, FRG

There has been a worldwide increase in systemic fungal infections caused by both primary pathogenic and opportunistic fungi. Predisposing factors for the latter group include neoplasms of the hemopoietic system in combination with granulocytopenia, immunosuppressive measures, cytostatic drugs, or increasing use of broad spectrum antibiotics (most frequently a combination of these factors is involved). The rising number of opportunistic fungal infections in neutropenic cancer patients has become a source of major concern. Postmortem examinations have shown that more than half of the deaths attributed to infection were due to disseminated fungal infections [1, 2]. *Candida* and *Aspergillus* species are the major pathogens. Most recently it has been reported [3] that recipients of T cell depleted allogeneic transplants - a new technique for prevention of graft-versus-host disease - have an even higher incidence of invasive fungal infection than those without T cell depletion early after transplantation.

Unfortunately, the early diagnosis of serious fungal invasion is exceedingly difficult in these patients, since the manifestations of infection are ill-defined and the organisms can only rarely be isolated from blood cultures. Therefore, fungal prophylaxis as well as empirical antifungal therapy early in the course of fever of unknown origin seems mandatory [2], particularly in those neutropenic patients who remain febrile despite broad spectrum antibiotic treatment. There is no optimal regimen to prevent systemic candidal infections. Nonabsorbable antifungal agents such as amphotericin B, nystatin, and ketoconazole reduce the gastrointestinal tract colonization due to *Candida* species significantly; however, their true prevention capacity is difficult to prove [4]. Ketoconazole has several major disadvantages in this connection because it may select some most dangerous yeasts such as *Torolopsis glabrata* or *Candida tropicalis* [5]. It is ineffective against *Aspergillus* species. Prevention of aspergillosis consists mainly in the isolation of patients in laminar air flow units because it is considered to be acquired by air-borne transmission.

---

* I am grateful to Dr. N. H. Georgopapadakou, Chief of the Scientific Laboratories of the Dept. of Chemotherapy, Hoffmann-La Roche Inc., Nutley, New Yersey, U.S.A. for many suggestions and some of the Figures.

Recent Results in Cancer Research, Vol. 108

Table 1. Anticandidals in use or undergoing clinical trials

Polyenes	Base analogues	Azoles
Amphotericin B Nystatin	5-Fluorocytosine	Miconazole Econazole Clotrimazole Ketoconazole
		Itraconazole (R 51211) Vibunazole (Bay-n-7133) ICI 153,066 Terconazole

Even if a fungal infection is diagnosed, treatment options are limited to a small number of drugs (Table 1), and the chances of successful treatment are slim. Although amphotericin B was discovered in 1953, it remains the most effective drug available for the treatment of systemic fungal infections; unfortunately it is also very toxic. Polyenes are characterized (Fig. 1) by a series of conjugated double bonds - the lipophil region - associated with a central macrolide ring which is closed by internal ester. Their mode of action involves binding to the sterols in the cell membrane, resulting in increased permeability, leakage of cytoplasmic content, and cell death. They are clinically useful because polyenes have a higher affinity to ergosterol, the major sterol in fungi, than to cholesterol, the chief sterol of mammalian cells. Nephrotoxicity limits the dose per injection and the total dose of amphotericin B. The damage is maximal in the renal tubules. The injury is primarily due to anoxia leading to altered function of the proximal tubules and increased permeability of their cell membranes. This event causes increased adsorption of chloride in distal tubules and, finally, a reduction in the rate of glomerular filtration. This process is salt dependent: depletion of sodium increases, and repletion with sodium chloride diminishes or even reverses nephrotoxicity, as shown in vivo by Heidemann et al. [6, 7] using 150-300 mval NaCl/day. The appropriate dose per injection is best established by monitoring serum levels of amphotericin B, which should be 2-2.5 μg/ml 1 h after the dose delivery [8]. Daily therapy is not necessary, because the half-life of amphotericin B in humans is about 24 h, and fungi replicate slowly. Moreover, alternate day therapy (1 mg/kg body weight) provides respite to the kidneys. Infusion of amphotericin B over 4-6 h is clinically, pharmacokinetically, and economically unsound [9]. Delivery of each dose over 45-60 min results in less severe immediate adverse reactions that occur once only after the dose has been given. A higher gradient is attained, favoring passage of amphotericin B from the blood compartment to the sites of infection. When given in combination with other drugs, e.g., 5-fluorocytosine, amphotericin B potentiates their effect because of synergism [10]. Since the doses of amphotericin B can be reduced when combining it with other fungistatics, its toxicity is diminished.

An exciting new development is liposomal amphotericin B, the incorporation of amphotericin B into sonicated liposomes made of egg phospholipids [11]. This has significantly reduced toxicity as compared to free amphotericin B and works even in those patients pretreated unsuccessfully with free amphotericin B [12], al-

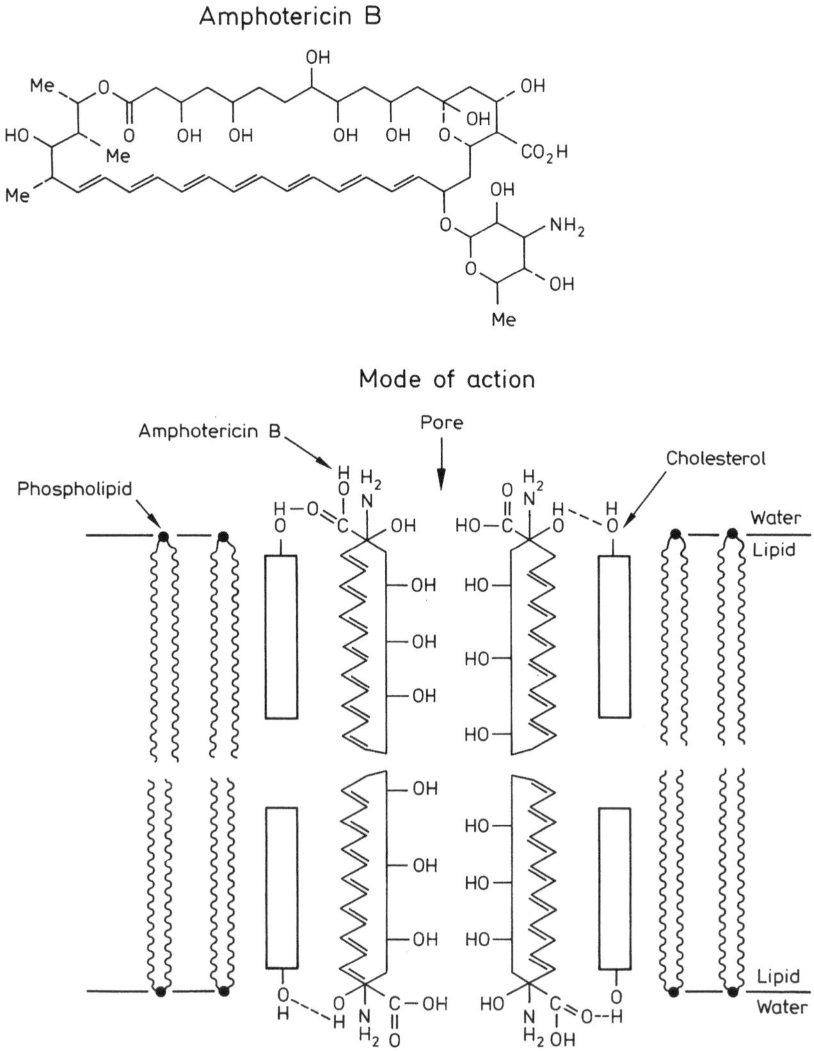

Fig. 1. Amphotericin B and its mode of action

though it is not yet available commercially. Azoles are characterized by a free imidazole or triazole ring bound through a C-N bond to an aromatic ring (Fig. 2). Their mode of action involves inhibition of ergosterol biosynthesis at the ^{14}C demethylation step [13]. The effect is only fungistatic. Miconazole also interacts with the cell membrane directly, but a higher concentrations. The effect then is fungicidal. The newer azoles such as ketoconazole, vibunazole, and itraconazole are orally active and less toxic; however, absorption requires a pH of 5.Azoles have been successfully used in the treatment of superficial candidal infections; they are not very active in systemic candidiasis. Since ketoconazole is a powerful inhibitor of adrenal steroid hormone synthesis, and particularly of testosterone [14], it is currently being investigated for its antihormonal effect in prostatic cancer.

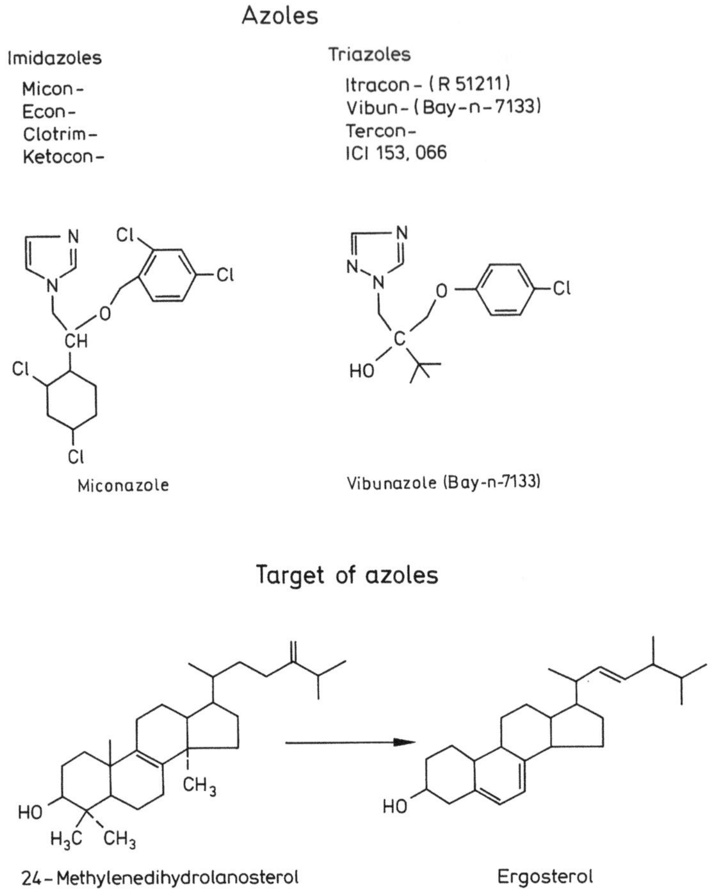

Fig. 2. Azoles and their targets

Potential anticandidals include inhibitors of other steps of ergosterol biosynthesis, as indicated in Fig. 3. They are inhibited by allylamines, 15-azasterols, and morpholino derivates. The reason ergosterol biosynthesis remains an attractive target despite its close similarity to cholesterol biosynthesis is that yeast has no uptake system for made-up sterols [15].

Chitin and glucan are both essential for the structure of the candidal envelope and have no counterpart in the mammalian cell. Inhibitors of chitin biosynthesis are the polyoxins; however, they have poor anticandidal activity due to the lack of penetrability into yeast. In contrast, inhibitors of glucan biosynthesis, echinocandins and papulacandins (Fig. 4), have good anticandidal potency and therefore are currently being tested in clinical trials.

Neutropenic cancer patients, particularly those suffering from hematological neoplasms, are at very high risk for herpesvirus infections as well as fungal infections. This is due to the defect in cell-mediated (= T cell) immunity associated with the disease itself and, in addition, to better control of serious bacterial infec-

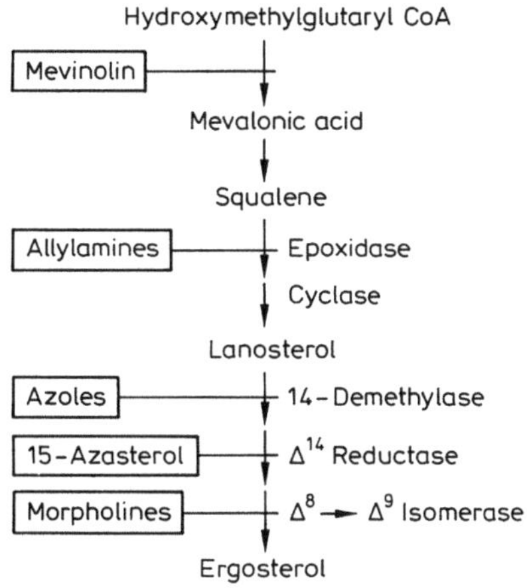

Fig. 3. Ergosterol biosynthesis and inhibitor targets

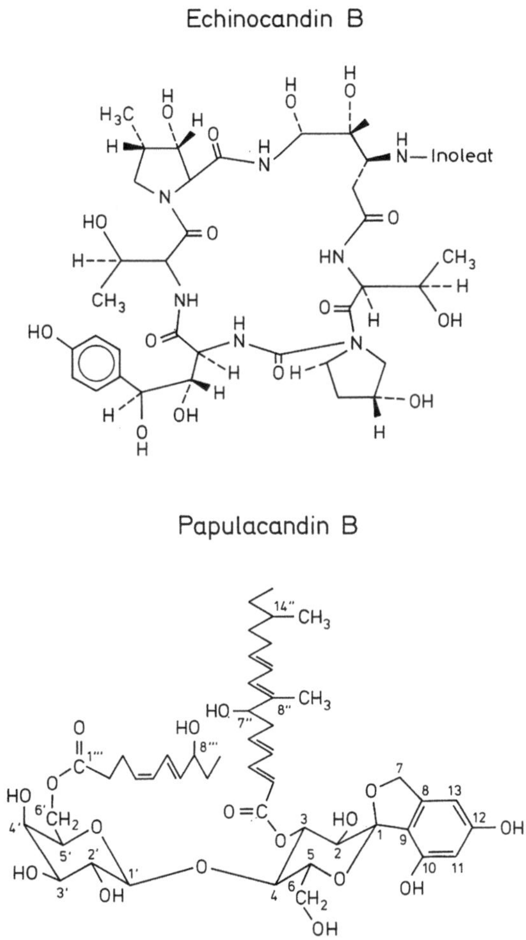

Fig. 4. Echinocandin B and papulocandin B

tions which previously were lethal. As shown in Table 2, herpesviruses reactivate in allogeneic bone marrow transplant (BMT) recipients in a certain sequence and a high proportion of patients [16]. Cytomegalovirus (CMV) infections, particularly when causing interstitial pneumonitis, are clinically most relevant because they are one of the major causes of death in BMT recipients. No effective antiviral drugs are available for CMV infections, but intravenous hyperimmune globulin proved of benefit in both preventing [17] and treating [18] CMV pneumonitis in these patients.

Acyclovir (ACV) and vidarabine are at present the only antiviral drugs licensed for herpes simplex virus (HSV) and varicella zoster virus (VZV) infections. As shown in a comparative trial recently [19], ACV seems to be the more effective drug. Although significantly more nephrotoxic, it is less hematotoxic. It is also the drug of choice for prevention of HSV infections in severely immunocompromised patients during the treatment period. However, when ACV is discontinued, infections may develop at the same frequency as in a placebo group, indicating no effect on the latent virus [20].

Fluoroiodoaracytosine (Fig. 5) has potent in vitro activity against HSV, VZV, CMV, and EBV but its in vivo therapeutic capacity is not very impressive, showing some side-effects like myelosuppression and vomiting.

Preliminary clinical studies have suggested that foscarnet (Fig. 6) is effective in diminishing the severity of generalized CMV infections when given intravenously at 2-8 g/day [21].

Structurally related to ACV is dihydroxypropoxymethylguanine (Fig. 7). As compared to ACV, it is ten fold more potent in vitro [22] and seems to be quite specific against CMV [23]. Because of this and the high clinical importance of

Table 2. Sequence in reactivation of viral infections after allogeneic BMT

HSV	42%	0- 20 days (peak: 18)
EBV	60%	14- 21 days (peak: 17)
CMV		40- 80 days (peak: 50)
VZV		100-160 days (peak: 130)

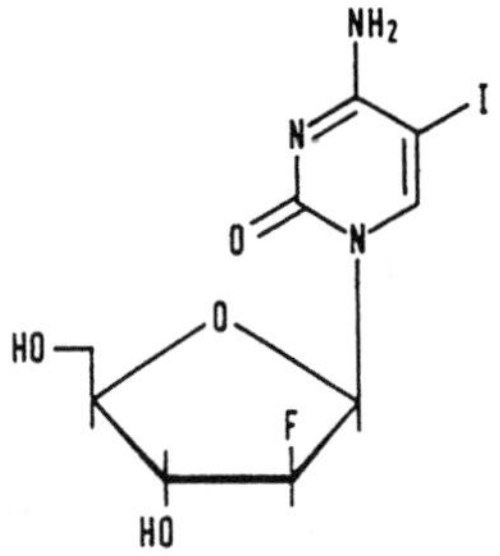

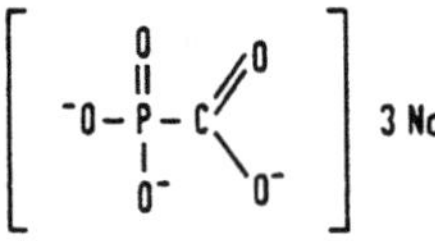

Fig. 5 *(left).* Structural formula of fluoroiodoaracytosine

Fig. 6 *(right).* Structural formula of foscarnet

CMV infections in immunocompromised cancer patients, several clinical trials have been initiated to assess its prophylactic and therapeutic value in CMV-infected patients.

Bromovinyldeoxyuridine (BVDV) (Fig. 8) is the most potent and most selective of all anti-HSV and -VZV agents that are currently being investigated for their therapeutic potential [20]. Its potendy in inhibiting viral replication is superior to that of ACV. Upon initiation of oral BVDU treatment (7.5 mg/kg/day), formation of new HSV-1 and VZV lesions was arrested in severely immunocompromised patients, including BMT recipients, within 1 day [24]. BVDU has several advantages over ACV in the oral treatment of VZV infections (Table 3) and is still effective when treatment is started after prolonged duration of infection even if the infection is not responsive to ACV.

The early diagnosis of viral infections in these patients is difficult, and serological tests are time consuming, results reaching the clinician either when diagnosis is clinically obvious or it is too late to alter the outcome. Unfortunately, not all antiviral chemotherapeutic agents work on latent viral infections, and prevention of outbreak can be achieved only during administration of the drug. Because of severe site-effects, their prophylactic use is rather limited.

The better the biochemistry of fungi and viruses is understood, the easier it will be to employ drugs to combat these targets successfully. Quite a few promising compounds are at present under investigation and being tested in clinical settings.

Summary

The increasing number of opportunistic fungal infections in neutropenic cancer patients has become of major concern. Postmortem examinations have shown that more than half of the deaths attributed to infection were due to disseminated fungal infections. Candida species are the major pathogens. Unfortunately, the early diagnosis of serious fungal invasion is exceedingly difficult in these patients, since the manifestations of infection are ill-defined and the organisms can only rarely be isolated from blood cultures. Therefore, empirical antifungal therapy in febrile patients early in the course of disease appears necessary to prevent fungal superinfections and to control clinically undetected fungal invasion. Even if a fungal infection is diagnosed, treatment options are limited to a small number of drugs, and the chance of successful treatment is slim. Amphotericin B remains the most effective drug for systemic fungal infection; however, it is also the most toxic antimicrobical in use. Reduction of its toxicity and, simultaneously, improvement of its effectiveness can be achieved by incorporation into liposomes, although liposomal amphotericin B is not yet available commercially. The newer azoles, such as ketoconazole, vibunazole, and itraconazole are orally active and less toxic. Azoles have been successfully used in the treatment of superficial candidal infections; they are not very active in systemic candidiasis. Inhibitors of the cell wall biosynthesis of candida species include inhibitors of chitin and glucan biosynthesis. Echinocandins and papulacandins interfer with the glucan synthesis and show good anticandidal activity. Their therapeutic potential is currently being explored in clinical trials. Neutropenic patients and particularly bone marrow transplant (BMT) re-

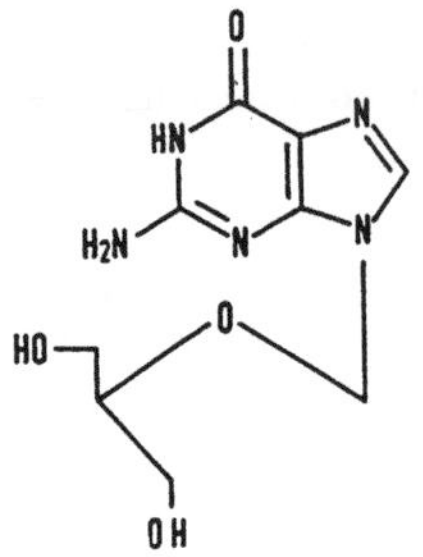

Fig. 7. Structural formula of dihydroxypropoxymethylguanine

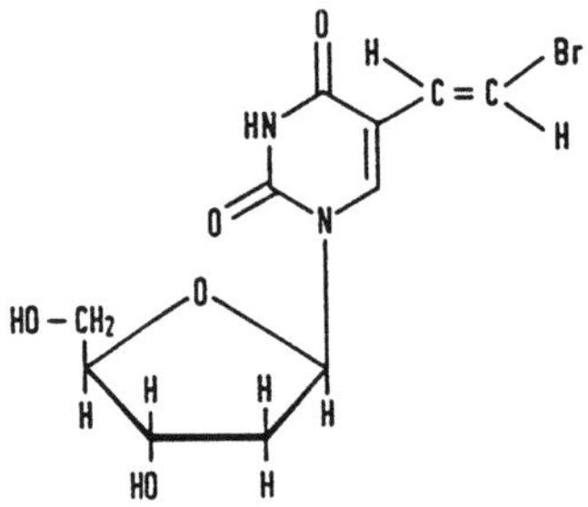

Fig. 8. Structural formula of bromovinyldeoxyuridine

Table 3. BVDU vs. ACV. (De Clercq [20])

1. BVDU is more potent than ACV against VZV replication in vitro
2. BVDU is more effective than ACV in simian varicella virus model in vivo
3. BVDU is better absorbed than ACV when administered perorally
4. BVDU is less immuno- and myelotoxic than ACV
5. BVDU is still effective when treatment is initiated after prolonged duration of the disease, even if unresponsive to ACV

cipients are, in addition to fungal infections, at very high risk for herpesvirus infections: herpes simplex virus (HSV) 0–20 days after BMT, cytomegalovirus (CMV) 40–80 days after BMT, varicella zoster virus (VZV) 100–160 days after BMT, and Epstein-Barr virus (EBV) 14–21 days after BMT. Acyclovir and vidarabine are, at present, the only antiviral drugs available for HSV and VZV infections, acyclovir apparently being the more effective. It is also the drug of choice for prevention of HSV infections in severely immunocompromised, i.e., BMT, patients. Bromovinyldeoxyuridine seems to be suitable for systemic treatment of HSV-1 and VZV infections in these patients. Its potency in inhibiting HSV-1 and VZV replication is superior to that of ACV, and in therapeutic doses it is nontoxic to hematopoietic progenitor cells. Moreover, it is also well absorbed when given orally. No antiviral drug can be recommended for treatment of CMV and EBV infections. Several other new drugs such as fluoroiodoaracytosine, dihydroxypropoxymethylguanine, and foscarnet show promising effectiveness against CMV both in vitro and in clinical phase I studies.

References

1. Sang YC, Hong YC (1979) Opportunistic fungal infection among cancer patients: a ten year autopsy study. Am J Clin Pathol 72: 617
2. Pizzo PA, Robichaud KJ, Gill FA, Witebsky FG (1982) Empiric antibiotic and antifungal therapy for cancer patients with prolonged fever and granulocytopenia. Am J Med 72: 101
3. Pirsch JD, Maki DG (1986) Infections after T-cell-depleted marrow transplants. Ann Intern Med 104: 619
4. de Gregorio MW, Lee WMF, Ries CA (1982) Candida infections in patients with acute leukemia: ineffectiveness of nystatin prophylaxis and relationship between oropharyngeal and systemic candidiasis. Cancer 50: 2780
5. Meuniers-Carpentier F, Van den Heule B, Klastersky J (1982) Prevention and therapy of fungal infections. 3rd Int Symp Ther Acute Leukem Abstr p 116
6. Gerkens JF, Branch RA (1980) The influence of sodium status and furosemide on canine acute amphotericin B, nephrotoxicity. J Pharmacol Exp Ther 214: 306
7. Heidemann H, Kirch W, Gerkens J, Branch R (1983) Salzbeladung verringert Amphotericin B-induzierte Nephrotoxizität. Verh Dtsch Ges Inn Med 89, Am J Med 75: 476
8. Fields BT, Bates JM, Abernathy RS (1971) Effect of rapid intravenous infusion on serum concentrations of amphotericin B. Appl Microbiol 22: 615
9. Hoeprich PD (1984) Selected aspects of the clinical use of amphotericin B. Proc IV Mediterr Congr Chemother, p 700
10. Bennett JE, Dismukes WE, Duna RJ et al (1979) A comparison of amphotericin B alone and combined with flucytosine in the treatment of cryptococcal meningitis. N Engl J Med 301: 126
11. Lopez-Berestein G, Melita R, Hopfer R et al. (1983) Treatment and prophylaxis of disseminated infection due to Candida albicans in mice with liposome-encapsulated amphotericin B. J Infect Dis 147: 939
12. Sculier JP, Coune A, Meunier F et al (1985) Pilot study of amphotericin B entrapped into sonicated liposomes in cancer patients with mycotic complications. Cancer Immunol Immunother 23 [Suppl]: A 64, no 255
13. Ragsdale NN (1977) Inhibitors of lipid synthesis. In: Siegel MR, Sisler HD (eds) Antifungal compounds, vol 2. Decker, New York, p 333
14. Pont A, Williams PL, Loose DS et al. (1982) Ketoconazole blocks adrenal steroid synthesis. Ann Intern Med 97: 370
15. Georgopapadakou NH (1984) Anticandidals: Prospects and problems. Proc IV Mediterr Congr Chemother, p 699
16. Saral R (1985) Herpesvirus infections in bone-marrow transplant recipients (abstr). Symp Chemother Herpesvirus Infect, Heidelberg
17. Kubanek B, Ernst P, Ostendorf P et al. (1985) Preliminary data of a controlled trial of intravenous hyperimmune globulin in the prevention of cytomegalovirus infection in bone marrow transplant recipients. Transplant Proc 17: 468
18. Blacklock HA, Griffith P, Stirk P et al. (1986) Cytotect treatment of cytomegalovirus pneumonitis after matched allogeneic bone marrow transplantation (Abstr no 22), EMBT European Meeting for Bone Marrow Transplantation, Courmayeur, March 1986
19. Shepp DH, Dandliker PS, Meyers JD (1986) Treatment of variecella-zoster virus infection in severely immunocompromised patients. N Engl J Med 314: 208
20. De Clercq E (1985) Problems and new aspects of antiviral treatment: herpesvirus infections in immunosuppressed patients. In: Jehn U (ed) Infections in cancer patients, Zuckschwerdt, Munich, p 91
21. Öberg B (1983) Antiviral effects of phosphonoformate (PFA). Pharmacol Ther 19: 387

22. Cheng YC, Huang ES, Lin JC et al. (1983) Unique spectrum of activity of DHPG against herpes virus in vitro and its mode of action against herpes simplex virus type 1. Proc Natl Acad Sci USA 80: 2767
23. Tyms AS, Davis JM, Jeffries DJ et al. (1984) BWB759 U, an analogue of acyclovir, inhibits human cytomegalovirus in vitro. Lancet 2: 924
24. Tricot G, de Clercq E, Boogaerts MA et al. (1986) Oral bromovinyl-deoxyuridine therapy for herpes simplex and varicella-zoster virus infections in severely immunosuppressed patients. J Med Virol 18: 11

Aspects of Infections in Children with Cancer

C. Viscoli

Department of Infectious Diseases, G. Gaslini Institute, University of Genova,
Via 5 Maggio 39, 16147 Genova, Italy

Introduction

There is no doubt that the last decade has witnessed an incredible improvement in the treatment of neoplastic diseases. This is true of not only primary treatment of tumors but also supportive care of patients. In this setting, however, infections remain a major problem because of their significant morbidity and mortality, as well as the impediment they frequently pose to the accomplishment of the antineoplastic therapy.

Combination chemotherapy with its attendant risk of neutropenia is no longer limited to the treatment of leukemias and lymphomas, but is also part of the therapeutic protocols for the treatment of solid tumors, especially in pediatrics; as a consequence, the number of subjects at high risk of developing infection is increasing. Furthermore, massive antitumor therapy followed by allogeneic or autologous bone marrow transplantation (BMT) is becoming a standard procedure for the treatment of certain types of cancer, resulting in a further widening of the infective problem in clinical oncology.

In this paper we will review some aspects of infections in cancer patients, paying particular attention to pediatric problems.

Children and Adults

The increasing impact of bacterial, fungal, viral, and protozoal infections concerns both pediatric and adult oncology, but it is currently believed that children have a better prognosis than adults as regards infections.

The problem has recently been dealt with by Mario Rossi on behalf of the EORTC International Antimicrobial Therapy Cooperative Group in the setting of its last prospective and randomized therapeutic trial [1].

Over a 2-year period, this trial, the fourth that our group has conducted during the last 10 years, has compared the therapeutic effectiveness of the combination of azlocillin, an extended-spectrum penicillin, and amikacin, with that of a combination of ceftazidime, a third-generation cephalosporin, and the same aminoglycoside, given either for 3 days or as a long-course therapy.

Recent Results in Cancer Research, Vol. 108

Out of 871 evaluable patients there were 184 children (i.e., patients less than 15 years old) and 687 adults. Within the two groups, the underlying diseases, the percentage of bacteremias (based on the overall number of episodes) and their etiology, the response to early empirical protocols, and the final outcome were considered.

As expected, a statistically significant difference in the distribution of the underlying diseases was found. Children had a relatively higher number of acute lymphoblastic leukemias than adults and a relatively lower number of other neoplastic conditions. The percentage of acute nonlymphoblastic leukemias was the same in both age groups. Chronic leukemias were prevalent in the adult group.

In contrast, no statistically significant difference was seen in the percentage of bacteremias, counting all febrile episodes (23% and 26%, respectively). Concerning the difference in the distribution of the causative pathogens (gram-positive and gram-negative), it is worthwhile to note the slightly higher number of gram-positive isolates in childhood bacteremias; this phenomenon, even if statistically nonsignificant, supports the already known claim that gram-positive cocci are more likely to be the leading pathogens of nosocomial infections in pediatric rather than in adult services [2].

Although a statistically significant difference was seen in the overall response to empirical treatments (73% in children and 64% in adults; $P=0.02$), there was no imbalance in the response rate of microbiologically documented infections and bacteremias. Surprising findings were, by contrast, observed regarding mortality. Children seemed to have a significantly lower overall mortality rate than adults (3% vs 19%, $P<10^{-6}$) and a significantly lower infectious mortality (2% vs 8%; $P<0.003$). While the different overall mortality might possibly be explained by varying distributions of underlying diseases, the explanation for the lower infectious mortality observed in children is still less evident.

Many factors may actually affect the outcome of infections in cancer patients. Although the development of granulocytopenia is the single most important factor, its duration and the functional integrity of the phagocyte reserves must also be taken into consideration [3]; other factors include the amount and specificity of circulating antibodies, the integrity of cell-mediated functions and of skin and mucosal barriers, the presence of heavy colonization and the virulence of the causative pathogens [4, 5, 6, 7, 8]. All these factors are likely to be influenced by the underlying disease and its treatment.

It is therefore credible that children and adults develop similar infectious complications when exposed to similar risks but that concurrent factors, such as those previously mentioned, can modify the final outcome of the complication. In conclusion, it is conceivable that children may be physically more able to overcome the many factors that may affect survival.

The Role of Central Intravenous Catheters

Indwelling right atrial Silastic catheters, by breaching the barrier between the internal and external environment, may facilitate the entrance of microorganisms into the bloodstream. This type of vascular approach has become particularly popular, especially in pediatric oncology, as it frees the young patient from the discomfort of repeated venipunctures and at the same time allows the administration of medications, blood products and large volumes of fluids, as is required for the modern treatment of neoplastic diseases [9].

These devices, while directed toward improving the treatment of the underlying disease and the patient's quality of life, may create problems related to infection control. When an infectious episode develops in a neutropenic cancer patient, clear signs identifying the source of the infection are frequently lacking and it is consequently difficult to determine where the primary localization of the infection is and whether or not the catheter is involved [10].

In our institution, from August 1983 to July 1986, 157 single lumen central catheters (Broviac type) were inserted in 145 children affected with various neoplastic diseases. The median time for which catheters remained inserted (catheter course) was 171 days (2-647), giving an overall duration of 30533 days.

While fitted with catheters, all patients received one or more courses of chemotherapy and radiotherapy, with the subsequent development of 387 episodes of granulocytopenia (PMN $< 1000/mm^3$), which lasted from 4 to 150 days (median 13 days). Fever (157 episodes) complicated 102 of 157 catheter courses.

According to EORTC criteria [11], of these 157 febrile episodes 79 (50%) were defined as microbiologically documented infections (MDIs), 57 (36%) with and 22 (14%) without bacteremia, 31 (20%) as clinically documented infections and 47 (30%) as possible infections. All MDIs were then evaluated to see whether they were related to the catheter. The following Definitions of catheter-related infections were used:

1. Microbiologically documented bacterial abscess or cellulitis localized at the exit site, in the subcutaneous tunnel, or at the entrance of the catheter in the neck blood vessel
2. Bacteremias in which microorganisms were isolated only in blood cultures taken from the i.v. catheter and not in blood cultures simultaneously taken from a peripheral vein
3. Bacteremias in which the same microorganism (identical biotype and susceptibility pattern) was simultaneously isolated from blood cultures and from swabs taken from the catheter insertion site and from the catheter hub; in cases in which the catheter was removed the tip was also cultured
4. The existence of a temporal relationship between manipulations of the catheter, the onset of chills and fever, and the isolation of a microorganism from blood culture taken during the episode, suggesting that manipulation of the catheter released microorganisms into the bloodstream.

According to these definitions a catheter-related infection (CRI) was found in 21 of 79 episodes (27%), while 32 of the infections were clearly unrelated to the catheter (CURI = catheter-unrelated infection). In the remaining 26 cases (33%) we were unable to detect any primary clinical localization of the infection (SUI = source unknown infection); we are therefore unable to exclude the possibility that at least some of the SUIs were related to an occult infection localized at the catheter. Of major interest for practical purposes, despite the small numbers, was the finding that only 10 of the 21 (48%) CRIs occurred during neutropenia

Table 1. Distribution of microorganisms in catheter-related, catheter-unrelated, and source-unknown infections (numbers in parentheses are percentages)

Microorganisms	Catheter-related infections	Catheter-unrelated infections	Source-unknown infections
Gram-positive	18 (78)	18 (47)	12 (43)
Gram-negative	3 (13)	17 (45)	10 (36)
Fungi	2 (9)	3 (8)	6 (21)
Total[a]	23 (100)	38 (100)	28 (100)

[a] Ten polymicrobial infections.
Statistical evaluation of the distribution of causative pathogens: $P=0.03$ χ^2 test).

(<1000 PMN/mm^3) compared to 28/32 (88%) CURIs and 25/26 (96%) SUIs (χ^2 test, $P=0.00007$. Fisher's exact test: CRI vs CURI, $P=0.002$; CRI vs SUI, $P=0.00001$; CURI vs SUI $P=0.24$).

Gram-positive cocci (65% staphylococci) were predominant in CRIs (Table 1), and there were 10 polymicrobial infections. Controversy exists about the need for catheter removal in this kind of infection. This creates a troubling dilemma which forces a decision taking into account the enormous benefit provided by these devices and the relative difficulty inherent in their replacement. In our institution 12 of the 21 (57%) CRIs were treated successfully with antibiotics alone without removing the catheter; this finding confirms reports by other centers [12, 13, 14, 15].

In conclusion, Silastic central catheters are considered indispensable in the management of children with cancer. However, one must be aware that their use is associated with a significant risk of infection. Therefore, our present protocol is, on one hand, not to insert Broviac catheters unless they are essential for the treatment of the underlying disease and, on the other hand, not to remove them unless their etiological involvement with the infection is unequivocally documented (i.e., we do not remove them in SUIs) and the antibiotic therapy has proven unsuccessful. Our present indications for insertion are acute nonlymphoblastic leukemias at onset or at relapse, relapsed acute lymphoblastic leukemia or lymphoma, B cell leukemia or lymphoma, solid tumors undergoing aggressive chemotherapy, autologous bone marrow transplantation and any other condition if it is accompanied by particularly poor venous access.

Changing Pattern of Infecting Organisms

The pattern of infecting organisms has changed during the last 5 years and in some centers gram-positive bacteria, which were prevalent in the 1950s and early 1960s, have again become the most common infecting pathogens [16, 17, 18, 19]. This is confirmed in an unquestionable manner by a review of the results of the

Table 2. Relative role of gram-positive and gram-negative organisms in causing single-agent bacteremias in EORTC trials I–IV (numbers in parentheses are percentages)

	Overall	Gram-positive	Gram-negative
Trial I	145	42 (29)	103 (71)
Trial II	111	37 (33)	74 (67)
Trial III	141	58 (41)	83 (59)
Trial IV	219	90 (41)	129 (59)
		$P = 0.01$	

Table 3. Etiology of single-agent bacteremias in a pediatric population affected with neutropenia and cancer (numbers in parentheses are percentages)

Years	Overall	Gram-positive	Gram-negative
1982–1984	62	41 (66)	21 (34)
1985–1986	22	17 (77)	5 (23)
Overall	84	58 (69)	26 (31)
		$P = 0.4$	

four trials that the EORTC group has performed during the last 10 years [11, 20, 21, 22, 23].

As shown in Table 2, the percentage of gram-positive bacteremias (as against gram-negative) rose from 29% and 33% in trials 1 and 2 (1975–1980) to 41% in trials 3 and 4 (1980–1985); this increase was statistically significant ($P = 0.01$).

In controlled studies, the increasing role of gram-positive organisms in causing bacteremias seems even more evident in pediatric populations [24, 25, 26, 27]. In our institution, which is exclusively pediatric, two studies performed during the last 5 years show that gram-positive microorganisms cause 69% of all single-agent bacteremias and that from 1982 to 1986 their role appeared to increase, though this was not statistically significant ($P = 0.4$), from 66% to 77% [17, 18, 27] (Table 3).

At least four factors must be mentioned in order to explain the increasing percentage of gram-positive bacteremias and their high prevalence in pediatric populations:

1. The already mentioned increasingly wide use of central catheters, which probably facilitates colonization by means of the skin flora
2. The progressive shifting of the spectrum of action of cephalosporins from gram-positive to gram-negative bacteria
3. The use of prophylactic regimens (oral non absorbable antibiotics) directed prevalently toward gram-negative bacteria
4. Children often carry gram-positive cocci in their oral and pharyngeal flora

Therapeutic Controversies

Some therapeutic controversies stem directly from the previous observations. The increasing role of gram-positive organisms and their frequent resistance to methicillin and oxacillin have induced some investigators to suggest the inclusion of an anti-gram-positive drug in the early empirical antibiotic regimens [28, 29, 30]. This suggestion is indirectly supported by the results of the fourth EORTC trial, which showed that in single gram-positive bacteremias, the overall response to the empirical protocols was particularly low, especially compared with the previous trials (41% in trial IV vs 75% in trial I, performed in the mid-1970s). The seriousness of this finding was, however, mitigated by the lack of increase in mortality rate [22, 23]. Contemporarily, other investigators have claimed that single agent therapy with a third-generation anti-pseudomonas cephalosporin (ceftazidime) could be as effective as standard combinations for the treatment of suspected infections in neutropenic cancer patients, thus allowing reduction of aminoglycoside-related toxicity [31, 32, 33, 34]. As reported by Thierry Calandra on behalf of the Group [35], the same conclusion did not result from the EORTC trial IV. In this study, in fact, the combination of ceftazidime and a short course of amikacin (3 days, six doses) performed significantly worse in single gram-negative bacteremias than a full course of both antibiotics; this effect applied especially to patients with profound and prolonged granulocytopenia (patients who had less than 100 PMN/mm^3 throughout the therapy). It is however, important to note that NCI and EORTC studies are hardly comparable, as they employ different methods and probably reflect different situations.

In our pediatric institution, as already mentioned above, gram-positive organisms are prevalent as the cause of MDIs and bacteremias, and there is a low incidence of "difficult" gram-negative organisms, such as *Pseudomonas* spp. and *Acinetobacter* spp. Moreover, as previously stated, children seem to have a better physical integrity than adults, thus probably allowing less aggressive antibiotic therapies. These considerations prompted us to start a randomized, prospective trial comparing ceftazidime plus amikacin, our so-called historic protocol, with ceftazidime, as a single anti-gram-negative drug, plus vancomycin, for early empirical anti-gram-positive coverage, in the treatment of suspected infections in neutropenic children with cancer (children undergoing bone marrow transplantation, being more severely immunocompromised, were excluded from the study). Blood levels of amikacin and vancomycin were monitored. So far 109 patients have been enrolled in the study. Of 98 evaluable patients, 50 received ceftazidime plus amikacin (C+A) and 48 ceftazidime plus vancomycin (C+V).

Fourteen of 50 patients (28%) had prolonged and severe neutropenia (less than 100 PMN/mm^3 for at least 10 days after randomization) in the C+A group and 17/48 (35%) in the C+V group ($P = 0.56$). The median duration of granulocytopenia (<1000 PMN/mm^3) was 8 days in the C+A group and 10 days in the C+V group. There were no statistically significant differences in age, sex, and underlying disease between the two groups. Twenty of 50 patients (40%) had MDIs in the C+A group (12 bacteremias) and 18/48 (38%) in the C+V group (10 bacteremias). As far as the response to the allocated regimens is concerned (Table 4), no statistically significant difference has so far been observed between the

Table 4. Outcome of 98 suspected and documented infections in neutropenic children with cancer treated with two different antibiotics regimens (numbers in parentheses are percentages)

	C+A	C+V	*P*
Response at day 4			
Overall	33/50 (66)	36/48 (75)	0.45
In MDI	12/20 (60)	11/18 (61)	0.79
In PPG	6/14 (43)	10/17 (59)	0.60
Final response[a]			
Overall	45/50 (90)	45/48 (94)	0.38
In MDI	17/20 (85)	17/18 (94)	0.34
In PPG	12/14 (86)	15/17 (88)	0.62
Mortality			
Overall	5/50 (10)	3/48 (6)	0.38
First episode	4/50 (8)	0/48 (0)	0.06
Second episode	1/50 (10)	3/48 (6)	0.29

C+A, ceftazidime+amikacin; *C+V,* ceftazidime+vancomycin; *MDI,* microbiologically documented infections; *PPG,* profound and prolonged granulocytopenias (patients with PMN count $<100/\text{mm}^3$ for at least 10 days after randomization).

[a] Cases which improved after protocol therapy was modified are included.

two protocols; however there seems to be a trend toward greater effectiveness of C+V.

Taking into account all randomized patients (109), it is notable that no one who received C+A developed side effects relatable to antibiotics, while 19/54 (35%) of those who received C+V complained of skin rashes and chills ($P=0.000007$).

Concerning failures, it must be underlined that in the C+A group, out of eight patients affected with MDIs who did not respond to this regimen, five (all with gram-positive infections, with the paradoxical exception of one case of *P. aeruginosa* necrotizing pharyngitis) responded to the subsequent addition of vancomycin. In the C+V group, five of ten staphylococcal infections failed to respond to this regimen and patients improved only after the addition of a third antibiotic.

The preliminary conclusions we draw from this still on-going study are therefore as follows:

1. In our hands, there seems to be a trend toward a better general outcome with the early use of vancomycin in combination with ceftazidime; this requires statistical confirmation
2. The use of vancomycin is associated with mild but bothersome side effects
3. It is likely that, in empirical therapy, the fastest response can be achieved by means of a triple antibiotic combination, comprising vancomycin, ceftazidime, and amikacin, but if we take into account only survival this approach will result in overtreatment

Conclusions

Owing to the development of new clinical and microbiological conditions as well as the discovery and marketing of new antibiotics a continuous research effort is required to assess the best management of infections in cancer patients. The conclusions of such clinical trials must be immediately transferred to the daily assistance of cancer patients, in order not only to reduce mortality due to infection, but also to improve the quality of life, the compliance with antineoplastic therapies and, eventually, the prospects of treatment of the underlying disease. However, it is likely that only multicenter trials will enable the study of an appropriate number of cases and therefore provide meaningful conclusions and useful guidelines. Concerning children and adults, it is doubtful whether the existing differences are so important as to justify different therapeutic approaches. Therefore, the problem needs to be studied further.

Summary

There are some differences between pediatric and adult cancer patients in terms of the problem of infection but it is doubtful whether such discrepancies justify different therapeutic approaches. For example, according to the results of EORTC trial IV, children seem to show lower overall (3% vs 19%) and infectious (2% vs 8%) mortality than adults, probably due to differences in underlying diseases and to a basic better physical integrity.

Central intravenous catheters appear to be indispensable in the modern management of neoplastic diseases, especially in pediatric oncology.

A prospective study performed in our institution on 157 Broviac catheters, has shown:

1. Of all microbiologically documented infections, occurring in children undergoing cancer chemotherapy and radiotherapy, 27% are related to the catheter
2. Gram-positive cocci are the leading pathogens (78%) of such infections
3. Catheter-related infections often occur in non-neutropenic patients
4. Such infections can be successfully treated without removing the intravenous device

The experience of the EORTC Cooperative Group and of other centers throughout the world shows that gram-positive cocci are increasingly being isolated as the cause of infections in cancer patients. This phenomenon is probably multifactorial in origin and appears to be more evident in pediatrics. For example, in our institution, during the last 5 years gram-positive organisms have caused 69% of all bacteremias. Moreover, these organisms, while responding poorly to the presently used empirical antibiotic regimens, seem not to be as aggressive as gram-negative organisms and cause lower mortality. There is therefore controversy over whether or not to include anti-gram-positive coverage in early empirical regimens. In our institution, a pilot study comparing ceftazidime + amikacin (C + A) and ceftazidime + vancomycin (C + V) seems to show an overall advantage for C + V. This advantage, however, is not statistically significant. One finding to be pointed out is that five of ten staphylococcal infections failed to respond to C + V and that in these cases a third antibiotic had to be added. Therefore, it is likely that, at least in institutions in which methicillin-resistant staphylococci are prevalent, a triple antibiotic empirical regimen will provide the best coverage, but this can result in overtreatment. However, only prospective, randomized and multicenter trials will be able to answer such questions definitely.

Acknowledgements. The author is a member of the Data Review Committee of EORTC International Antimicrobial Therapy Cooperative Group. Data presented are in part the results of personal studies and in part those of EORTC cooperative studies. The author would like to thank all members of EORTC group and in particular Dr. Mario Rossi from Milan and Dr. Thierry Calandra from Lausanne for having kindly provided some data for the study on children and adults and the study on gram-negative bacteremias respectively. The author is also endebted to the medical and laboratory staff and the nurses of G. Gaslini Children's Hospital for their assistance.

References

1. EORTC-International Antimicrobial Therapy Cooperative Group (1986) Empiric therapy in febrile neutropenic patients: different responses in children and adults (abstract). 26th Interscience conference on antimicrobial agents and chemotherapy, New Orleans, September 28 - October 1, 681
2. Cooper RG, Sumner C (1970) Hospital infection data from a children's hospital. Med J Aust 2: 1110-1113
3. Bodey GP, Buckley M, Sathe JS, Freireich EJ (1966) Quantitative relationships between circulating leucocytes and infection in patients with acute leukemia. Ann Intern Med 64: 328-340
4. Ziegler EF, McCutchan JA, Fierer JA (1982) Treatment of Gram-negative bacteremia and shock with human antiserum to a mutant *Escherichia coli.* N Engl J Med 307: 1225-1230
5. Peter G, Pizzo PA, Robichaud KJ, Visconts ER, Farman EN, Zinna SH (1979) Possible protective effect of circulatory antibodies to the shared care glycolipid of Enterobacteriaceae in children with malignancy (abstract). Soc Pediat Res 13: 466
6. Schimpff SC, Young VM, Greene WH, Vermeulen GD, Moody MK, Wiernik PN (1972) Origin of infection in acute non-lymphocytic leukemia: significance of hospital acquisition of potential pathogens. Ann Intern Med 77: 704-714
7. Schimpff SC, Greene WH, Young VM et al. (1974) Significance of *Pseudomonas aeruginosa* in the patient with leukemia or lymphoma. J Infect Dis 130: 24-31

8. Kurrle E, Bhaduri S, Krieger D et al. (1981) Risk factors for infections of the oropharynx and the respiratory tract in patients with acute leukemia. J Infect Dis 144: 128-136
9. Kingston JE, Fowler PC, Jackson DB, Potter V, Malpas JS (1985) Experience with central intravenous catheter in a pediatric oncology unit. Eur Pediatr Hematol Oncol 2: 29-34
10. Pizzo PA (1981) Infectious complications in the child with cancer. I. Pathophysiology of the compromised host and the initial evaluation and management of the febrile cancer patient. J Pediatr 98: 341-354
11. EORTC International Antimicrobial Therapy Project Group (1978) Three antibiotic regimens in the treatment of infections in febrile granulocytopenic patients with cancer. J Infect Dis 137: 14-29
12. Pizzo PA, Commers J, Cotton D, Gress J, Hathorn J, Hiemenz J, Longo D, Marshall D, Robichaud KD (1984) Approaching the controversies in antibacterial management of cancer patients. Am J Med 76: 436-449
13. Abraham JL, Mullen JL (1982) A prospective study of prolonged central venous access in leukemia. JAMA 248: 2868-2873
14. Prince A, Heller B, Levy J, Heird W (1986) Management of fever in patients with central vein catheters. Pediatr Infect Dis 5: 20-24
15. Hiemenz J, Skelton J, Pizzo P (1986) Perspective on the management of catheter-related infections in cancer patients. Pediatr Infect Dis 5: 6-11
16. Pizzo P, Ladisch S, Simon RM, Gill F, Levine AS (1978) Increasing incidence of Gram-positive sepsis in cancer patients. Med Pediatr Oncol 5: 241-244
17. Viscoli C, Perlino GF, De Bernardi B, Fabbri A, Massimo L, Terragna A (1985) Infections in children with cancer. Ital J Pediatr 11: 37-43
18. Viscoli C, Perlino GF, Moroni C, Ferrea G, Fabbri A, Haupt R, Massimo L, Terragna A (1984) Gram-positive infections in pediatric cancer patients (abstract). 3rd International symposium on infections in the immunocompromised host, Toronto, June 24-28: 136
19. Wade JC, Schimpff SC, Newman KA, Wiernik PH (1982) *Staphylococcus epidermidis:* an increasing cause of infection in patients with granulocytopenia. Ann Intern Med 97: 503-508
20. EORTC International Antimicrobial Therapy Project Group (1983) Combination of amikacin and carbenicillin with or without cefazolin as empirical treatment of febrile neutropenic patients. J Clin Oncol 1: 597-603
21. EORTC International Antimicrobial Therapy Project Group (1986) Prospective randomized comparison of three antibiotic regimens for empirical bacteremic infections in febrile granulocytopenic patients. Antimicrob Agents Chemother 29: 263-270
22. Klastersky J (1986) Concept of empiric therapy with antibiotic combinations: indications and limits. Am J Med 80 [suppl 5c]: 2-12
23. EORTC International Antimicrobial Therapy Cooperative Group (1986) Gram-positive septicemias in cancer patients (abstract). 26th Interscience conference on antimicrobial agents and chemotherapy, New Orleans, September 28-October 1: 679
24. Kosmidis HV, Lusher JM, Shope TC, Ravindranath Y, Dajani AS (1980) Infections in leukemic children: a prospective analysis. J Pediatr 96: 814-819
25. Nachman JB, Honig GR (1980) Fever and neutropenia in children with neoplastic disease. An analysis of 158 episodes. Cancer 45: 407-412
26. Pizzo PA, Robichaud KJ, Wesley R, Commers JR (1982) Fever in the pediatric and young adult patient with cancer. A prospective study of 1001 episodes. Medicine 61: 153-165
27. Viscoli C, Moroni C, Garaventa A, Dini G, Mori P, Ferrea G, Massimo L, Terragna A (1986) Ceftazidime + amikacin versus ceftazidime + vancomycin as initial empiric treatment of febrile episodes in neutropenic children (abstract). 4th International symposium on infections in the immunocompromised Host, Ronneby Brunn (Sweden), June 15-19: 120
28. Sorrell TC, Packman DR, Shanker S, Foldes M, Munzo R (1982) Vancomycin therapy for methicillin resistant *Staphylococcus aureus*. Ann Intern Med 97: 344-350

29. Jadeja L, Bolivar R, Fainstein V, Keating M, McCredie K, Hay M, Bodey G (1984) Piperacillin plus vancomycin in the therapy of febrile episodes in cancer patients. Antimicrob Agents Chemother 26: 295-299
30. Karp J, Dick J, Angelopulos C, Charache P, Greene L, Burke P, Saral R (1986) Empiric use of vancomycin during prolonged treatment induced granulocytopenia. Randomized, double blind, placebo-controlled clinical trial in patients with acute leukemia. Am J Med 81: 237-242
31. Morgan G, Duerden BI, Lilleyman JS (1983) Ceftazidime as a single agent in the management of children with fever and neutropenia. J Antimicrob Chemother 12 [suppl A]: 347-351
32. Fainstein V, Bodey G, Elting L et al. (1983) A randomized study of ceftazidime compared to ceftazidime and tobramycin for the treatment of infections in cancer patients. J Antimicrob Chemother 12 [suppl A]: 101-110
33. Donnelly JP, Marcus RE, Goldman JM, Cohen J, Worsley AM, Catovsky D, Darrel JH, Want SV, Jalton JAD (1985) Ceftazidime as first line therapy for fever in acute leukemia. J Infect 11: 205-215
34. Pizzo PA, Hathorn JW, Hiemenz J, Browne M, Commers J, Cotton D, Gress J, Longo D, Marshall D, McKnight J, Rubin M, Skelton J, Thaler M, Wesley R (1986) A randomized trial comparing ceftazidime alone with combination antibiotic therapy in cancer patients with fever and neutropenia. N Engl J Med 315: 552-558
35. EORTC International Antimicrobial Therapy Cooperative Group (1986) Amikacin short or full course plus ceftazidime versus amikacin plus azlocillin for Gram-negative rod bacteremia in granulocytopenic cancer patients (abstract). 26th Interscience conference on antimicrobial agents and chemotherapy, New Orleans, September 28-October 1: 247

Selective Decontamination of the Digestive Tract and Fungal Infection in Acute Leukemia Patients

I. Günther, U. Kaben, H. Dunker, R. Brijmohan-Günther, and H. Konrad

Abteilung für Hämatologie, Klinik für Innere Medizin, Wilhelm-Pieck-Universität, Ernst-Heydemann-Straße, 2500 Rostock, GDR

There is substantial evidence in the literature that fungal infections are increasing in frequency [2, 6, 7, 11, 12]. Thus in recent years the frequency of major fungal infections documented at autopsy in leukemia patients has risen to 38% [5, 14]. The causes are intensified cytostatic treatment, severe and long-term granulocytopenia, mucosal lesions, the type of antibiotic prescribed, and the duration of the antibiotic therapy and of hospitalization [7]. These factors have favored the emergence of increasingly diversified, potentially pathogenic microorganisms. Most infections originate from the patients own digestive tract and are caused by aerobic gram-negative bacilli and gram-positive cocci. Major fungal infections occur less frequently, are difficult to treat, and are often fatal. Their lethality has varied between 50% and 100% over the last 10 years [6, 7, 8, 12, 16]. Consequently it is necessary to prevent proliferation and subsequent invasiveness from the gastrointestinal tract of fungi and yeasts. This can be accomplished not only by treatment with antifungal drugs alone, but also with the help of ecological control of fungal proliferation [15].

The best approach to preventive treatment and maintenance of the ecosystem is selective decontamination (SD) of the digestive tract. SD is based on the concept of colonization resistance (CR). The CR of the digestive tract is a physiological barrier which controls colonization by exogenous, potentially pathogenic bacteria and fungi. The purpose of SD is to eradicate these potentially pathogenic organisms during granulocytopenia without affecting the anaerobic microflora and viridans group streptococci responsible for CR. The importance of CR, especially as far as fungi are concerned, has been demonstrated by van der Waaij. The most common fungal pathogens in granulocytopenic patients are *Candida* and *Aspergillus* species. There are differences between *Candida* and *Aspergillus* as regards source, port of entrance, and clinical manifestation [15]. SD drugs suppress *Candida* species only since they mostly grow in the digestive tract. SD antifungals exert no influence on *Aspergillus* because *Aspergillus* spore formations colonize the mucous membranes of the nose, paranasal sinus, and bronchial tree [16].

Recent Results in Cancer Research, Vol. 108

Table 1. Patient characteristics

No. of patients (f/m)	108	(60/48)
Age (yrs), median (range)	48.2	(16-79)
Myeloid leukemia	73	
Nonmyeloid leukemia	20	
Blast crisis (CML)	15	
No. of treatment periods	138	
1st remission induction course	96	
2nd remission induction course	29	
3rd remission induction course	13	
Duration (days)		
- of treatment periods	78.1	(20-193)
- of granulocytopenia $<0.5 \times 10^9$/liter	40.3	(21- 94)
- of granulocytopenia $<0.1 \times 10^9$/liter	25.2	(11- 68)
- of thrombocytopenia $<5 \times 10^9$/liter	10.6	(0- 59)

Materials and Methods

The characteristics of the patients who were treated in our hospital between 1981 and 1986 are shown in Table 1. We analyzed 108 cases and 138 treatment periods. To induce remission of acute myeloid leukemia we administered 6-thioguanine, cytosine arabinoside, and daunorubicin (TAD regime), together with oncovin and prednisolone in two or three phases. Patients with nonmyeloid leukemia were treated with a regimen of oncovin, daunorubicin, prednisolone, and L-asparaginase. For the second remission induction course we employed the TAD or COAP (cyclophosphamide, oncovorin, cytosine arabinoside, prednisolone) regime, or a combination involving cyclophosphamide, methotrexate, and 6-mercaptopurine. Patients who were older than 60 years received the COAP regime or cytosine arabinoside. Patients with blastic crisis were treated with Oncovin and prednisolone or the ViDaP (oncovin, daunorubicin, prednisolone), COAP, or TAD regime. The intensified chemotherapy resulted in severe granulocytopenia below 0.1×10^9/liter granulocytes over 25.2 days. For prevention of infection we used an SD design including antibacterial (trimethoprim 480 mg/daily, sulfamerazine 720 mg daily, and polymyxin 0.25 g daily) and antifungal (4-6 million IU nystatin daily, in the form of lozenges, plus topical measures) components. SD was started before the cytostatic treatment. The SD drugs were given orally and for as long as patients were granulocytopenic. Microbiological surveillance was carried out once a week with bacteriological and mycological cultures from fecal samples and oral washings. Mycological cultures were performed semiquantitatively. We evaluated specific antibodies with cell agglutination by using *Candida albicans* blastospores as well as immunodiffusion in agar gel with somatic *Candida* antigen. We designated fungal infections as either major (deep, invasive, disseminated, systemic, or organ mycosis) or minor (thrush, stomatitis, glossitis, pharyngitis, tonsillitis, and eosophagitis).

Table 2. Indications for antimycotic therapy in 19 granulocytopenic patients with acute leukemia

	No.
Persistent fever (38.5 °C) despite antibiotics	19
Duration of antibiotic treatment >8 days	19
Thrush	5
Oral lesions	9
Pulmonal infiltrates	7
Candida cell agglutination titer ⩾ 1:640	14
Immunodiffusion positive	13
Blood cultures positive (*Candida*)	2

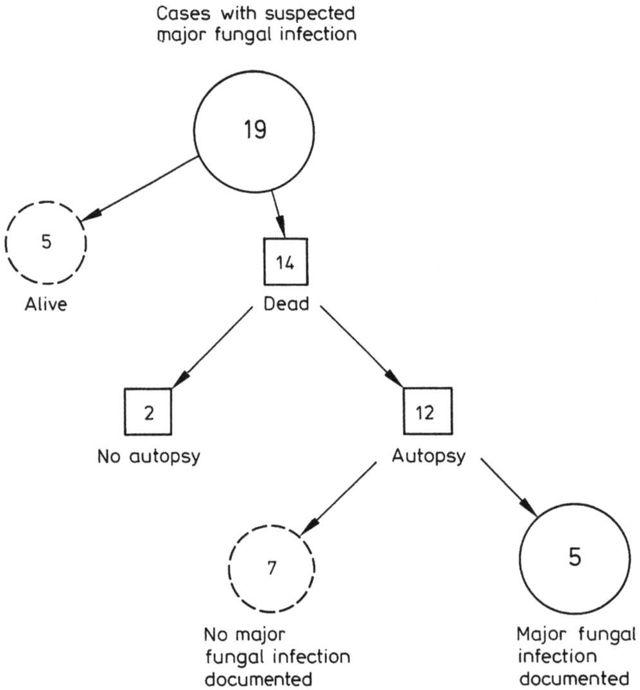

Fig. 1. Outcome of antimycotic therapy

Results

Nineteen granulocytopenic patients had persistent fever despite administration of broad spectrum systemic antibiotics for 10 days. The antibiotic treatment was given in a double combination with gentamicin and ampicillin or oxacillin, azlocillin, or cefotiam. The SD drugs were continued. The findings in these patients are listed in Table 2. After a test dose of 1 mg amphotericin B we treated our patients every second day with 5–40 mg, reaching a total dosage of up to 600 mg. We also gave 8–10 g 5-fluocytosine p.o. daily. The duration of antimycotic treatment ranged from 10 to 49 days. Of the 19 patients treated, 14 died. Autopsies were per-

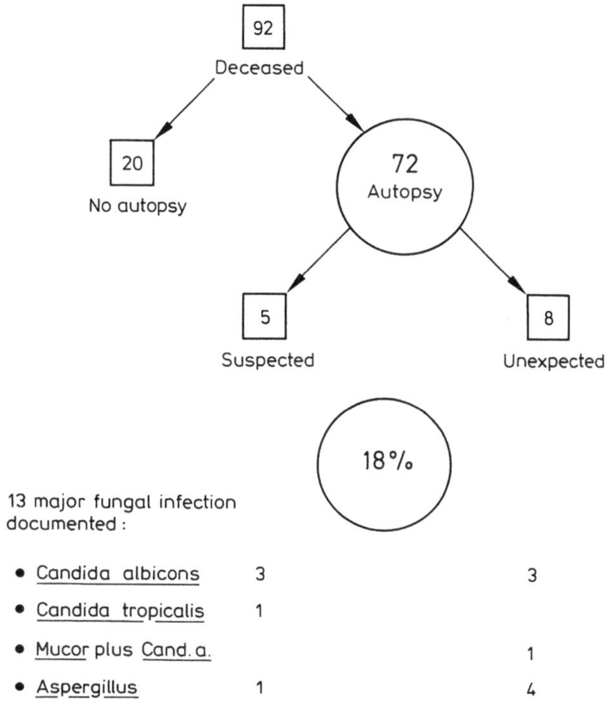

Fig. 2. Findings at autopsy

formed on 12. In five cases we registered major fungal infections. There was no evidence of major fungal infection in seven cases (Fig. 1). In a total of 72 autopsies, 13 major fungal infections were documented; this is equivalent to 18% (Fig. 2). We correlated the pathological findings of major fungal infections with the clinical signs. Fungal infections were found more often during second and third courses of remission induction than during the first course. The longer lesions of the oropharyngeal mucosa were present, the more often we found fungal infections. In order to correlate the mycological culture findings with the actual fungal infections, we classified the latter into three groups: clinically suspected fungal infection, pathologically documented fungal infection, and patients without fungal infection. Our culture findings showed no correlation with the groups. We found an increased cell agglutination titre (CAT, >1:160) as well as precipitating antibodies in all three groups. Suspicion of fungal infection arose in the first group in 12 patients, in the second group in 4 patients, and in the third group in 12 patients.

Discussion

Prevention of yeast overgrowth in the digestive tract is advisable in the compromised patient to reduce yeast infection [2]. De Vries showed a significant reduction of yeast cell concentration in the feces and on throat swabs after using nystatin 6 million IU/daily or amphotericin B 2 g daily. Since she noticed poor compliance

Table 3. Fungal infection in SD patients (first and second) induction courses, clinical results)

Author	No. of patients	Frequency of fungal infection		
		Major and minor	*Candida*	*Aspergillus*
Sleijfer et al. 1980	58	5	5	
de Vries-Hospers 1984	102	3	2	1
Kurrle et al. 1984	125	15	14	1
Kurrle et al. (EORTC) 1986	140	12	12	
Total	425	35 (8.2%)	33	2

of patients treated with nystatin, she changed to amphotericin B [3]. The frequency of major fungal infections reported by the EORTC – Gnotobiotic Project Group is presented in Table 3. During the treatment of 425 patients they found fungal infections clinically in 8.2% [4, 9, 10, 13]. A number of clinical symptoms are suggestive of major fungal infection. Most patients with fungal infection, however, do not have these alarming symptoms (Gold 1984). The physician should suspect fungal infection if a patient develops persistent fever which is resistant to the usual antibiotic therapy regime, especially if mucocutaneous candidal lesions, saprophytic mucosal foci, or pulmonary infiltrates are present [11, 12]. The presence of precipitating antibodies to cytoplasmic antigens of *Candida albicans* can be a useful adjunct in the diagnosis of major fungal infection [7]. Precipitin, however, can often be detected in serum from hospitalized patients in the absence of overt fungal infection. The serological findings could be false-positive or false-negative [1]. Since laboratory findings and clinical signs do not give reliable indications of fungal infections, empirical amphotericin B therapy has become very useful [8, 12]. When Pizzo and Klastersky began early empirical use of amphotericin B in fever of unknown origin in granulocytopenic patients, they were able to reduce the lethality and frequency of major fungal infections at autopsy from 50% to 12%. The combination of amphotericin B and 5-fluocytosin is still the therapy of choice for fungal infection in granulocytopenic patients. Unfortunately, the side-effects and the toxicity of amphotericin B are worrisome. However, these disadvantages are usually manageable and reversible. Low doses of steroids or meperidine have been reported to be frequently effective in abolishing or reducing immediate toxic reactions such as shaking chills and fever [7]. The optimal duration of amphotericin B therapy is still not clear. Pizzo has emphasized that such patients should be treated until they have achieved an accumulative dose of 1–2 g. A tendency toward an increase in aspergillosis during the last 10 years has been reported. The ratio between candidosis and aspergillosis is about 3:2 [5, 6, 7, 16]. The most common mode of infection by *Aspergillus* is the inhalation of spores. Because of the air-borne transmission and the landing site of the spores the most appropriate prophylactic measure seems to be isolation of patients in units such as laminar air flow rooms, equipped with a system filtering the air. This is quite a sophisticated approach and not yet suited for general clinical practise. The next best approach may be the topical application of antifungal agents, e.g., aerosols or nasal spray of amphotericin B [16].

Conclusion

Selective decontamination may represent the way forward in reducing the morbidity and lethality not only of bacterial but also of major fungal infections. It is advisable to start the antifungal drugs as early as possible and a few days before the antibacterial prophylaxis. The antifungals must be given in an adequate dosage and for a long enough period. Systemic antibiotics should be given in order to maintain the colonization resistance. The adherence of *Candida* cells to the oropharyngeal mucosa is an essential step in candidal infection. The blocking of receptors for yeast adherence is therefore an important mechanism of antifungal activity [15].

Summary

For prevention of infection we used an SD design including antibacterial (trimethoprim 480 mg/daily, sulfamerazine 720 mg/daily, and polymyxin 0.25 mg/daily) and antifungal (4-6 million IU nystatin/daily) components. We analyzed retrospectively 138 treatment periods in 108 patients. The intensified chemotherapy resulted in severe granulocytopenia below 0.1×10^9/liter over 25.2 days. In 19 patients there was suspicion of major fungal infection; therefore they were given amphotericin B and 5-fluocytosine. Fourteen of them died; major fungal infections were documented in 5 cases. In 18% of all the deceased we found major fungal infections. There was a correlation between fungal infection, the late stages of the hematological malignancy, and the lesions on the oropharyngeal mucosa. However, in terms of the serological and culture findings no correlation appeared to exist between the group with and the group without fungal infection. The SD regime is meant to suppress the *Candida* cell concentration in the digestive tract but has no influence on *Aspergillus* in the respiratory tract.

References

1. Armstrong D, Gersten M (1982) Laboratory diagnosis of fungal and parasitic diseases in patients with neoplastic disease. In: Klastersky J (ed) Infection in cancer patients, Raven, New York, pp 55-72
2. De Gregorio MW, Lee WMF, Ries CA (1982) *Candida* infections in patients with acute leukemia: ineffectiveness of nystatin prophylaxis and relationship between oropharyngeal and systemic candidiasis. Cancer 50: 2780-2784
3. De Vries-Hospers HG, Mulder NH, Sleijfer DT, van Saene HK (1982) The effect of amphotericin B lozenges on the presence and number of *candida* cells in the oropharnyx of neutropenic leukemia patients. Infection 10: 71-75
4. De Vries-Hospers HG, Sleijfer DT, Mulder NH, Nieweg HO, van der Waaij D (1984) Selective decontamination of the digestive tract as a method of infection prevention in granulocytopenic patients; a follow-up study in 102 patients. In: Sibinga CT et al. (eds) Transplantation and blood transfusion. Martinus Nijhoff, Boston, pp 65-72
5. Donhuijsen J, Samandari S (1985) Tiefe Mykosen bei Leukämien und malignen Lymphomen. Dtsch Med Wochenschr 110: 903-907
6. Ezdinli EZ, O'Sullivan DD, Wasser LP, Kim U, Stutzman L (1979) Oral amphotericin for candidiasis in patients with hematological neoplasms. JAMA 242: 258-260

7. Gold JWM (1984) Opportunistic fungal infections in patients with neoplastic disease. Am J Med 76: 458-463
8. Klastersky J (1983) A cooperative trial of empiric treatment in febrile neutropenic patients. In: Spitzky HH et al. (eds) 13th International congress of chemotherapy. Vienna 28th August 2nd September 1983, Vienna, part 71, pp 33-35
9. Kurrle E, Krieger D, Vanek E, Heimpel H (1984) Selektive Dekontamination als Verfahren einer Infektionsprophylaxe bei Patienten mit akuten Leukämien. Fortschr Antimikrobiellen Antineoplast Chemother 3-6: 997-1003
10. Kurrle E, Dekker AW, Gaus W, Haralambie E, Krieger D et al. (1986) Prevention of infection in acute leukemia: prospective randomized study on the efficacy of adsorbable and non-absorbable antimicrobial drugs. Infection 14: 226-232
11. Meunier-Carpentier F (1984) Chemoprophylaxis of fungal infections. Am J Med 76: 652-656
12. Pizzo PA, Robichand KJ, Gill FA, Witebsky FG (1982) Empiric antibiotic and antifungal therapy for cancer patients with prolonged fever and granulocytopenia. Am J Med 72: 101-111
13. Sleijfer DT, Mulder NH, de Vries HG, Gidler V, Nieweg HO, van der Waaij D, van Saene HKF (1980) Infection prevention in granulocytopenic patients by selective decontamination of the digestive tract. Eur J Cancer Clin Oncol 16: 859-869
14. Stahel RA, Vogt P, Schüler G, Rüttner JR, Frick P, Oelz O (1983) Systemische Pilzinfekte bei hämatologischen Neoplasien. Schweiz Med Wochenschr 113: 44-46
15. van der Waaij D (1982) Gut resistance to colonization: clinical usefulness of selective use of orally administered antimicrobial and antifungal drugs. In: Klastersky J (ed) Infections in cancer patients. Raven, New York, pp 73-85
16. Warren RE, Warnock DW (1982) Clinical manifestation and management of aspergillosis in the compromised patient. In: Warnock DW, Richardson MD (eds) Infection in the compromised patient. Wiley, pp 119-153

Management of Treatment Side-Effects

Controlling Emesis in Patients Receiving Cancer Chemotherapy

R. J. Gralla, M. G. Kris, L. B. Tyson, and R. A. Clark

Solid Tumor Service, Department of Medicine, Memorial Sloan-Kettering Cancer Center, 1275 York Avenue, New York, NY 10021, USA

Over the past several years, the appropriate use of antiemetics has increased, as has the ability to control chemotherapy-associated nausea and vomiting. With greater use of chemotherapy and with the development of newer agents in which emesis is a major side-effect, the need for improved control of nausea and vomiting has become an important consideration in medical oncology and in supportive care. The primary objective of this paper is to provide a practical guide that discusses some of the major issues in the antiemetic approach to the patient receiving chemotherapy.

Important areas to discuss include (a) different types of emesis, (b) patient characteristics that may affect emetic control, (c) the patterns of emesis associated with different chemotherapy drugs, (d) the mode of action of antiemetics, (e) the active available antiemetics, and (f) antiemetic regimens.

Emetic Syndromes

In patients receiving chemotherapy, three types of emesis have been identified. Careful attention to which problem is to be treated or prevented is significant in that the cause of and the treatment for the problem may differ. These emetic syndromes include acute chemotherapy-induced emesis, delayed emesis, and anticipatory emesis. An additional problem is that patients may have emesis for reasons other than their chemotherapy, such as that induced by pain medications, bronchodilators, other medications, or by tumor-related problems, including intestinal obstruction. In these instances, adjustment of medications or treatment of the complications of the tumor may be more important than the selection of the proper antiemetic drug. Most antiemetic studies have investigated acute chemotherapy-induced emesis. This will be the major topic of discussion, with separate sections to follow concerning the latter two emetic problems.

Recent Results in Cancer Research, Vol. 108

Table 1. Important factors in the approach to the patient receiving cancer chemotherapy

Patient characteristics:	- Prior chemotherapy experience
	- Alcohol usage history
	- Age
Chemotherapy:	- Emetic potential of the drug
	- Dosage and schedule
	- Route of administration
	- Time of onset of emesis (especially: cyclophosphamide)
	- Consideration individually of each drug in combinations
Antiemetics:	- Dosage and schedule
	- Route of administration
	- Combination regimen

Patient Characteristics and Emesis

Several aspects of a patient's prior experience or characteristics may influence emetic outcome. Studies to date have indicated that the patient's age, alcohol intake history, and prior emesis with chemotherapy are factors of importance, as outlined in Table 1. The patient's age is relevant not so much because it directly affects the control of emesis as because there is a greater tendency for younger patients to experience acute dystonic reactions when receiving antiemetics with dopamine receptor blocking as the mechanism of action [1]. This category of antiemetics includes such valuable agents as substituted benzamides, butyrophenones, and phenothiazines. In a report summarizing the experience of nearly 500 patients receiving metoclopramide, the incidence of trismus or torticollis was only 2% in those over age 30; by contrast a 27% occurrence was reported in younger patients [1, 2]. In addition, when dopamine blocking antiemetics are given on several consecutive days, dystonic reactions are also more common [2]. This can be of particular importance for younger patients in that several regimens for malignancies of this age group utilize chemotherapy on a daily schedule.

Three studies have indicated that emesis is more easily controlled in patients with chronic heavy alcohol usage histories (>100 g/day - or approximately five mixed drinks) that in those without this past experience [3, 4]. In the one prospective evaluation, in 52 patients receiving high-dose cisplatin and an appropriate combination antiemetic regimen, 93% of those with the high alcohol history had no emesis as opposed to 61% ($P<0.01$) of the other patients [3].

Poor control of emesis with past courses of chemotherapy predisposes a patient to unsatisfactory antiemetic results with subsequent similar chemotherapy. One trial in which patients received their initial treatment with the same antiemetic noted that major control was three times more likely in those who had not previously had chemotherapy [5]. Whether this is due to the development of conditioned anticipatory emesis or to other possible factors is not clear.

Table 2. The potential of commonly used chemotherapy agents to induce emesis

High potential	Moderate potential	Low potential
Cisplatin	Carmustine	Etoposide
Dacarbazine	Lomustine	Mitomycin C
Dactinomycin	Doxorubicin	Methotrexate
Mechlorethamine	Daunorubicin	5-Fluorouracil
Cyclophosphamide	Cytarabine	Hydroxyurea
	Procarbazine	Bleomycin
		Vinblastine
		Vincristine
		Chlorambucil

Chemotherapeutic Agents and Emesis

The differences in the potential of various chemotherapeutic drugs to result in emesis are given in Table 2. In general, the agents most often associated with emesis also induce the greatest severity of this side-effect. Differences occur among patients and even among treatment courses in the same patient.

Both the drug dose and the route of administration can affect the incidence of nausea and vomiting (Table 1). With most agents, emesis begins between 1 and 2 h after starting chemotherapy, in patients who have not previously received chemotherapy. A most important exception to this pattern occurs with cyclophosphamide. When cyclophosphamide is given intravenously in high doses, the onset of emesis is usually delayed until 9–18 h after chemotherapy [6]. This factor emphasizes two important principles. First, to be effective, an antiemetic regimen must consider the potential of the chemotherapeutic drug to cause emesis and its individual pattern in so doing. Second, when combination chemotherapy is used, each of the drugs must be individually considered. Thus, a regimen that is effective against cisplatin may not be well designed for the patient receiving cyclophosphamide in that the blood levels of the antiemetic agent may be too low to prevent the late onset of cyclophosphamide-induced emesis.

The mechanism by which chemotherapy induces emesis is still not completely understood, although the studies of Borison have been revealing [7]. Studies support the hypothesis that reflex-induced emesis is caused by stimulation of receptors in the central nervous system or in the gastrointestinal tract. Receptor areas have been identified that affect a vomiting center in the lateral reticular formation of the medulla, which then coordinates the act of vomiting. An important area also located in the medulla is the chemoreceptor trigger zone (CTZ), in the area postrema. This receptor region is sensitive to chemical stimuli from both the blood and the cerebrospinal fluid. Chemotherapeutic agents or their metabolites may stimulate receptors in the CTZ, such as dopamine receptors. Impulses generated in the CTZ and transmitted to the vomiting center may then lead to the initiation of emesis. Neuroreceptors in the gastrointestinal tract, which has afferents to the vomiting center, may also play a role in chemotherapy-induced nausea and vomiting.

Antiemetic agents that block neuroreceptors in the CTZ, the vomiting center, or in the gastrointestinal tract may be useful in preventing or controlling emesis.

Antiemetic Agents

Several antiemetic agents have been shown to be safe and effective (see Table 3). In that no agent is ideal, and since many trials indicate that appropriate combinations of agents can be more useful than a single drug, a familiarity with a few of the more active agents is essential. Among the best studied of the more effective agents are those that exert their activity by blocking dopamine receptors. These include such classes and agents as: (a) substituted benzamides (metoclopramide), (b) butyprophenones (haloperidol and droperidol), and (c) phenothiazines (prochlorperazine and chlorpromazine). Additionally, corticosteroids (dexamethasone and methylprednisolone) are effective agents, and benzodiazepines and cannabinoids may also have a role.

Table 3. The doses and administration of a number of frequently used antiemetic agents

Antiemetic agent	Route	Dose range	Frequency of administration
Substituted benzamide:			
Metoclopramide	Intravenous	1-3 mg/kg	Every 2 h
	Oral[a]	1-3 mg/kg	Every 2-4 h
Butyrophenones:			
Haloperidol	Intravenous	1-3 mg	Every 2-6 h
	Oral	1-2 mg	Every 3-6 h
Droperidol	Intravenous	0.5-2 mg	Every 4 h
Corticosteroids:			
Dexamethasone	Intravenous/oral	4-20 mg	Once only, or every 4-6 h
Methylprednisolone	Intravenous	250-500 mg	Once only, or every 4-6 h
Phenotiazines:			
Prochlorperazine	Oral	5-10 mg	Every 2-4 h
	Rectal	25 mg	Every 4-6 h
	Intramuscular/intravenous	10-20 mg	Every 3-6 h
Chlorpromazine	Oral	25-50 mg	Every 3-6 h
	Intramuscular/intravenous	25 mg	Every 3-6 h
Benzodiazepine:			
Lorazepam	Intravenous	1-2 mg/m^2	Every 4 h
Cannabinoid:			
THC	Oral	5-10 mg/m^2	Every 3-4 h

[a] Using investigational 50- and 100-mg tablets.

Substituted Benzamides

The most commonly used drug of this class is metoclopramide. A recent pharmacological study demonstrated that efficacy was correlated with the establishment of high blood levels (> 850 ng/ml) of metoclopramide in patients receiving cisplatin [8]. Also of importance is maintenance of an adequate level of this antiemetic at the time of emetic vulnerability through the use of an appropriate dosing schedule. In preventing emesis induced by cisplatin or by cyclophosphamide plus doxorubicin, metoclopramide administration every 2 h (beginning shortly before chemotherapy) appears to be the most effective schedule. Doses and schedules of metoclopramide are outlined in Tables 3 and 4.

Random-assignment studies have shown that in respect of cisplatin-induced emesis, metoclopramide is superior, or at least equivalent, to all other antiemetic agents with which it has been compared [9, 10, 11, 12, 13, 14]. Several reports have indicated useful activity against the emesis associated with a number of other chemotherapeutic agents [15, 16, 17].

High oral doses of metoclopramide (using 50- and 100-mg tablets) can result in therapeutic blood levels and can be highly effective [17, 18, 19]. A recent trial comparing similar high doses and schedules of oral metoclopramide with the same agent given intravenously, in patients receiving cisplatin 60 mg/m^2, reported similar results in both arms of the study. Emesis was completely controlled in half of the patients while two-thirds achieved a major response (two or fewer emetic episodes) [18].

The side-effects commonly associated with metoclopramide include mild sedation, dystonic reactions (age-related, as discussed above), akathisia (restlessness), and diarrhea (which may be an effect of specific chemotherapeutic agents, such as cisplatin) [1, 9, 20]. In general, the side-effects are easy to control or prevent. Akathisia is easily prevented or treated with a benzodiazepine, and dystonic reactions can be dealt with similarly or with diphenhydramine. As will be discussed in the section on combinations of antiemetics, dexamethasone in addition to metoclopramide both improves efficacy and reduces diarrhea.

Butyrophenones

Haloperidol and droperidol were shown in initial trials to be active antiemetics [21, 22]. In that substantial differences have not been demonstrated between these two butyrophenones, most of the comments below will refer to studies conducted with haloperidol. A formal study comparing haloperidol with metoclopramide in patients receiving cisplatin reported that both antiemetics are effective, although a trend toward greater activity was seen with metoclopramide [13]. Doses of 1–3 mg haloperidol given intravenously every 2–6 h have been most commonly used (Table 3); the higher doses and more frequent schedules have more often been associated with better results. Toxicity commonly includes sedation, dystonic reactions, and akathisia, with hypotension occasionally being observed.

Phenothiazines

The unsatisfactory results observed with oral and intramuscular phenothiazines encouraged new studies to examine other classes of agents, different administration schedules, and higher dosage regimens. Structure-activity studies indicated that variations of the side chain at position 10 of the phenothiazine ring affect the antiemetic properties of these drugs [23]. Agents such as prochlorperazine would be predicted to have greater activity than other commonly used phenothiazines, such as chlorpromazine. This predicted difference, however, has not been established in patients receiving chemotherapy.

Prochlorperazine given in typical oral and intramuscular doses in random-assignment trials has been found to be less active than metoclopramide [9] or dexamethasone [24], and equivalent to or less active than tetrahydrocannabinol [25, 26, 27]. A more recent study using intravenous prochlorperazine in comparison with metoclopramide was indicated more encouraging results [28]. There are two problems with this trial which should be considered: (a) an imbalance in the arms of the study (concerning additional cyclophosphamide with the late onset of emesis), and (b) failure to evaluate adequately the incidence of orthostatic blood pressure changes, an important side-effect of phenothiazines with major implications for outpatient usage. Other side-effects are similar to those listed for haloperidol.

Corticosteroids

Although several theories exist, the antiemetic mechanism of action of corticosteroids remains unclear. Several open studies and random-assignment trials have confirmed their utility [11, 12, 24, 29, 30, 31, 32]. Dexamethasone doses have generally been in the range of 4–20 mg per dose. In the majority of trials in which a corticosteroid has been added to an effective agent of another class, improved antiemetic efficacy for the combination has resulted.

Toxicity has generally been mild with short courses of dexamethasone or methylprednisolone. There has been no indication of a lessening of chemotherapeutic effect through the use of steroids as antiemetics. With the low degree of toxicity and with a different mechanism of action than other agents, corticosteroids are ideal candidates for use in combination antiemetic regimens.

Benzodiazepines and Cannabinoids

Recent studies have indicated that benzodiazepines can be useful additions to antiemetic regimens. Trials with lorazepam have shown a high degree of patient acceptance with a marked decrease in akathisia and anxiety. Additionally, lorazepam may add a small degree of objective antiemetic efficacy [33]. In a phase I trial only modest major antiemetic activity was observed, but the subjective benefits appeared to make it an agent worth considering for use in combination [34]. A major difficulty in evaluating this agent's true activity is that it produces a dose-related memory loss [33, 34].

Most cannabinoid trials have included delta-9-tetrahydrocannabinol (THC); two synthetic cannabinoids, nabilone and levonantradol, have also been tested clinically [35, 36, 37, 38]. THC has been tried at many doses with differing schedules. Doses in the range of 5–10 mg/m^2, every 3–4 h, orally, appear to be among the most useful [10, 35, 39]. In general, THC has been found to be superior to placebo, and equivalent to or superior to oral prochlorperazine [25, 26]. Similar results have been reported with nabilone [37]. Side-effects have been frequent but generally manageable; they have included sedation, dry mouth, orthostatic hypotension, ataxia, dizziness, a "high," and euphoria or dysphoria. The role of the cannabinoids remains unclear. It is apparent that such agents as metoclopramide and corticosteroids are superior and have fewer side-effects [10, 40].

Antiemetic Combinations

Trials of single agents have indicated which are the most effective antiemetics and which are most likely to be compatible with other active drugs. Guidelines for effective combination regimens include: (a) regimens should combine agents that have different mechanisms of activity and do not have overlapping toxicities; (b) the drugs should be active as single agents, with the optimal doses, best route of administration, and proper schedules having been previously established; (c) agents added to the combination may be useful if they lessen the side-effects of the regimen or if they reduce other toxicities of the chemotherapy (see Table 4).

Several recent studies have compared the activity of metoclopramide with the combination of metoclopramide plus a corticosteroid. In each of these studies, the combination of the two active antiemetics has been superior to the single agent [32, 41, 42, 43]. In addition to improved antiemetic efficacy with the steroid plus metoclopramide, the incidence of diarrhea was significantly reduced. An open study combining a butyrophenone with a corticosteroid also reported favorable results [44].

At our institution the preferred regimen for patients receiving high doses of cisplatin (120 mg/m^2) has been as follows: metocloramide 3 mg/kg i.v. at 30 min before cisplatin and at 90 min after the start of the cisplatin, plus dexamethasone 20 mg i.v. at 40 min before cisplatin, plus diphenhydramine 50 mg i.v. at 35 min before chemotherapy. The cisplatin, following hydration and mannitol, is administered over 20 min. Given the subjective benefits seen with lorazepam, a recent study investigated the combination of metoclopramide plus dexamethasone plus either lorazepam or diphenhydramine, in a random-assisignment design. The doses of the agents were as listed above, with the lorazepam given at 1.5 mg/m^2 i.v. Both arms of the study had similar objective antiemetic efficacy, with over 60% of patients having complete control and nearly 90% having major control. The lorazepam-containing regimen, however, was favored due to improved subjective results, with reduced anxiety and akathisia [33].

Table 4 outlines recommended regimens, and alternatives, for use with a variety of chemotherapeutic drugs. These regimens have all been tested, either in formal comparison studies or in open trials. It is clear from this table that in nearly

Table 4. Examples of and approach fo combination antiemetics in patients receiving some specific chemotherapy regimens

General approach:	Neurotransmitter blocking agent - *plus* - Corticosteroid - *plus* - Benzodiazepine or antihistamine
Chemotherapeutic agent	*Antiemetic regimen*
Cisplatin[a]:	
>99 mg/m^2	Methoclopramide 3 mg/kg i.v.[b], 30 min before and 90 min after chemotherapy + Dexamethasone 20 mg i.v.[c], 40 min before chemotherapy + Lorazepam 1.5 mg/m^2 i.v., 35 min before chemotherapy
40–70 mg/m^2	Metoclopramide 2 mg/kg i.v.[b], 30 min before and 90 min after chemotherapy + Dexamethasone (as above)[c] + Lorazepam (as above) *or:* Diphenhydramine 50 mg i.v., 35 min before chemotherapy
<40 mg/m^2	Metoclopramide 1–2 mg/kg i.v.[b] (schedule as above) + Dexamethasone (as above)[c] + Lorazepam or diphenhydramine (as above)
Cyclophosphamide + doxorubicin combinations	Metoclopramide 2 or 3 mg/kg p.o., every 2 h × 3 doses, then every 4 h × 3 doses *or* Metoclopramide 3 mg/kg i.v., every 2 h × 2 doses, then 40 mg p.o. every 3 h × 4 *or* Metoclopramide 2 mg/kg i.v., every 2 h × 3 doses, then 40 mg p.o. every 3 h × 3 - *plus* - Dexamethasone 20 mg i.v.[c] (as for cisplatin) - *plus* - Diphenhydramine 50 mg i.v. or p.o., with the first and then every other metoclopramide dose
Dacarbazine	As for cisplatin, 40–70 mg/m^2

[a] Cisplatin total dose given over 15–30 min in these studies. A longer period of cisplatin administration might require more antiemetic doses.
[b] Alternative choice: haloperidol 3 mg i.v.
[c] Alternative choice: methylprednisolone 250–500 mg i.v.

all instances, unless an agent is contraindicated for a specific patient, combinations are recommended.

Chemotherapy regimens which involve several consecutive days of treatment present a special problem in controlling emesis. The antiemetics which block dopamine receptors appear to result in a greater incidence of dystonic reactions when given on multiple consecutive days. Of additional interest is the observation that when agents such as cisplatin or dacarbazine are given over several days, the emesis gradually lessens. The regimen currently being investigated at our institution in patients receiving cisplatin at 25-33 mg/m^2/daily for 3-4 days, has gradually decreasing doses of antiemetics. Patients are given dexamethasone at 20 mg i.v., 30 min before chemotherapy on each day. Metoclopramide is given at 2 mg/kg at 30 min before cisplatin, also. On the first and second treatment days, the same metoclopramide dose is repeated 90 min after cisplatin; on the third day, the metoclopramide dose is repeated but only at 1 mg/kg, and no repeat dose is given on the fourth day. Diphenhydramine 50 mg i.v. is given with the first metoclopramide dose each day. The study is still in progress, but initial results are encouraging in patients over age 30.

Other Emetic Problems

Anticipatory Emesis

Anticipatory emesis is defined as nausea or vomiting, often beginning before the administration of chemotherapy, in patients with poor control of emesis with past chemotherapy. As this is a conditioned response, the hospital environment or other treatment-related associations may trigger its onset. The administration of the chemotherapy itself may bring on this response, not only as a chemical stimulus but also as a psychological factor. The stronger the likelihood of emesis, and the poorer the control, the greater is the chance of developing anticipatory emesis [45].

Treatment of this problem is important; however, its prevention is probably more successful. The difficulties of anticipatory emesis underscore the importance of giving the most effective antiemetics with the initial course of emesis-producing chemotherapy. Several reports have indicated that behavior therapy can be helpful for patients with anticipatory emesis [46, 47]; however, patients with this problem will need effective control of emesis with the next chemotherapy administration if further anticipatory emesis is to be avoided.

Delayed Emesis

Delayed emesis is defined as nausea or vomiting beginning 24 h or more after chemotherapy administration. This is a particular problem with major sources of emesis such as high-dose cisplatin. A recent natural history study observed that delayed emesis is less severe than emesis which occurs acutely, but that it still causes significant difficulties with hydration and nutrition as well as contributing to a lowered activity level. Although delayed emesis occurs less often in those patients who have complete emetic control on the day of chemotherapy, it still can occur in this group. The majority of patients treated with cisplatin at doses greater than 100 mg/m^2 experience some degree of delayed emesis, with the onset being most frequent 48-72 h after chemotherapy [48]. Two preliminary open trials have indicated that steroid plus metoclopramide or prochlorperazine combinations may be useful in controlling this problem [49, 50]; formal comparison studies are now being conducted.

Conclusion

Controlling emesis is an ideal situation for the collaboration of the skills and experiences of physicians and nurses who are oncology speciallists. While new agents could be helpful, better application of the available techniques would likely result in major improvements in patient care. This goal requires a knowledge of the more active drugs, experience with their use in combination, and consideration of the emetic problem of each patient.

There are some specific areas in which improvements in antiemetic treatment would be most helpful. With the predisposition to dystonic reactions in younger patients and in those receiving consecutive daily chemotherapy, control of emesis remains difficult. A new agent with activity not exerted through dopamine receptors might solve these problems. Currently, several agents meeting this requirement are in various stages of development. Effective approaches for delayed emesis would be most welcome; the results of ongoing trials may improve the management of this problem.

It is important that new studies are accurately interpreted. Precision in evaluation techniques is mandatory if accurate results are to be obtained. Additionally, attention to the differing patient characteristics and to specific emetic patterns of individual chemotherapeutic agents must be considered in the design of trials.

The control of emesis is one of many important topics in the supportive care of patients with cancer. The considerable research efforts of the past 5-10 years in this area have resulted in improvements; the application of these findings is a responsibility of all of us in clinical oncology.

References

1. Kris MG, Tyson LB, Gralla RJ, et al. (1983) Extrapyramidal reactions with high-dose metoclopramide. N Engl J Med 309: 433
2. Allen JC, Gralla RJ, Reilly C et al. (1985) Metoclopramide: dose-related toxicity and preliminary antiemetic studies in children receiving cancer chemotherapy. J Clin Oncol 3: 1136-1141
3. D'Acquisto RW, Tyson LB, Gralla RJ et al. (1986) The influence of a chronic high alcohol intake on chemotherapy-induced nausea and vomiting. Proc Am Soc Clin Oncol 5: 257
4. Sullivan JR, Leyden MJ, Bell R (1983) Decreased cisplatin induced nausea and vomiting with alcohol ingestion. N Engl J Med 309 (13): 796
5. Gralla RJ, Braun TJ, Squillante A et al. (1981) Metoclopramide: initial clinical studies of

high dosage regimens in cisplatin-induced emesis. In: Poster D (ed) The treatment of nausea and vomiting induced by cancer chemotherapy. Masson, New York, pp 167-176
6. Fetting JH, Grochow LB, Folstein MF et al. (1982) The course of nausea and vomiting after high-dose cyclophosphamide. Cancer Treat Rep 66: 1487-1493
7. Borison HL, McCarthy LE (1983) Neuropharmacology of chemotherapy induced emesis. Drugs 25: 8-17
8. Meyer BR, Lewin M, Dreyer DE et al. (1984) Optimizing metoclopramide control of cisplatin-induced emesis. Ann Intern Med 100: 393-395
9. Gralla RJ, Itri LM, Pisko DE et al. (1981) Antiemetic efficacy of high-dose metoclopramide: randomized trials with placebo and prochloperazine in patients with chemotherapy-induced nausea and vomiting. N Engl J Med 305: 905-909
10. Gralla RJ, Tyson LB, Borden LB et al. (1984) Antiemetic therapy: a review of recent studies and a report of a random assignment trial comparing metoclopramide with delta-9-tetrahydrocannabinol. Cancer Treat Rep 68: 163-172
11. Frustaci S, Tumolo S, Tirell U et al. (1983) High-dose metoclopramide versus dexamethasone in the prevention of cisplatin induced vomiting. Proc ASCO 2: 87
12. Aapro MS, Plezia PM, Alberts DS et al. (1983) Double-blind crossover study of the antiemetic efficacy of high-dose dexamethasone vs high-dose metoclopramide. Proc. ASCO 2: 93
13. Grunberg SM, Gala KV, Lampenfeld M et al. (1984) Comparison of the antiemetic effect of high-dose intravenous metoclopramide and high-dose intravenous haloperidol in a randomized double-blind crossover study. J Clin Oncol 2: 782-787
14. Richards PD, Flaum MA, Batemen M et al. (1986) The antiemetic efficacy of secobarbital and promazine compared to metoclopramide, diphenhydramine, and dexamethasone. A randomized trial. Cancer 58: 959-962
15. Strum SB, McDermed JE, Opfell RW et al. (1982) Intravenous metoclopramide. An effective antiemetic in cancer chemotherapy. JAMA 247: 2683-2686
16. Tyson LB, Clark RA, and Gralla RJ (1982) High-dose metoclopramide; control of dacarbazine-induced emesis in a preliminary trial. Cancer Treat Rep 66: 2108
17. Gralla RJ, Tyson LB, Clark RA et al. (1985) An all oral combination antiemetic regimen of patients receiving cytoxan + adriamycin + vincristine (CAV). Proc Am Soc Clin Oncol 4: 267
18. Anthony LB, Krozely MG, Woodward NJ et al. (1986) Antiemetic effect of oral versus intravenous metoclopramide in patients receiving cisplatin: a randomized double-blind trial. J Clin Oncol 4: 98-103
19. Garnick MB (1983) Oral metoclopramide and cisplatin chemotherapy. Ann Intern Med 99: 127
20. Von Hoff DD, Schilsky R, Reichert CM et al. (1979) Toxic effects of cis-dichlorodiamineplatinum (II) in man. Cancer Treat Rep 63: 1527-1531
21. Grossman B, Lessin LS, and Cohen P (1979) Droperidol prevents nausea and vomiting from cis-platinum. N Engl J Med 301: 47
22. Neidhart J, Gayen M, and Metz E (1980) Haldol is an effective antiemetic for platinum and mustard induced vomiting when other agents fail. ProcASCO 21: 365
23. Wampler G (1983) The pharmacology and clinical effectiveness of phenothiazines and related drugs for managing chemotherapy-induced emesis. Drugs 25: 35-51
24. Markman M, Sheidler V, Ettinger DS et al. (1984) Antiemetic efficacy of dexamethasone. Randomized, double-blind, crossover study with prochlorperazine in patients receiving cancer chemotherapy. N Engl J Med 311: 549-552
25. Frytak S, Moertel CG, O'Fallon J et al. (1979) Delta-9-tetrahydrocannabinol as an antiemetic in patients treated with cancer chemotherapy: a double comparison with prochlorperazine and a placebo. Ann Intern Med 91: 825-830
26. Sallan SE, Cronin CM, Zelen M et al. (1980) Antiemetics in patients receiving chemotherapy for cancer: a randomized comparison of delta-9-tetrahydrocannabinol and prochlorperazine. N Engl J Med 302: 135-138

27. Orr LE, McKerman JF, Bloone B (1980) Antiemetic effect of tetrahydrocannabinol. Arch Intern Med 140: 1431-1433
28. Carr BI, Bertrand M, Browning S et al. (1985) A comparison of the antiemetic efficacy of prochlorperazine and metoclopramide for the treatment of cisplatin-induced emesis: a prospective randomized double-blind study. J Clin Oncol 3: 1127-1132
29. Aapro MS, and Alberts DS (1981) High-dose dexamethasone for prevention of cisplatinum induced vomiting. Cancer Chemother Pharmacol 7: 11-14
30. Lee BJ (1981) Methylprednisolone as an antiemetic. N Engl J Med 3034: 486
31. Cassileth PA, Lusk EJ, Torri S et al. (1983) Antiemetic efficacy of dexamethasone therapy in patients receiving cancer chemotherapy. Arch Intern Med 143: 1347-1349
32. Kris MG, Gralla RJ, Tyson LB et al. (1985) Improved control of cisplatin-induced emesis with high-dose metoclopramide and with combinations of methoclopramide, dexamethasone, and diphenhydramine. Results of consecutive trials in 255 patients. Cancer 55: 527-534
33. Kris M, Clark R, Gralla R et al. (1986) Randomized double-blind antiemetic (AE) trial comparing combinations of metoclopramide, dexamethasone and lorazepam (MDL) in 120 patients (PTS) receiving cisplatin (DDP). Proc Am Soc Clin Oncol 5: 251
34. Laszlo J, Clark RA, Hanson DC et al. (1985) Lorazepam in cancer patients treated with cisplatin: a drug with antiemetic amnestic and anxiolytic effects. J Clin Oncol 3: 864-869
35. Vincent BJ, McQuistion DJ, Einhorn LH et al. (1983) Review of cannabinoids and their antiemetic effectiveness. Drugs 25: 52-62
36. Tyson LB, Gralla RJ, Clark RA et al. (1985) Phase I trial of levonantradol in chemotherapy-induced emesis. Am J Clin Oncol 8: 528-532
37. Herman TS, Einhorn LH and Jones SE (1979) Superiority of nabilone over prochlorperazine as an antiemetic in patients receiving cancer chemotherapy. N Engl J Med 300: 1295-1297
38. Steele N, Gralla RJ, Braun DW Jr (1980) Double-blind comparison of the antiemetic effects of nabilone and prochlorperazine on chemotherapy-induced emesis. Cancer Treat Rep 64: 219-224
39. Chang AE, Shiling DJ, Stillman RC et al. (1979) Delta-9-tetrahydrocannabinol as an antiemetic in patients receiving high-dose methotrexate: a prospective randomized evaluation. Ann Intern Med 91: 819-824
40. Venner P, Bruera E, Drebit D et al. (1986) Intensive treatment scheduling of nabilone (N) plus dexamethasone (DM) vs. methoclopramide (M) plus DM in cisplatinum (CP)-induced emesis. Proc Am Soc Clin Oncol. 5: 253
41. Allan SG, Cornbleet MA, Warrington PS et al. (1984) Dexamethasone and high-dose metoclopramide: efficacy in controlling cisplatin-induced nausea and vomiting. Br Med J 289: 878-879
42. Rosell R, Abad-Esteve A, Ribas-Mundo M et al. (1985) Evaluation of a combination antiemetic regimen including IV high-dose metoclopramide, dexamethasone, and diphenhydramine in cisplatin-based chemotherapy regimens. Cancer Treat Rep 69: 909-910
43. Roila F, Tonato M, Basurto C et al. (1986) Antiemetic activity of high doses of metoclopramide (MTC) combined with methylprednisolone (P) vs. MTX alone in cisplatin treated cancer patients (PTS). A randomized double blind trial of the Italian Oncology Group for Clinical Research (GOIRC). Proc Am Soc Clin Oncol 5: 263
44. Mason BA, Dambra J, Grossman B et al. (1982) Effective control of cisplatin-induced nausea using high-dose steroids and droperidol. Cancer Treat Rep 66: 243-245
45. Wilcox PM, Fetting JH, Nettesheim KM et al. (1982) Anticipatory vomiting in women receiving cyclophosphamide, methotrexate and 5-FU (CMF) adjuvant chemotherapy for breast carcinoma. Cancer Treat Rep 66: 1601-1604
46. Morrow GR (1982) Prevalence and correlates of anticipatory nausea and vomiting in chemotherapy patients. JNCI 68: 585-588
47. Morrow GR, Morrell C (1982) Behavioral treatment for the anticipatory nausea and vomiting induced by cancer chemotherapy. N Engl J Med 307: 1476-1480

48. Kris MG, Gralla RJ, Clark RA et al. (1985) Incidence, course, and severity of delayed nausea and vomiting following the administration of high-dose cisplatin. J Clin Oncol 3: 1379-1384
49. Strum S, McDermed J, Abrahano-Umali R et al. (1985) Management of cisplatin (DDP)-induced delayed-onset nausea (N) and vomiting (V): preliminary results with two drug regimens. Proc Am Soc Clin Oncol 4: 263
50. Clark R, Kris M, Tyson L et al. (1986) Antiemetic (AE) trials to control delayed vomiting (V) following high-dose cisplatin (DDP). Proc Am Soc Clin Oncol 5: 257

Corticosteroids as Antiemetics

M. S. Aapro*

Division d'Onco-Hématologie, Hôpital Cantonal Universitaire de Genève,
24, Rue Micheli-du-Crest, 1211 Genève 4, Switzerland

Although several antiemetic agents can exert some control of cancer chemotherapy-related nausea and vomiting, none is totally effective. As in many other instances of medical treatment, combinations of drugs will probably prove the best means of controlling the situation. We need agents that can be safely combined and that provide at least an additive protective effect. This paper demonstrates that corticosteroids are a significant addition to antiemetic therapy.

Preliminary Observations

Many tumors are treated with steroid-containing combination chemotherapy. In some instances it has been possible to observe that cycles containing prednisone are better tolerated (as in the original MOPP for Hodgkin's disease [1]. Several pilot studies showed that corticosteroids could exert a protective effect against chemotherapy-induced emesis [2, 3, 4, 5]. Most of these observations were based on patients with a history of severe emesis during previous courses of chemotherapy. This approach is interesting, as anticipatory nausea and vomiting might have decreased the effectiveness of corticosteroids [6]. The fact that they were actually found to have some efficacy was thus very encouraging. Furthermore, it shows that one can find an effective antiemetic treatment in this particular setting. Many other noncontrolled studies have been reported since then, but we will not review these.

Randomized Studies

Comparison of Corticosteroids with Other Agents or Placebo

Baker et al. [2] were the first to conduct a study of this nature. Of 20 patients in a double-blind crossover study who received additional antiemetics, 14 were considerably "helped" by the addition of dexamethasone, as compared to placebo. The

* Doctor P. Huber provided major encouragement in the writing of this chapter, which would never have been achieved without the secretarial skills of Ms. L. Clement.

Recent Results in Cancer Research, Vol. 108

Table 1. Controlled studies of corticosteroids as antiemetics

Type	Ref.	Author, journal	Patients	Agent(s)	Chemotherapy	Results
O	10	Breau et al. Presse Med, 1983	35	Methylprednisolone 2 mg/kg/d, d1 to d6	Cisplatin 20 mg/m² + others × 5 d	80% cycles ⩽ 2 ep. vomiting
			35	Medication p.r.n.		6% cycles ⩽ 2 ep. vomiting
DB	11	Cassileth et al. Arch Intern Med, 1983	26 25	Dexamethasone 10 mg i.v., 0 h Placebo (prochlorperazine p.r.n.)	Mainly CMF, no cisplatin	83% no V 57% no V
O	12	Kolaric and Roth Tumori, 1983	30	Placebo	Cisplatin 30 mg/m²	13% no V
			29	Thiethylperazine 20 mg i.v. −30 min		11% no V
			31	Methylprednisolone 250 mg i.v. −120 min		32% no V
DB	13	Aapro et al. J Clin Oncol, 1984	27	Dexamethasone 8 mg p.o. hs 4 mg p.o. q 4 h × 6, 10 mg i.v. 0 h, taper off d2 and 3	Cisplatin ⩾ 50 mg/m²	11% no V
				crossover		Patients prefer dexamethasone
				Metoclopramide 110 mg p.o. hs 75 mg p.o. q 4 h × 6, 75 mg i.v. 0 h		19% no V
O	14	Cognetti et al. Eur J Cancer, 1984	35	Dexamethasone 8 mg i.m. −24, −12 h 10 mg i.v. at chemotherapy +6, +12 h: 8 mg i.m.	Cisplatin 50 mg/m²	20% no V 4.4 h nausea
				crossover		Patients prefer dexamethasone
				Metoclopramide 1 mg/kg: 0, +1, +2, +4 h		26% no V 3.1 h nausea
O	15	Giaccone et al. Tumori, 1984	16	Methylprednisolone 250 mg i.v. × 4	Cisplatin ⩾ 50 mg/m² + other	20% no V
			26	Metoclopramide 40 mg i.v. × 2		20% no V
DB	16	Markman et al. N Engl J Med, 1984	42	Dexamethasone 20 mg i.v. −0.5 h 10 mg p.o. q 6 h × 4 post	Only 2/42 cisplatin	69% no V
				crossover		
				Prochlorperazine 10 mg i.v., same schedule		40% no V
DB	17	Dana et al. Am J Clin Oncol, 1985	16	Dexamethasone 10 mg i.v. −0.5 h 4 mg i.v. q 4 h × 6	Cisplatin 100 mg/m²	3/16 no V 5.6 h nausea
				crossover		No preference
				Placebo		2/16 no V 11.8 h nausea

Table 1 *(continued)*

Type	Ref.	Author, journal	Patients	Agent(s)	Chemotherapy	Results
DB	18	D'Olimpio et al. J Clin Oncol, 1985	32	Dexamethasone 20 mg i.v. −2 h and +3, +6, +9, +12 h	Cisplatin, dose?	28% no V 0.5 h nausea 25% unacceptable N/V
			32	Placebo		21% no V 3.5 h nausea 53% unacceptable N/V
O	19	Frustaci et al. Cancer Chemother Pharmacol, 1986	25	Dexamethasone 8 mg i.v. −0.5 h and q 3 h × 4 post	Cisplatin 120 mg/m²	(mean V): dexamethasone (9.4) metoclopramide (5)
			17	crossover	Cisplatin 60 mg/m²	Dexamethasone (4), metoclopramide (2.3); patients prefer metoclopramide
			25	Metoclopramide 2 mg/kg i.v. −0.5 h and +1.5, +3.5, +5.5, +8.5 h	Cisplatin 60 mg/m² + other chemo	Dexamethasone (13.6), metoclopramide (8.9)
DB	20	Ibrahim et al. Eur J Cancer, 1986	40	Dexamethasone 20 mg i.v. −0.5 h and 10 mg i.v. +1.5, +3.5, +5.5, +8.5 h	No cisplatin	58% no V
				crossover		Patients prefer dexamethasone
				Metoclopramide 1 mg/kg, same schedule		28% no V
O	21	Shinkai et al. Jpn J Clin Oncol, 1986	11	Dexamethasone 16 mg −0.5 h and 8 mg +1.5, +3.5, +5.5 h	Cisplatin 80 mg/m² + other	55% 0–2 episodes
			18	Metoclopramide 2 mg/kg, same schedule		67% 0–2 episodes
			11	Metoclopramide	Cisplatin 120 mg/m²	27% 0–2 episodes
			12	Metoclopramide + dexamethasone		92% 0–2 episodes
O	22	Niijima et al. Gan To Kagaku Ryoho, 1986	21	Methylprednisolone, dose?		
			18	Metoclopramide	Cisplatin, dose?	Methylprednisolone significantly "better"
			21	Droperidol		

DB, double-blind; *O*, open; *N*, nausea; *V*, vomiting.

Table 2. Corticosteroids combined to other antiemetics (controlled studies)

Type	Ref.	Author, journal	Patients	Agent(s)	Chemotherapy	Results
DB	23	Gathercole et al. Oncol Nurs F, 1982	20	Prochlorperazine 25 mg p.o.	Several, no cisplatin	30% "good score"
				crossover		
				Prochlorperazine + dexamethasone 10 mg i.v.		70% "good score"
				Prochlorperazine + dexamethasone 10 mg i.v.		70% "good score"
SB	24	Bruera et al. Cancer Treat Rep, 1983	26	Metoclopramide 40 mg i.v. −0.5 h, 20 mg i.v. +6, +12, +18 h	Refractory to prior metoclopramide	Median 18 episodes
				crossover		
				Metoclopramide + dexamethasone 24 mg i.v. 0, +3, +6 h		Median 5 episodes
DB	25	Colbert et al. J Clin Oncol, 1983	19	ACTH i.m. −24, −12, 0 h + chlorpromazine 50 mg i.m. −0.5 h	Cisplatin 80-100 mg/m² + others	42% no V
			18	Chlorpromazine + placebo		6% no V
DB	26	Allan et al. Br Med J, 1984	45	Metoclopramide 5 mg/kg i.v. −0.5 h	Cisplatin 30-100 mg/m²	26% no N/V
				crossover		
				Metoclopramide + dexamethasone 20 mg i.v.		43% no N/V
O	27	Donovitz et al. Gynecol Oncol, 1984	19	Droperidol 1 mg i.v. 0, +1, +2, +3, +4, +5, +6 h	Cisplatin 50 mg/m² + others	12% no V 5.9 h nausea
				Metoclopramide 1 mg/kg −0.5, +2.5, +5.5, +8.5, +11.5 h		
				crossover		
				Droperidol as above and methylprednisolone 500 mg i.v. −2, +4, +10, +16 h		21% no V 2.4 h nausea
O	28	Panza et al. Cancer Treat Rep, 1984	40	Methylprednisolone 125 mg i.m. 0 h, 40 mg i.m. +4 h	Cisplatin 80 mg/m²	7% 0-1 episode
			40	Chlorpromazine 6.5 mg i.m. q 4 h × 4		19% 0-1 episode
			40	Methylprednisolone + chlorpromazine		34% 0-1 episode
DB	29	Benrubi et al. Gynecol Oncol, 1985	9	Methylprednisolone 250 mg i.v.	Cisplatin, dose? + others	4% no V
			11	Metoclopramide 1.5 mg/kg −1, +1, +3 h		30% no V
			9	Both		68% no V

Table 2 *(continued)*

Type	Ref.	Author, journal	Patients	Agent(s)	Chemotherapy	Results
DB	30	Ell et al. Oncology, 1985	11	Metoclopramide 1 mg/kg −1, +1, +3, +5, +7 h	Cisplatin 60 mg/m^2	70% no V
				crossover		
				Metoclopramide + methylprednisolone 250 mg i.v. 0, +2, +4, +6 h		90% no V
			18	Same design metoclopramide	Cisplatin 120 mg/m^2	27% 0–1 episode
				crossover		
				Metoclopramide + methylprednisolone		82% 0–1 episode
SB	31	Strum et al. J Clin Oncol, 1985	16	Metoclopramide 2.0 mg/kg i.v. −0.5, +2, +4 h	Cisplatin 50–100 mg/m^2 + others	50% no V
			14	Metoclopramide + dexamethasone 20 mg i.v., same schedule		Patients prefer metoclopramide + dexamethasone 50% no V
SB	32	Becouarn et al. Eur J Cancer, 1986	24	Metoclopramide 1 mg/kg +0.5, +2, +4 h	Cisplatin 75–100 mg/m^2	13% no V
			23	Metoclopramide + methylprednisolone 1 mg/kg, same schedule		50% no V
O	33	Fujii et al. Gan To Kagaku Ryoho, 1986	12	Metoclopramide + droperidol	Cisplatin 120 mg/m^2 (?)	13% no V
			12	Same + methylprednisolone		44% no V
DB	34	Rhinehart et al. Prog Clin Biol Res, 1986	14	Metoclopramide 2 mg/kg Diphenhydramine 0.4 mg/kg −0.5, +1.5, +3.5, +5.5, +8.5 h	Plat 60–100 mg/m^2	
				crossover		Dexamethasone improves results ($P<0.01$)
				Same + dexamethasone 0.06 mg/kg, same schedule		
O	35	Senn et al. Dtsch Med Wochenschr, 1986	25	Metoclopramide 50 mg orally −2, +2, +6 h	Cisplatin	32% no N/V
			33	Metoclopramide + prednisone 25 mg orally, same schedule		39% no N/V

DB, double-blind; *SB*, single-blind; *O*, open; *N*, nausea; *V*, vomiting.

difficult evaluation of antiemetic results [7, 8] has led us to show in Table 1 only the percentages (when available) of patients with *no* nausea or vomiting. Total protection is probably the real goal [9]. As can be seen, of 13 studies (10-22), six [10, 11, 12, 16, 20, 22] have found corticosteroids to be of significant benefit to the patients. All these positive studies included patients whose chemotherapy contained no or low-dose (less than 50 mg/m^2) cisplatin. It is remarkable that even patients who seemed not to benefit from the antiemetic effect of corticosteroids preferred the double-blind crossover study arm that contained these agents [13, 14, 30].

Corticosteroids Added to Other Antiemetic Agents

Some data from 13 reports [23-35] on the effectiveness of corticosteroids in combination with other antiemetic agents are shown in Table 2. Overall, 11 are positive, leading us to conclude that corticosteroid-based antiemetic combinations provide significantly better control of chemotherapy-induced nausea and vomiting than do non-steroid-based combinations.

Corticosteroids as Antiemetics in Children

Two pilot studies [36, 37] have shown that it is possible to use corticosteroids to control emesis in pediatric oncology (Table 3).

Corticosteroids as Antiemetics in Radiation Therapy

A Medline search has failed to provide any data related to this topic.

Table 3. Corticosteroids as antiemetics in children

Type	Ref.	Author, journal	Patients	Agent(s)	Chemotherapy	Results
O	36	Ise et al. Gan To Kagaku Ryoho, 1982	18	Methylprednisolone 125 mg i.v. q 6 h × 4	Various	89% "effective"
			23	Domperidone 0.4 mg/kg i.v. × 1		52% "effective"
			21	Metoclopramide 10 mg i.v. post chemo		17% "effective"
O	37	Mehta et al. J Pediatr, 1986	10	Methylprednisolone 4 mg/kg pre chemo	No Cisplatin	4/10 no N/V safety study
			10	Chlorpromazine 0.5 mg/kg	All had had severe N/V	3/10 no N/V

O, open; *N*, nausea; *V*, vomiting.

Limitations to the Use of Corticosteroids as Antiemetics

Obviously, even when used for a very short period, corticosteroids can decompensate a diabetes or induce a psychosis. It may also be that they can reactivate a duodenal or gastric ulcer, although this is debatable. Use of active antiulcer agents should allow the use of corticosteroids in patients who need them. Long-term use of corticosteroids has been shown to have many other side-effects which should not be limiting factors in the antiemetic setting. It is probable that there is no significant hypothalamic-pituitary adrenal suppression, even after a 4-week course of treatment with methylprednisolone [38].

Some people have expressed concern over the possible immunosuppressive effects of corticosteroids [39, 40]. Most antitumor chemotherapies are immunosuppressive. Furthermore, there are some data showing that the addition of corticosteroids does not modify the antitumor effectiveness of cisplatin. Our results are actually in favor of an additive antitumor effect, which is not significant, either in a mouse model or in vitro [41].

Side-effects of Corticosteroids as Antiemetics

There has been one report of hyperglycemia [5]. Other side-effects have included insomnia, euphoria, and anxiety; these are no more frequent than with prochlorperazine, which induces significantly more somnolence [16]. Facial flush has been reported by several authors. At least three papers have mentioned pharyngeal or perineal itch [11, 13, 23], which has recently been emphasized and may be vehicle or formulation related [42–44].

Mechanism of Action

There is no explanation for the effectiveness of corticosteroids in the control of chemotherapy-induced emesis. It has been suggested that they might act on the prostaglandin pathway [3], but there is no increase of plasma prostaglandins in patients submitted to cisplatin [45]. It is also possible that corticosteroids act on the chemoreceptor trigger zone, either modifying capillary permeability or stabilizing some membrane or intracellular components (lysosomes)?

What is at least clear is that many authors report that steroid treatment confers a general sense of well-being. It is possible that the effect of steroids is more psychological in nature, as it has been shown that many techniques affecting the patients' psyche can modify their tolerance to the emetic action of chemotherapy [6].

Dose Schedule of Corticosteroids as Antiemetics

As can be observed from Tables 1–3, there is considerable variation in the dose schedules used in different studies. When corticosteroids are used as single agents, one author has seen a possibly better response with high doses [46].

We had thought that steroids should be started several hours before chemotherapy [47]. Also, we used to taper off doses of steroids over 2 days, as some patients complained of myalgias or recurrent vomiting after abrupt discontinuation [5]. In fact these procedures are necessary only for a minority of patients.

Conclusion

There are considerable data indicating that corticosteroids can decrease the severity of chemotherapy-related emesis. Used on a very short-term basis they should have no major side-effects, if one is careful with patients suffering from diabetes, gastrointestinal ulcers, or prior psychotic reactions. Corticosteroids are best used at low doses to enhance the antiemetic efficacy of other drugs [48]. The effective low dose of corticosteroids remains to be determined.

References

1. Winokur SM, Baker JJ et al. (1981) Dexamethasone in the treatment of nausea and vomiting from cancer chemotherapy. J Med Assoc Ga 70: 263-264
2. Baker JJ, Lockey JL et al. (1979) Nabilone as an antiemetic. N Engl J Med 301: 728
3. Rich NM, Abdulhayoglu G, Disaia PJ (1980) Methylprednisolone as an antiemetic during cancer chemotherapy - a pilot study. Gynecol Oncol 9: 193-198
4. Lee BJ (1981) Methylprednisolone as an antiemetic (letter). N Engl J Med 304: 486
5. Aapro MS, Alberts DS (1981) High-dose dethamexasone for prevention of cisplatin-induced vomiting. Cancer Chemother Pharmacol 7: 11-14
6. Morrow GR, Morrel C (1982) Behavioral treatment for the anticipatory nausea and vomiting induced by cancer chemotherapy. N Engl J Med 307: 1476-1480
7. Pater LJ, Willan AR (1984) Methodologic issues of antiemetics. J Clin Oncol 2: 484-487
8. Olver IN, Simon RM, Aisner J (1986) Antiemetic studies: a methodological discussion. Cancer Treat Rep 70: 555-563
9. Bennett JM, Byrne P et al. (1985) A randomized multicenter trial of cyclophosphamide, novantrone and 5-fluorouracil (CNF) versus cyclophosphamide, adriamycin and 5-fluorouracil (CAF) in patients with metastatic breast cancer. Inv New Drugs 3: 179-185
10. Breau JL, Israel L et al. (1983) Efficacité de la méthylprednisolone dans la prévention des vomissements dus aux chimiothérapies par sels de platine dans un essai randomisé. Presse Med 12: 2058
11. Cassileth PA, Lusk EJ et al (1983) Antiemetic efficacy of dexamethasone therapy in patients receiving cancer chemotherapy. Arch Int Med 43: 1347:1349
12. Kolaric K, Roth A (1983) Methylprednisolone as an antiemetic in patients on cis-platinium chemotherapy. Results of a controlled randomized study. Tumori 69: 43-46
13. Aapro MS, Plezia PM et al. (1984) Double-blind crossover study of the antiemetic efficacy of high-dose dexamethasone versus high-dose metoclopramide. J Clin oncol 2: 466-471
14. Cognetti F, Pinnaro P et al. (1984) Randomized open cross-over trial between metoclopramide (MCP) and dexamethasone (DXM) for the prevention of cisplatin-induced nausea and vomiting. Eur J Cancer Clin Oncol 20: 183-187
15. Giaccone G, Donadio M et al. (1984) Comparison of the antiemetic effect of high-dose intravenous metoclopramide in the prophylactic treatment of cis-platin-induced nausea and vomiting. Tumori 70: 237-241

16. Markman M, Sheider V et al. (1984) Antiemetic efficacy of dexamethasone. Randomized, double-blind, crossover study with prochlorperazine in patients receiving cancer chemotherapy. N Engl J Med 311: 549-552
17. Dana BW, Everts EC, Dickison D (1985) Dexamethasone vs. placebo for cisplatin-induced emesis. A randomized cross-over trial. Am J Clin Oncol 8: 426-428
18. D'Olimpio JT, Camacho F et al. (1985) Antiemetic efficacy of high-dose dexamethasone versus placebo in patients receiving cisplatin-based chemotherapy: a randomized double-blind controlled clinical trial. J Clin Oncol 3: 1133-1136
19. Frustaci S, Grattoni E et al. (1986) Randomized crossover antiemetic study in cisplatin-treated patients. Comparison between high-dose i.v. metoclopramide and high-dose i.v. dexamethasone. Cancer Chemother Pharmacol 17: 75-79
20. Ibrahim EM, Al-Idrissi H-Y et al. (1986) Antiemetic efficacy of high-dose dexamethasone: randomized, double-blind, crossover study with high-dose metoclopramide in patients receiving cancer chemotherapy. Eur J Cancer Clin Oncol 39: 619-24
21. Shinkai T, Saijo N et al. (1986) Antiemetic efficacy of high-dose intravenous metoclopramide and dexamethasone in patients receiving cisplatin-based chemotherapy: a randomized controlled trial. Jpn J Clin Oncol 16: 279-287
22. Niijima T, Isurugi K et al. (1986) Randomized cross-over study on the effects of methyprednisolone, metoclopramide and droperidol on the control of nausea and vomiting associated with cis-platinum chemotherapy. Gan To Kagaku Ryoho 13: 2376-2382
23. Gathercole F, Connolly N, Birdsell J (1982) The use of dexamethasone (Hexadrol) as an antiemetic in association with chemotherapy for neoplastic disease. Oncol Nurs Forum 9: 17-19
24. Bruera E, Roca E et al. (1986) Improved control of chemotherapy induced emesis by the addition of dexamethasone to metoclopramide in patients resistant to metoclopramide. Cancer Treat Rep 67: 381-383
25. Colbert N, Izrael V et al. (1983) Adrenocorticotropic hormone in the prevention of cisplatin-induced nausea and vomiting. J Clin Oncol 1: 635-639
26. Allan SG, Cornbleet MA et al. (1984) Dexamethasone and high-dose metoclopramide efficacy in controlling cisplatin-induced nausea and vomiting. Br Med J 289: 878-879
27. Donovitz GS, O'Quinn AG et al. (1984) Antiemetic efficacy of high-dose corticosteroids and droperidol and metoclopramide. Gynecol Oncol 18: 320-325
28. Panza N, de Cesare M et al. (1984) Methylprednisolone and chlorpromazine alone or in combination for the control of cisplatin-induced emesis. Cancer Treat Rep 68: 1310-1311
29. Benrubi GI, Norvell M et al. (1985) The use of methylprednisolone and metoclopramide in control of emesis in patients receiving cis-platinum. Gynecol Oncol 21: 306-313
30. Ell C, Konig HJ et al. (1985) Antiemetic efficacy of moderately high-dose metoclopramide in patients receiving varying doses of cisplatin. Controlled comparison with a combination of methylprednisolone and metoclopramide. Oncology 42: 354-357
31. Strum SB, McDermed JE et al. (1985) High-dose intravenous metoclopramide versus combination high-dose metoclopramide and intravenous dexamethasone in preventing cisplatin-induced nausea and emesis: a single-blind crossover comparison of antiemetic efficacy. J Clin Oncol 3: 245-251
32. Becouarn Y, Nguyen B et al. (1986) Improved control of cisplatin-induced emesis with a combination of high doses of methylprednisolone and metoclopramide: a single-blind randomized trial. Eur J Cancer Oncol 22: 1421-1424
33. Fujii M, Kiura K et al. (1986) Randomized crossover trial of the antiemetic effects obtained with metoclopramide and droperidol versus those obtained with metoclopramide, droperidol and methylprednisolone in patients receiving cis-platinum chemotherapy. Gan To Kagaku Ryoho 13: 2562-2567
34. Rhinehart SN, Dugan WM et al. (1986) The value of dexamethasone when added to combination drug therapy in the prevention of cisplatin-induced nausea and vomiting, evaluated by time-lapse video technology. Prog Clin Biol Res 216: 407-416

35. Senn HJ, Kohler M et al. (1986) Prevention of nausea and emesis during cytostatic therapy. Antiemetic efficacy of high-dosage oral metoclopramide without and with prednisone. Dtsch Med Wochenschr 11: 129-135
36. Ise T, Ohira A et al. (1982) Clinical evaluation of antiemetics for vomiting due to cancer chemotherapy in children. Gan To Kagaku Ryoho 9: 1108-1118
37. Mehta P, Gross S et al. (1986) Methylprednisolone for chemotherapy-induced emesis: a double-blind randomized trial in children. J Pediatr 108: 774-776
38. Levitt M, Sharma RN et al. (1979) Normal metyrapone response after 1 month of high-dose methylprednisolone in cancer patients: a phase I study. Cancer Treat Rep 63: 1327-1330
39. Haid M (1981) Steroid antiemesis may be harmful. N Engl J Med 304: 1237
40. Grundwald HW, Rosner F (1984) Dexamethasone as an antiemetic during cancer chemotherapy. Ann Intern Med 101: 398
41. Aapro MS, Alberts DS, Serokan R (1983) Lack of dexamethasone effect on the antitumor activity of cisplatin. Cancer treat Treat Rep 67: 1013-1017
42. Baharav E, Harpaz D et al. (1986) Dexamethasone-induced perineal irritation. N Engl J Med 314: 515
43. Allan SG, Leonard RCF (1986) Dexamethasone antiemesis and side-effects. Lancet 1: 1035
44. Thomas VL (1986) More on dexamethasone-induced perineal irritation. N Engl J Med 314: 1643
45. Stephen LC, Rine J et al. (1981) The role of prostaglandins in the excessive nausea and vomiting after intravascular cis-platinum therapy. Gynecol Oncol 12: 89-91
46. Drapkin RL, Sokl GH et al. (1982) The antiemetic effect and dose response of dexamethasone in patients receiving cis-platinum (Abstr). Proc Am Soc Clin Oncol 1: 64
47. Kessler JF, Alberts DS et al. (1986) An effective five-drug antiemetic combination for prevention of chemotherapy-related nausea and vomiting. Experience in eighty-four patients. Cancer Chemother Pharmacol 282-286
48. Mark GK, Richard JG et al. (1985) Improved control of cisplatin-induced emesis with high-dose metoclopramide and with combinations of metoclopramide, dexamethasone, and diphenhydramine. Results of consecutive trials in 255 patients. Cancer 55: 527-534

Hypnotherapy as Antiemetic Treatment in Cancer Chemotherapy

A. A. Fortuin

The Netherlands Cancer Institute, 1083 HD Amsterdam, The Netherlands

In this paper some general information about hypnosis will be given and a few case histories will be presented to illustrate how hypnosis can be used in cancer patients complaining of nausea and vomiting. Finally a short description will be given of a research program in the Netherlands Cancer Institute where we are comparing the effects of hypnosis and progressive muscle relaxation in reducing nausea and vomiting caused by cytostatic drugs.

What Is Hypnosis?

Hypnosis has been given various definitions. Since no one has discovered exactly how it works, we can only describe the effects. Hypnotic subjects seem much more open to suggestions from the hypnotist than they would be in a waking state. Hypnotic subjects appear extremely attentive to what the hypnotist is saying and become less aware of other stimulation, such as noises in an adjacent room. They have a heightened ability to fantasize and an increased openness to focusing and distraction techniques (e.g., guided imagery).

It is imperative to remove all of the most common misconceptions about hypnosis before attempting an induction procedure. The most prevalent of these is that the subject is asleep or in an unconscious state. This is not true. A person in trance will be more alert than when in a normal waking state! Another misconception concerns the so-called surrender of the will, or the belief that weak-minded persons make the best hypnotic subjects.

Not everyone can be hypnotized equally well. About 15% of the population can be hypnotized very well, 70% score an average talent for hypnosis, whereas 15% are difficult to hypnotize. With cancer patients an average level of talent is sufficient to use hypnosis to some extent. This means that 85% of these patients may benefit from hypnosis.

Recent Results in Cancer Research, Vol. 108

Hypnotherapy for Treatment of Nausea and Vomiting Caused by Cytostatic Drugs

Nausea and vomiting are frequent and unpleasant side-effects of cancer chemotherapy. These side-effects are sometimes of such a serious nature that the patient prefers to stop the chemotherapy. Post-treatment nausea and vomiting are caused by irritation of the vomiting center by the cytostatic agent. It is a curious fact, however, that about 45% of the patients treated with chemotherapy also complain of anticipatory nausea and/or vomiting before treatment starts again. The development of *anticipatory* nausea and emesis is gradual, usually first appearing some time after the third or fourth course of treatment and escalating in severity during subsequent courses [1, 2].

The occurrence of anticipatory nausea and vomiting can be conceptualized as a classically condition response. The patient experiences an involuntary adverse reaction, i.e., severe nausea (the unconditioned response) in response to chemical agents (the unconditioned stimulus), which becomes associated with aspects of the environment (conditioned stimuli) surrounding the administration of chemotherapy. Eventually these conditioned environmental stimuli come to produce the nausea (conditioned response) [3]. Thus, through repeated association with chemotherapy and its aversive after-effects, previously neutral stimuli (e.g., the sights, sounds, and smells of the treatment environment) can produce anticipatory nausea/emesis.

Anxious and depressive patients tend to suffer sooner from anticipatory nausea and vomiting than nonanxious and nondepressive patients. Patients who reported either unsuccessful attempts to cope with side-effects or no attempts at all had greater distress than those who were successful. There is also a connection between feelings of fear just before and sensations of taste during the injection, and anticipatory nausea and vomiting [4].

As stated before, "conditioning" plays an important role in anticipatory nausea and vomiting. It can therefore be expected that hypnosis or relaxation techniques may be particularly successful in controlling anticipatory nausea and vomiting.

How Is Hypnosis Introduced to a Cancer Patient?

During the first consultation the patient is informed about hypnosis and misconceptions about the technique are discussed. He is told that hypnosis is not a treatment against cancer and that possible spread of the disease will not be masked by the use of hypnosis. It is made clear to the patient that hypnosis can be a means of influencing his well-being; that it gives him the possibility of more self-control within the given situation. In order to gain an impression of the way the patient is experiencing his disease, he is asked to tell something about himself, his private situation, his occupation, and his medical history. We also talk at great length about his special interests, hobbies, and pleasant events. It is our experience that by introducing hypnosis in this way the initial barriers to its acceptance by the patient can be minimized.

A test trance induction is followed by a description of a pleasant scene about which the patient has spoken. After deduction (ending of trance), the patient is asked if other components should be added or subtracted from the scene. Another trance induction with the adapted version of the pleasant scene takes place, this time recorded on cassette. He is given suggestions for well-being and ego strengthening. It is also suggested that it will become increasingly easier to reach deep relaxation with the help of hypnosis if he practices regularly. Every patient gets a cue for self-hypnosis, for instance taking a deep breath in the case of nausea. For a small number of patients nausea itself can be a cue for self-hypnosis! As a posthypnotic suggestion the patient is told that the vomiting can be very serious at certain times, but these will be followed by a period of growing rest and relaxation in which he will be able to get sufficient energy for his recovery.

Clinical patients often undergo aggressive chemotherapy. Hypnosis during the infusion period may have a surprising effect on the patient's sense of well-being. This can be illustrated by means of two case histories: one in which age *re*gression was employed and another where age *pro*gression worked best.

1. Age Regression

A 20-year-old man with osteosarcoma was referred because of strong vomiting responses to chemotherapy. During the introductory phase he spoke about his holidays at his grandparents' farm when he was about 9 years old. He was allowed to milk the cows, made cheese himself, and looked after the rabbits. Again and again he enjoyed the beautiful surroundings.

After the trance induction the surroundings of the farm were described - the pure air and the clear brook in which he played. In order to increase the value of reality and to obtain an age regression the past tense is changed into the present at a certain moment: "... you really feel like playing with the rabbits, just go to the hutches and get one out. You are walking to your own place on the brook and you're lying down with the bunny on your belly. It is so nice and quiet, it feels so good to have this little warm rabbit on your belly, which you can stroke gently ..." The response was striking: the vomiting stopped, he became very relaxed, and ultimately fell asleep. The words nausea and vomiting were avoided, and in this indirect way unpleasant sensations in his stomach area were replaced by a relaxed warm feeling. Although the patient's hypnotic talents were important indeed, his motivation played a very significant role. The situation had become so threatening that he seized any opportunity for increasing his well-being.

2. Age Progression

A young mother with advanced melanoma was very nauseated before receiving the chemotherapy and vomited severely during the injection of DTIC.

She had a 2-year-old son. In order to induce an age progression, while she was in trance it was suggested to her that she was taking her son to primary school for the first time; in other words, it was suggested to her that her son was a 6-year-old boy rather than a toddler. Under hypnosis she reported what the child was wearing, what the tram ride to school was like, what the new teacher looked like, and what her son's reactions were to the new surroundings.

The fact that she was totally absorbed was evident when she answered the question: "How many sandwiches did you make him?" "Four!"

During the administration of the chemotherapy she ceased to vomit. When she used self-hypnosis on the way to the hospital the nausea she previously felt disappeared as well.

The use of age progression has the important advantage that it implies "survival," which makes it possible to influence the expectations for the future.

Hypnotherapy and Progressive Muscle Relaxation for Treatment of Nausea and Vomiting Caused by Cytostatic Drugs: A Comparative Study

Several studies have reported the use of hypnosis and progressive muscle relaxation (PMR) for control of anticipatory and post-treatment nausea and vomiting in cancer patients receiving chemotherapy. Most of these studies have involved case histories or descriptions of small groups of patients. Frequently, data regarding the specific cancer type or the chemotherapeutic drugs have not been reported. In those studies in which groups of patients were compared, the composition of the groups was heterogeneous. Patients had different types of cancer, were in different stages of illness, and were treated with different chemotherapeutics.

In 1986, a comparative study was begun in the Netherlands Cancer Institute to examine the effectiveness of hypnosis and PMR in controlling treatment-related nausea and vomiting. To be able to interpret the study results more clearly, it was considered necessary to employ a relatively homogeneous patient group. Patients with *breast cancer* treated with chemotherapy at the outpatient medical oncology clinic are being studied. The following eligibility criteria are used as the basis for recruitment into the study:

1. Treatment with cytostatics (adjuvant therapy Cytoxan, methotrexate, 5-fluorouracil, or Cytoxan, adriamycin, and 5-fluorouracil in combination)
2. Patients must indicate nausea and/or vomiting due to administration of chemotherapy
3. Patients must have two or more chemotherapy sessions planned

In order to obtain consent, patients are informed, in general terms, of the purpose and the procedures of the study. They are randomly assigned to one of three treatment arms:

1. Standard pharmacological treatment with antiemetic drugs
2. PMR therapy
3. Hypnotherapy

The principal aim of the study is to investigate the effect of hypnosis and PMR on nausea and vomiting caused by cytostatic drugs. If necessary all patients can receive antiemetics according to a standard antiemetic protocol (chlorpromazine 25 mg one to three times a day).

After randomization, a short baseline questionnaire is administered. In this questionnaire we ask patients to report their feelings of nausea and vomiting before, during, and after the chemotherapy session. We inquire into their quality of life during the rest period, the situation in the therapy room, and so on.

An appointment is made for those assigned to one of the experimental conditions with either the PMR therapist or the hypnotherapist. No further contact is made with those in the control group until the next chemotherapy session. All patients are contacted by phone by a trained interviewer, who collects follow-up questionnaire data. Patients are followed for a maximum of six therapy sessions. At the end a final evaluation takes place.

While it is too early to provide results from the study, our first impressions suggest that neither PMR nor hypnotherapy has a dramatic effect on nausea and vomiting per se. However, both techniques seem to have a significant impact on the way in which patients are affected by these side-effects. They appear to be more relaxed during chemotherapy sessions and to have fewer problems in general with relaxing and sleeping.

References

1. van Dam FSAM, Kanis JW, ten Bokkel Huinink WW, Hanewald GJFP (1986) Misselijkheid en braken voorafgaand aan de toediening van cytostatica. *Ned Tijdschr Geneeskd* 130: 1479-1481
2. Andrykowski MA, Redd WH, Hatfield AK (1985) Development of anticipatory nausea: a prospective analysis. J Consult Clin Psychol 53: 447-454
3. Burish TG, Carey MP (1986) Conditioned averse responses in cancer chemotherapy patients: theoretical and developmental analysis. J Consult Clin Psychol 54: 593-600
4. Nerenz D, Leventhal H, Easterling DV, Love PR (1986) Anxiety and drug taste as predictors of anticipatory nausea in chemotherapy. J Clin Oncol 4: 224-233

Fighting Alopecia in Cancer Chemotherapy

R. A. Joss, J. Kiser, S. Weston, and K. W. Brunner

Institut für Medizinische Onkologie, Inselspital, Universität Bern, 3010 Bern, Switzerland

Hairstyle is an integral part of our personal identity. Hair contributes greatly to our physical appearance and throughout the ages the luxuriously adorned scalp has been an object of admiration associated with virility, male strength, and female beauty. Alopecia - a well known and feared side-effect of cancer chemotherapy - threatens the integrity of a patient's self-image and can be psychologically devastating. Ocassionally, patients may reject a cytostatic treatment because of their inability to accept hair loss.

After a brief review of the physiology of the normal hair and the effects of chemotherapy on hair growth, we will discuss possibilities for supporting the patient with hair loss and measures to prevent alopecia.

Physiology of Normal Hair Growth

In animals hair is an important means of protection from cold, heat, and mechanical damage and serves as a means of social communication and camouflage. In men hair has lost most of these vital functions, but it is still of prominent social and psychological significance.

There are approximately 100000 hairs on the scalp [21]. Each hair consists of the hair bulb, containing the germinative cells, the hair root, and the hair shaft or hair fiber. The proliferation of the germinative cells in the hair bulb pushes the hair from the root up through the scalp surface. The final product is a strand of tightly compacted keratin, consisting of an outer layer, the cuticula, a middle layer, the cortex, and an inner layer, the medulla. The cortex contains the melanin granula.

Hair grows in a tricyclic manner. During anagen the mitotic activity of the germinative cells of the hair bulb produces an average daily growth of 0.35 mm. This period lasts from 2 to 6 years. About 85% of the follicles are actively growing whereas the remaining 15% are in the phase of involution (catagen) or dormancy (telogen). During catagen, the hair root is separated from the hair bulb, the pigment storage is terminated, and the club-shaped root end is pushed out from the bulb. About 1% of human scalp hair is in the catagen phase, lasting a few weeks.

Recent Results in Cancer Research, Vol. 108

During telogen, lasting for about 3-6 months, the mitotic activity is arrested. Hair growth is dependent on several factors such as age, sex, race, hormones, nutrition, and temperature, as well as the topographical location of the hair.

Clinical Aspects of Chemotherapy-Induced Alopecia

One of the most obvious sites of toxicity of cytostatic agents is the integument. Hair, nails, skin, and the mucous membranes are all affected and this toxicity may be of great psychological concern to the patient. Although these side-effects are generally considered more cosmetic than hazardous, at least mucous membrane ulceration and local tissue necrosis can lead to life-threatening medical complications.

Different cytostatic agents listed in Table 1 cause alopecia. The potential for epilation differs markedly among the listed agents. The effect depends not only on the drug itself but also markedly on the route of administration, the dosage, and the schedule used. High-dose, intermittent intravenous therapy is commonly associated with sudden and almost complete hair loss. Drugs given orally daily or on a weekly intravenous schedule at lower doses cause sinificantly less hair loss, even though the total dose may be large. There are also marked differences in the potential for alopecia between drugs belonging to the same generic class. For example, intermittent cyclophosphamide causes marked alopecia in almost all patients whereas intermittent thiotepa or chlorambucil causes little hair loss at comparable therapeutic or myelosuppressive dosages. Alopecia is often exacerbated by the concurrent administration of multiple agents that cause epilation. Furthermore, the degree of hair loss is dependent on different poorly defined individual patient characteristics such as sex, age, and performance status.

Usually the hair starts to fall out approximately 2-4 weeks after the initial dose of chemotherapy. To be noticeable approximately 50% of the hair must be shed. Regrowth of hair may occur despite continued treatment, with new scalp hair appearing in about 3-6 months, the normal duration of the telogen. Sometimes the new hair is different in color and/or texture from the original hair [10].

The psychological impact of chemotherapy-induced alopecia is not well understood. Since hair contributes greatly to physical attractiveness and to body image, alopecia might be expected to be distressing to patients, resulting in decreased social interaction. Wagner and Bye have administered a body image/social activity questionnaire to 77 cancer patients receiving chemotherapy [29]. Subjects with

Table 1. Potential for epilation of cytotoxic agents

High:	adriamycin, daunorubicin, cyclophosphamide, ifosfamide, etoposide, teniposide
Moderate:	methotrexate, nitrogen mustard, fluorouracil, vinblastine, vincristine, vindesine, epiadriamycin, mitoxantrone, mithramycin, mitomycin, actinomycin, hydroxyurea, procarbazine
Low:	BCNU, CCNU, streptozocin, busulfan, chlorambucil, melphalan, thiotepa, DTIC, cisplatin, mercaptopurine, thioguanine, cytosine arabinoside, bleomycin, L-asparaginase, hexamethylmelamine

alopecia were expected to have significantly lower scores than those without alopecia. However, there were no significant differences in mean body image scores or mean social activity scores. The authors reasoned that the negative effect of hair loss was minimized by adaptation to change in body image, thus suggesting that appropriate nursing interventions can facilitate this adaptation.

Physical and Psychological Care of the Patient Experiencing Chemotherapy-Induced Alopecia

According to the findings of Wagner and Bye outlined above, nurses and physicians must try to help the patient prepare for the sudden loss of their hair, thus minimizing the negative impact on the patient's self-image. Patients must be reassured that alopecia is not a sign of advancing disease but a temporary side-effect of treatment. When they are informed appropriately, most patients will accept alopecia in exchange for a reasonable change of tumor regression following treatment.

The practical information should include advice on:

- The probable onset, presentation, duration, severity, and reversibility of hair loss, the expected time of regrowth, and the possibility that the new hair may be of a different color and/or texture
- Special hair care with the use of soft brushes, mild shampoos, and avoidance of permanents, dyes, heated curlers, and hairdryers.
- Protection of the alopecic scalp from cold, heat, mechanical irritation, and exposure to the sun, including use of sunglasses and hats to protect the eyes if eyelashes and eyebrows are lost.
- Where and when to get a wig. The hair piece should be selected while the patient still has his own hair in order to match the color, style, and hair texture. Photographs of other patients wearing a wig usually help new patients overcome prejudices and help to demonstrate that wigs of excellent quality, with almost an identical appearance to normal hair, are available. Information on financial assistance or third-party coverage for wigs should be provided. One should check from time to time that the wig fits properly so that the skin is not wounded or abraded since skin breaks are a source of infections in the immunocompromised host.
- Alternatives to wigs in order to mask alopecia, such as colorful scarves and turbans for women, and hats, knitted caps, or sport caps for men.

Finally, patients should be encouraged to speak about their feelings encountered with hair loss. Some find it helpful to talk to other patients, who, having also experienced hair loss, have already found their own personal way to handle the problem.

Possibilities for Preventing Chemotherapy-Induced Hair Loss

There are at least three possible ways of preventing chemotherapy-induced hair loss:

- By temporary reduction of the blood flow to the scalp
- By drugs
- By pharmacological interventions

These possibilities will be discussed in further detail.

Prevention of Hair Loss by Temporary Reduction of the Blood Flow to the Scalp

As early as 1966 anecdotal reports described attempts to prevent cancer chemotherapy-induced hair loss by temporary reduction of blood flow to the scalp, thereby minimizing drug contact with hair follicles [27]. Since then tourniquets and hypothermia have been the two basic methods used to temporarily decrease blood supply to the scalp. These techniques are based on the assumption that a short reduction in the arterial blood supply to the scalp hair follicles during the time of the administration of the cytostatic drugs will protect the hair bulb from exposure to the antiproliferative agents. The utility of these techniques must be questioned when peak blood levels are not achieved rapidly (slow distribution, activation) or when active drug or metabolites remain in the circulation for prolonged periods (long half-life, extensive plasma binding, continuous infusion). Adriamycin and vincristine both have a short initial half-life of less than 30 min [8]. Patients treated with these drugs should therefore profit most from techniques protecting hair follicles from drug exposure. On the other hand, cyclophosphamide requires hepatic activation and has a plasma half-life of over 6 h; therefore a 30- to 60-min period of decreased blood flow to the scalp would not be expected to protect against hair loss [8].

Most of the more recent studies have focused on the prevention of adriamycin-induced alopecia by scalp hypothermia. An early study by Luce and co-workers achieved good protection against doxorubicin-induced alopecia in 12 of 15 patients by means of regional direction of chilled air to the scalp [17]. A few years later Edelstyn and co-workers reported a large, randomized pilot study exploring the value of Cryogel bags [9]. In 1979 Dean and co-workers published their experience with the prevention of adriamycin-induced hair loss with scalp hypothermia [5]. All 33 patients included in this trial were beginning adriamycin-cyclophosphamide chemotherapy. All patients except one were female. After insulation of the ears from excessive exposure to cold, ice packs consisting of crushed ice in two plastic bags were applied to cover the entire scalp. The "ice turban" was applied 5 min before each doxorubicin injection and left in place until 30 min after the injection, for a total of 35–40 min of scalp hypothermia. The outcome was evaluated by both the patient and the examining nurse before the initiation of chemotherapy and after the completion of each cycle of treatment. In addition to clinical assessments, routine serial photographs of the scalp were obtained and a graded rating scale of protection against hair loss was used. Of the 33 patients, 60% experienced good protection against hair loss throughout all cycles of treatment and did not usually require wigs. The degree of protection was clearly related to the adriamycin dose administered; thus 19 of 20 patients treated at adriamycin doses ≤ 50 mg achieved good protection whereas less than half of the patients receiving ≥ 60 mg adriamycin had satisfactory results.

This landmark paper induced a rapidly growing number of other nonrandomized and randomized trials, listed in Table 2. Comparisons between these different trials or between the experimental and a usual historical control group are difficult due to several confounding variables: there are differences in the techniques used to achieve scalp hypothermia; drugs and dose schedules are not identical; the ad-

Table 2. Effectiveness of temporary reduction of blood flow to the scalp in preventing loss of hair, as reported by different studies

Technique	Type of study	Evaluable patients	Epilating agents	Success rate (%)	Authors
Tourniquet	Nonrandomized concurrent control	31	ADM, CTX, VCR, VM	67	Pesce et al. [23]
Tourniquet	Randomized	3	ADM + different	100	Lovejoy [16]
Tourniquet	Nonrandomized concurrent control	5	ACT, CTX, VCR, MTX	0	Maxwell [19]
Thermocirculator	Nonrandomized historical control	12	ADM, CTX, VCR, MTX	66	Guy et al. [12]
Hypothermia	Uncontrolled	28	ADM, VCR, VDS	78	Anderson et al. [1]
Hypothermia	Nonrandomized concurrent control	72	ADM, CTX, VCR, MTX, FU, DDP	72	Belpomme et al. [2]
Hypothermia	Nonrandomized historical control	33	ADM, CTX	61	Dean et al. [5]
Hypothermia	Randomized (crushed ice vs. Kold Kap)	35	ADM, CTX	57	Dean et al. [7]
Hypothermia	Randomized	40	ADM, VCR, FU, CLB, MTX	50	Edelstyn et al. [9]
Hypothermia	Nonrandomized historical control	24	ADM, VCR	42	Gregory et al. [11]
Hypothermia	Randomized	10	ADM, CTX	10	Kennedy et al. [13]
Hypothermia	Uncontrolled	281	ADM ± CTX ± different	61	Kiser et al. [14]
Hypothermia	Uncontrolled	60	ADM, CTX, VCR	0	Middleton et al. [20]
Hypothermia	Randomized	12	ADM + different	75	Satterwhite and Zimm [25]

ministered cumulative dose of a given drug varies considerably; other epilating agents are administered concurrently in a variety of doses and schedules; the methods of response assessment are not specified or vary between different trials; and small number of patients do not allow for valid statistical analysis.

A summary of the results achieved in these trials might be as follows:

- The effectiveness of scalp hypothermia in preventing adriamycin-induced hair loss has been proven in prospective, randomized controlled trials [25]
- When adriamycin is given as a single agent, 50%–70% of patients experience good to excellent protection
- The results are dependent upon the adriamycin dose schedule, with patients receiving single doses of adriamycin > 50 mg experiencing less protection [5, 14]
- Concurrent or subsequent application of other epilators such as cyclophosphamide compromise the effectiveness of scalp hypothermia
- The influence of impaired liver function on the success rate of scalp hypothermia is unclear even though it is conceivable that an impaired liver function alters the pharmacokinetics of adriamycin, thereby rendering scalp hypothermia less effective [1, 14]
- Males experience better protection than females [14]
- Patients with good performance status (WHO scale 0–1) experience better protection than patients with poor performance status (WHO scale 2–3) [14]
- Scalp hypothermia is generally well tolerated, with only about 2% of patients interrupting the procedure due to intolerance (headache, cold sensation, feeling of panic) [14]
- The incidence of scalp metastases among patients treated with scalp hypothermia has been of concern [6, 24]. Whereas one report suggested an incidence of 11% [20], most other studies have found an incidence of well below 1% [7, 14].

Based on these results one can define a group of patients in whom scalp hypothermia is indicated and offers a good chance of protection:

1. Patients undergoing an adriamycin containing chemotherapy with palliative intent or patients with solid tumors rarely metastasizing to the scalp
2. Patients not receiving other potent epilating agents (cyclophosphamide, etoposide, etc.) and not undergoing cranial irradiation
3. Patients with good performance status
4. Patients with normal hepatic function
5. Patients willing to spend the time necessary for scalp cooling.

Even though the indications for the prevention of hair loss by scalp hypothermia are fairly well defined and the methodology refined, at least two questions remain to be answered by well conducted, prospective randomized trials: What scalp temperature has to be achieved to obtain maximum protection? And what duration of scalp hypothermia will achieve maximum protection?

Prevention of Hair Loss by Drugs

Attempts to prevent chemotherapy-induced hair loss by drugs have been rare in the past. In 1985 Wood reported on the possible protective effect of α-tocopherol given in high doses to patients receiving adriamycin [31]. Of 16 patients (69%) receiving adriamycin plus 1600 IU alpha-tocopherol per day, 11 did not have alopecia. There was a correlation between the time that tocopherol was taken before the first dose of doxorubicin and subsequent hair loss, with a suggestion that the vitamin should be taken at least 72 h before the first dose of doxorubicin.

This uncontrolled trial has prompted at least two confirmatory studies. Martin-Jimenez et al. tested the hair loss preventing potential of α-tocopherol in a prospective nonrandomized trial in breast cancer patients receiving adjuvant chemotherapy with FAC (fluorouracil 500 mg/m^2 body surface area, adriamycin 50 mg/m^2, and cyclophosphamide 500 mg/m^2 given on the first day of every 3-week cycle for six courses) [18]. Thirteen patients received 1600 IU α-tocopherol orally each day starting 7 days before the beginning of adjuvant chemotherapy, whereas 12 patients served as controls. α-Tocopherol did not change the natural course of alopecia induced by chemotherapy with FAC, with 92% of the patients in the control group and 100% of the patients in the treatment group experiencing grade 3 alopecia after six courses of chemotherapy. In order to evaluate the contribution of the other drugs included in the combination (fluorouracil and cyclophosphamide), the authors analyzed simultaneously 28 operated breast cancer patients treated with intravenous cyclophosphamide (600 mg/m^2), methotrexate (60 mg/m^2), and fluorouracil (600 mg/m^2) on the first day of every 3-week cycle for six courses. None of these 28 patients had grade 3 alopecia after six courses of chemotherapy. The authors concluded that the efficacy of high-dose oral α-tocopherol in preventing alopecia induced by adriamycin seemed to be nonexistent. Another negative trial of α-tocopherol has been reported by Perez and co-workers [22].

Recently the topical application of minoxidil, an antihypertensive agent inducing hypertrichosis, has received extensive clinical evaluation for male pattern baldness and alopecia areata [28, 30]. A cosmetically acceptable response can be induced in about half of the patients [28, 30]. Minoxidil is a potent vasodilator with a direct action on arterial smooth muscle [3]. The mechanism for regrowth of hair with minoxidil is unknown. It has been postulated that locally increased cutaneous blood flow may account for the increase in hair growth (due to the potent small vessel vasodilating effect of the drug). Experimental findings suggest that minoxidil may prolong the anagen phase of hair growth and lengthen the time the cells can divide [4]. If, in fact, minoxidil induces increased hair growth by vasodilation, then this agent might be of limited value in the prevention of adriamycin-induced hair loss. However, the drug might be of value in stimulating the regrowth of hair after chemotherapy- or radiation-induced alopecia. If the minoxidil-induced hypertrichosis is due to stimulation of the mitotic activity of the hair follicles and a prolongation of the anagen phase of hair growth, then the drug might be of value as a protective agent in chemotherapy-induced alopecia. So far no clinical trials have been performed in cancer patients undergoing chemo- or radiotherapy.

Finally, another experimental study suggested that a preparation rich in the amino acid L-cystein and vitamin A (Gelacet) could protect rabbits from chemotherapy-induced alopecia [32]. Before undergoing clinical evaluation these experimental results should be reproduced in a confirmatory trial.

Prevention of Hair Loss by Pharmacological Interventions

The potential for prevention of hair loss by pharmacological interventions is largely underestimated by medical oncologists. This may in part be due to the fact that the proof of equipotency of two different treatments with one inducing less alopecia is time and resource consuming and bears little scientific merit. However, it would be of invaluable practical help if the patient and the physician could choose between treatments with similar antitumor activity but different potential for the induction of hair loss. A trial by the Swiss Group for Clinical Cancer Research is currently comparing two adjuvant chemotherapy regimens in breast cancer patients, where the only variable is the alkylating agent, i.e., cyclophosphamide is replaced by chlorambucil in the experimental regimen (CMF vs. LMF) [26].

Alteration of dose schedules and the development of analogues with a lesser potential for chemotherapy-induced hair loss are the two principal ways of preventing hair loss by pharmacological interventions. Alteration of the dose schedule has been used successfully with adriamycin. When given in high intermittent doses, this drug induces alopecia in almost all patients. The same drug given in lower weekly doses has a lesser potential for alopecia. The same is true for high, intermittent intravenous doses of cyclophosphamide or continuous, low oral doses of the same drug. Even drugs with a usually negligible potential for epilation when given in conventional dosages, such as melphalan, can cause frequent and severe alopecia when given in high dosages intravenously [15].

Varying agents of a given class display marked differences in their potential for causing alopecia. Whereas adriamycin has a high potential for the induction of hair loss, the analogue epiadriamycin and mitoxantrone (a drug closely related to the anthracyclines) induce less alopecia. The same is true for different alkylating agents (cyclophosphamide vs. chlorambucil, thiotepa, melphalan, etc.).

Conclusions

Alopecia occurring after the use of cytotoxic chemotherapy is perceived by many patients as a threat to their body image and often arouses anxiety. During recent years this side-effect of cancer chemotherapy has received increased attention and several methods are now available to prevent or mask alopecia. The most successful measure to prevent chemotherapy-induced hair loss is scalp hypothermia. However, this method is limited to a subset of patients, i.e., those receiving adriamycin-containing chemotherapies. Furthermore, a considerable number of patients still experience hair loss despite prophylactic scalp cooling. Currently no effective drugs are available to prevent chemotherapy-induced hair loss, but minoxidil might be a good candidate for further clinical evaluation. The potential of pharmacological interventions to prevent chemotherapy-induced alopecia is underestimated and deserves further clinical testing. Finally, patients should receive early practical information about wigs and head coverings to mask hair loss and should be reassured that alopecia is not a sign of advancing disease but a temporary side-effect of treatment.

References

1. Anderson JE, Hunt JM, Smith IA (1981) Prevention of doxorubicin-induced alopecia by scalp cooling in patients with advanced breast cancer. Br Med J 282: 423-424
2. Belpomme D, Mignot L, Grandjean M (1982) Prévention de l'alopécie des chimiothérapies anticancereuses par hypothermie du cuir chevelu. Nouv Presse Med 11: 929-931
3. Campese VM (1981) Minoxidil: a review of its pharmacological properties and therapeutic use. Drugs 22: 257
4. Cohen RL, Alvers ME, Weiss V (1984) Direct effects of minoxidil on epidermal cells in culture. J Invest Dermatol 82: 90-93
5. Dean JC, Salmon SE, Griffith KS (1979) Prevention of doxorubicin-induced hair loss with scalp hypothermia. N Engl J Med 301: 1427-1429
6. Dean JC, Salmon SE, Griffith KS (1980) Prevention of doxorubicin-induced hair loss. N Engl J Med 302: 921
7. Dean JC, Griffith KS, Cetas TC (1983) Scalp hypothermia: a comparison of ice packs and the Kold Kap in the prevention of doxorubicin-induced alopecia. J Clin Oncol 1: 33-37
8. Dorr RT, Fritz WL (1980) Cancer chemotherapy handbook. Kimpton, London
9. Edelstyn GA, MacDonald M, MacRae KD (1977) Doxorubicin-induced hair loss and possible modification by scalp cooling. The Lancet 2: 253-254
10. Gauci L, Serrou B (1980) Changes in hair pigmentation associated with cancer chemotherapy. Cancer Treat Rep 64: 193
11. Gregory RP, Cooke T, Middleton J (1982) Prevention of doxorubicin-induced alopecia by scalp hypothermia: relation to degree of cooling. Br Med J 284: 1674
12. Guy R, Parker H., Shah S (1982) Scalp cooling by thermocirculator. Lancet 1: 937-938
13. Kennedy M, Packard R, Grant M (1983) The effects of using Chemocap on occurrence of chemotherapy-induced alopecia. Oncol Nurs Forum 10: 19-24
14. Kiser J, Weston S, Büsching G (1987) Wann ist der Einsatz der Skalphypothermie wirklich sinnvoll? In: Unterstützende Pflege bei Krebspatienten. Glaus A, Senn HJ (eds) Springer, Berlin Heidelberg New York Tokio
15. Lazarus HM, Herzig RH, Graham-Pole J (1983) Intensive melphalan chemotherapy and cryopreserved autologous bone marrow transplantation for the treatment of refractory cancer. J Clin Oncol 1: 359-365
16. Lovejoy NC (1979) Preventing hair loss during adriamycin therapy. Cancer Nurs 2: 117-121
17. Luce JK, Raffetto RJ, Crisp I (1973) Prevention of alopecia by scalp cooling of patients receiving adriamycin. Cancer Chemother Rep 57: 108-109
18. Martin-Jimenez M, Diaz-Rubio E, Gonzalez Larriba JE (1986) Failure of high-dose tocopherol to prevent alopecia induced by doxorubicin. N Engl J Med 315: 894-895
19. Maxwell MB (1980) Scalp tourniquets for chemotherapy-induced alopecia. Am J Nurs 80: 900-903
20. Middleton J, Franks D, Buchanan RB (1985) Failure of scalp hypothermia to prevent hair loss when cyclophosphamide is added to doxorubicin and vincristine. Cancer Treat Rep 69: 373-375

21. Munro DD (1971) Disorders of hair. In: Fitzpatrick TB, Arndt KA, Clark WH et al. (eds) Dermatology in general medicine. McGraw-Hill, New York, pp 297-331
22. Perez JE, Macchiavelli M, Leone BA (1986) High-dose alpha-tocopherol as a preventive of doxorubicin-induced alopecia. Cancer Treat Rep 70: 1213-1214
23. Pesce A, Cassuto JP, Joyner MV (1978) Scalp tourniquet in the prevention of chemotherapy-induced alopecia. N Engl J Med 298: 1204-1205
24. Presser SE (1980) Prevention of doxorubicin-induced hair loss. N Engl J Med 302: 921
25. Satterwhite B, Zimm S (1984) The use of scalp hypothermia in the prevention of doxorubicin-induced hair loss. Cancer 54: 34-37
26. Senn HJ Unpublished data of the Swiss Group for Clinical Cancer Research.
27. Simister JM (1966) Alopecia and cytotoxic drugs. Br Med J 2: 1138
28. Storer JS, Brzuskiewicz J, Floyd H (1986) Review: topical minoxidil for male pattern baldness. Am J Med Sci 291: 328-333
29. Wagner L, Bye MG (1979) Body image and patients experiencing alopecia as a result of cancer chemotherapy. Cancer Nursing 2: 365-369
30. Weiss VC, West DP, Fu TS (1984) Alopecia areata treated with topical minoxidil. Arch Dermatol 120: 457-463
31. Wood LA (1985) Possible prevention of adriamycin-induced alopecia by tocopherol. N Engl J Med 312: 1060
32. Zografos E (1984) Medikamentöse Prophylaxemöglichkeiten der zytostatikabedingten Alopezie. Tierexperimentelle Arbeit. Krankenhausarzt 57: 620-622

Managing Side-Effects in Radiotherapy with Regard to the Gastrointestinal Tract

L. Franzén, U. Hellsing, R. Henriksson, and B. Littbrand*

Department of Oncology, University of Umeå, 901 85 Umeå, Sweden

Radiation treatment of neoplasms in the gastrointestinal tract is associated with a high frequency of side-effects. In the upper gastrointestinal tract the direct effect of irradiation is erythema, plaque formation, and in severe cases ulceration and bleeding [2]. The injuries are aggravated by the radiation damage to salivary glands and by the secondary decreased salivary flow [4, 8]. The altered salivation is also followed by dental caries. It is obvious that the patients suffer from discomfort in speaking, mastication, and swallowing.

Treatment affecting the radiosensitive intestinal mucosa - i. e. pelvic radiotherapy of neoplasms in the rectum, prostate, and urinary bladder - is characterized by the main symptom of diarrhea. The advantage of reducing the secondary diarrhea following mucosal damage is obvious, and during recent years interest has been focused on bile acid malabsorption [1, 3]. Indeed, manipulation of the fat intake and use of bile acid sequestering resins have been shown to be quite effective in preventing acute diarrhea induced by pelvic irradiation. However, these drugs are associated with a high rate of adverse effects [3].

For these reasons, we feel it is of interest to describe some of our efforts to minimize the side-effects following radiotherapy of the gastrointestinal tract. Measures include diet, the use of sucralfate (an aluminum hydroxide of sulfated sucrose), and minimizing the volume in radiation treatment.

Materials and Methods

Fifty-two patients were included in these investigations. They were irradiated in the head and neck region and in the pelvic region. The number of patients in the treatment groups, their age range, and the total dose of irradiation are presented in Table 1.

Radiotherapy was administered with 4 MV (Warian) at 80-cm source skin distance (SSD), 6 MV (Brown-Bowery) at SSD 100 cm, and 20 MV or different elec-

* The financial support provided by the Swedish Cancer Society is gratefully acknowledged.

Table 1. Details of the treatment groups

Localization	Treatment technique	Number of patients	Age range	Total dose (Gy)
Head-neck	Unilateral	16	22–80	50–68
Head-neck	Bilateral	21	28–78	50–68
Pelvic	Four-field	15	53–74	50–67

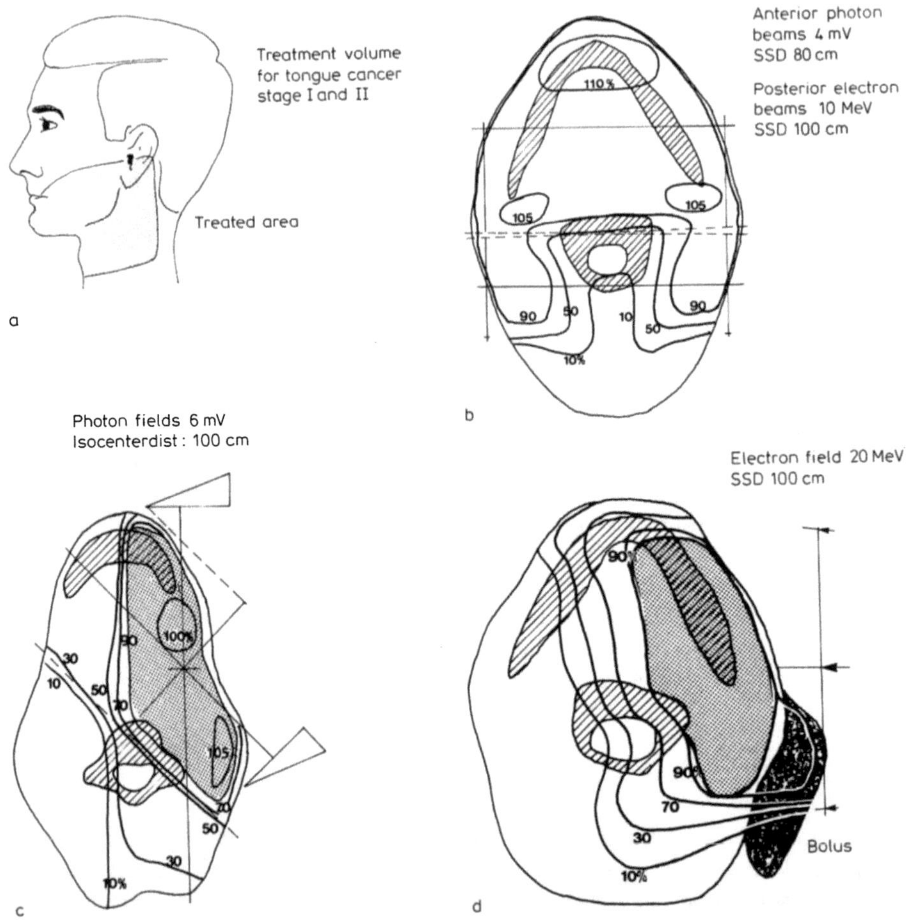

Fig. 1 a–d. The radiation treatment techniques used for head and neck cancer. **a** Field size unilateral treatment of tongue cancer stage I–II. **b** Cross-section of bilateral fields in a dose plan using photons and electrons in the head-neck region. **c** Cross-section of unilateral isocentric dose plan using photons. **d** Cross-section of unilateral dose plan with electrons

tron energies 16–20 MeV (Microtron, Sanditronix) at SSD 100 cm. The fraction schedule was five fractions per week with daily doses of 1.8–2.2 Gy. The different types of treatment modality for head and neck cancer are illustrated in Fig. 1. Pelvic irradiation was administered by the Microtrone 20 MV fotons, four-field technique, with a mean field size of 11 × 14 cm.

Saliva was collected before radiotherapy, and then weekly during therapy and when patients returned for follow-up. The saliva samples were stimulated parotid saliva selectively collected from the right and left parotid glands. Lashley cups were used to collect the saliva, and the saliva production was stimulated by salivary stimulating tablets. Approximately 1.5 ml saliva was collected from each gland.

Sucralfate Studies

The study was an open consecutive study conducted over 3 months. When the study started the first 15 patients planned for pelvic radiation were included. None had undergone pelvic surgery. Dose granulate of sucralfate (an alkaline aluminum hydroxide of sulfated sucrose) was dispensed to each patient when symptoms of diarrhea appeared at radiation doses of 12–35 Gy, with the instruction to ingest one dose package (1 g) dissolved in water four to eight times daily. Patients were instructed to ask for loperamide or diphenoxylate when they required symptomatic therapy for diarrhea. Two patients were excluded early in the study, one because of discomfort with meteorism in the stomach and one because of disagreement with the study design. Apart from these two patients, compliance was good, and no other unwarranted effects were observed. There was no significant weight loss. The patients' symptoms were registered during the radiotherapy. Each week the patients' daily frequency and stool consistency were recorded. The details of the bowel action from the calendar were converted to a diarrhea scale (Table 2). The study was terminated concomitantly with the radiotherapy. The general condition was followed throughout the treatment period, and the occurrence of symptoms such as nausea and vomiting was especially observed.

Another group of patients (55) had regular consultation with a dietitian, a dentist, and physicians during the treatment.

Results

Treatment of Head and Neck Cancer

With a unilateral mode of radiotherapy the contralateral salivary glands were protected from radiation damage (see Figs. 1, 2). The salivary flow was intact, whereas the parotid glands directly affected by the radiation displayed an extremely low salivary flow. The decrease in salivary flow was already evident within 1 week of commencement of treatment, while the nonirradiated glands displayed signs of increased activity. The immediate decrease in the salivary flow was also registered when both parotid glands were irradiated using the technique illustrated in

Table 2. Diarrhea scale

Scale	
0	No change in bowel habit ("normal")
1	Minor increase in frequency and soft stools
2	Increase in frequency and loose stools
3	Marked increase in frequency and watery stools

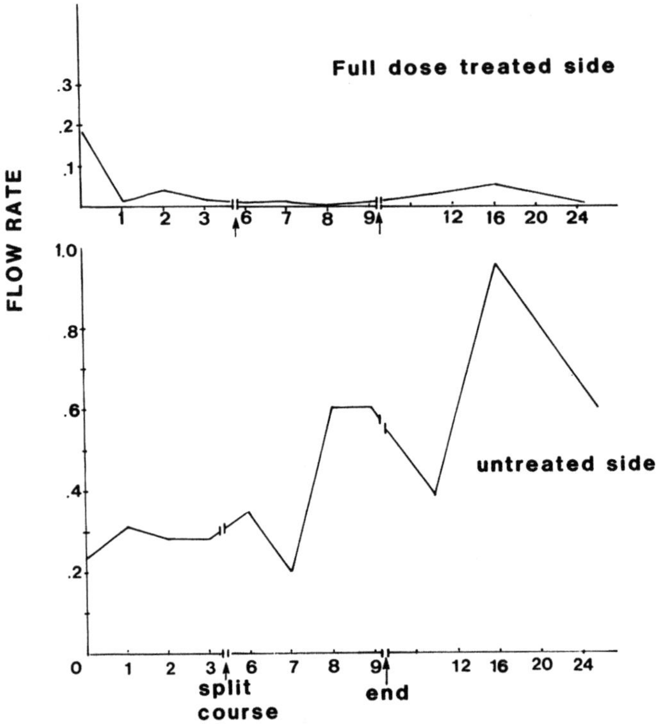

Fig. 2. Unilateral treatment. Salivary flow from parotid gland in the full treated side *(top)* and the contralateral untreated side *(bottom)*

Figs. 1b and 3. The mucosal damage and dental caries were also less frequently seen in the patients with unilateral radiation therapy compared to the patients treated bilaterally.

Treatment of Pelvic-Associated Cancer

The treatment with sucralfate significantly decreased the symptoms of diarrhea and the patients displayed only minor alterations in bowel habit even at the end of the radiation treatment (Table 3). All patients experienced a significant improve-

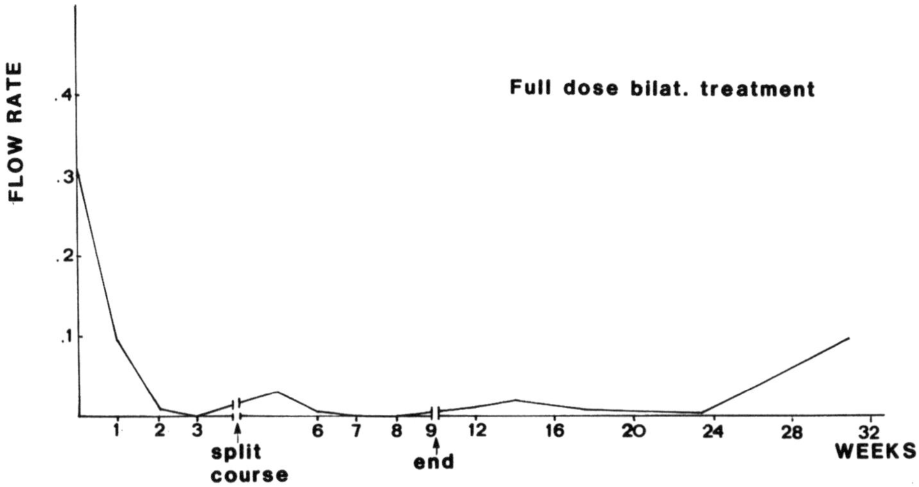

Fig. 3. Bilateral treatment. Salivary flow rate from both right and left parotid glands. Split course 3 weeks. *End*, end point of radiation treatment

Table 3. The diarrhea score (see Table 2) at the start of sucralfate treatment *(A)*, at the end of radiation therapy *(C)*, and in the middle between these two scoring events *(B)*

Number of patients	Diarrhea score, mean ± SE		
	A	B	C
15	1.3 ± 0.03	0.2 ± 0.004	0.5 ± 0.02

ment in gasatrointestinal function as compared to patients not receiving the drug. None of the patients required symptomatic therapy with loperamide or diphenoxylate.

Diet. Follow-up of a group of patients with regular consultations and strict advice regarding the necessity of a low fat intake had a clear effect on the discomfort of diarrhea.

Discussion

In recent years quality of life has become a crucial concept in the treatment of patients suffering from all grades of disease. The present study demonstrates some efforts to make radiotherapy more convenient for patients.

The results showed that the early adverse effects of radiotherapy could be significantly reduced by minimizing the treatment volume. By using the unilateral treatment technique in tongue cancer stages I and II, as compared to bilateral radiation fields, the contralateral salivary glands were protected and the oral mucosa less affected. Obviously, the comfort increased during as well as after the treatment period. The decrease in treatment volume caused no obvious deterioration in therapeutic success. It is of course a matter of controversy whether the uninvolved neck side should be irradiated or not. However, retrospective analysis of tongue cancer stages I and II [5] and malignant nasopharyngeal tumors [6] has suggested that prophylactic irradiation could have added very little or nothing to the curability while it would have caused increased radiation morbidity. In a medically well developed region with good possibilities for follow-up of all patients, prophylactic irradition of the neck does not always seem to be necessary or to be minimized in volume as much as is possible.

The present preliminary, open consecutive study suggested that the aluminum hydroxide complex of sulfated sucrose, sucralfate, could be of value in diminishing discomfort during radiation therapy to the gastrointestinal tract. The most pronounced-improvements seemed to be prevention of mucosal damage to the lower gastrointestinal tract and of the secondary appearance of diarrhea. Results have to be compared with the earlier observations that about 75% of patients receiving pelvic radiotherapy displayed diarrhea. Furthermore, we also observed that sucralfate seemed to decrease the oral mucositis and the discomfort in speaking and swallowing when treating head and neck cancer (unpublished data).

One can only speculate on which mechanism causes the protective effect of sucralfate. A plausible explanation could be that it protects the damaged mucosa from the effect of local irritants, as has been suggested in respect of its capacity to heal gastric ulcers [7]. The suggested cytoprotective properties [9] seem an acceptable explanation even for prevention of radiation - induced injury in both the upper and the lower gastrointestinal tract, although the binding capacity of bile salts [10] can also have an additive effect in preventing diarrhea. The advantages of using sucralfate are the simple means of administration and especially the low frequency of side-effects despite its extensive use [7]. However, before any conclusive remarks can be offered concerning the role of sucralfate, results from a recently started randomized trial using placebo in the control group of patints have to be evaluated.

Apart from the effect of sucralfate it was observed that straightforward recommendation of a low fat intake apparently resulted in improvement in diarrhea and a sense of solace during the treatment. This is at least partly dependent on minimizing bile acid malabsorption, which has been described as an important factor underlying the occurrence of disturbances in the lower gastrointestinal tract during pelvic radiotherapy.

Reduction in the duration of radiotherapy (e.g., avoiding split-course therapy with a rest period during treatment) is also a possibility if one can reduce the acute effect of the radiotherapy. By reducing treatment time the possibility of proliferation of the tumor cells during the treatment is decreased and an increased therapeutic ratio might be obtained.

In conclusion, with this presentation we have aimed to demonstrate some methods to minimize early and late complications of radiotherapy. It is obvious that it is of great importance to increase the quality of life of the treated patients. Furthermore, a reduction in the risk of complications can also make possible an increase in the total dose and/or a reduction in the duration of irradiation, which might increase the possibility of curing the patient with cancer by means of radiotherapy.

Summary

Three different means of diminishing discomfort during radiation therapy of the gastrointestinal tract are demonstrated and discussed:

1. Use of the smallest possible treatment volumes in medically well developed regions with good possibilities for follow-up of all patients.
2. Regular consultations, with advice concerning food intake and dental hygiene
3. Use of the drug sucralfate, which may improve tolerance against the radiation-induced damage to the gastrointestinal mucosa.

References

1. Andersson H, Bosaeus I, Nyström C (1978) Bile salt malabsorption in the radiation syndrome. Acta Radiol [Oncol] 17: 312
2. Beumer I, Curtis T, Harrison RE (1979) Radiation therapy of the oral cavity: sequelae and management. Head Neck Surg 1: 301
3. Chary S, Thomson DH (1984) A clinical trial evaluating cholestyramine to prevent diarrhea in patients maintained on low fat diets during pelvic radiation therapy. Int J Radiat Oncol Biol Phys 10: 1885
4. Eneroth CM, Henriksson CO, Jakobsson PÅ (1972) Effect of fractionated radiotherapy on salivary gland function. Cancer 30: 1147
5. Franzén L, Carlsöö B, Henriksson R, Littbrand B, Löfroth PO (1987) Evaluation of radiotherapy of tongue cancer. (Submitted)
6. Larsson LG, Seelig I (1976) Malignant nasopharyngeal tumours. Result of radiation therapy. Acta Radiol [Oncol] 15: 209
7. Martin F, Farley A, Gagnon M, Bensemona D (1982) Comparison of the healing capacities of sucralfate and limetidine in the short-term treatment of duodenal ulcer. Gastroenterology 82: 401
8. Mossman KL, Shatzman AR, Chencharick JD (1981) Effects of radiotherapy on human parotid saliva. Radiat Res 88: 403
9. Tamawski A (1984) Sucralfate: Is it more than just a barrier? Cytoprotection. Cur Concept Gastroenterol 1: 5
10. Tobiasson P, Stenstam M (1985) Effects of sucralfate and cholestyramine on bile acid absorption. Gastroenterology 88: 393

Principles and Potential of Palliative Surgery in Patients with Advanced Cancer

J. F. Forbes

Department of Surgical Oncology, Newcastle Mater Misericordiae Hospital, Waratah, NSW 2298, Australia

Although the majority of patients with advanced cancer are unlikely to be cured, recurrent or metastatic disease does not have to mean that a rapid or painful death is imminent. Palliative surgery aims to improve patients' quality of life without necessarily removing all tumor, as when malignancy is advanced there is less emphasis on specific tumor therapy and more on supportive care. Palliative surgery should be seen in this context - as a part of overall patient management aimed at reduction of symptoms and prolongation of useful life without curative intent. Palliative surgery for advanced cancer should follow sound principles of surgical oncology. These involve preoperative, operative, and postoperative patient care as well as surgery of particular complications. It must be remembered that patients with cancer might also have a nonmalignant surgical problem such as appendicitis that can be readily corrected, and this dictates that a careful, rapid, and thorough assessment be made to allow early aggressive and definitive surgery to be undertaken. It should never be assumed that a new clinical problem in a cancer patient is certainly due to the cancer. This is bad medicine and the basis of unnecessary suffering and mortality.

There is a paucity of scientific data and controlled trials to determine the proper role of palliative surgery for advanced cancer. Surgical interventions are consequently based largely on principles, experience, and instructive data from surgery in other settings, and hence new scientific investigations are required. Major problems encountered by patients with advanced cancer requiring a degree of palliative surgery are discussed in detail elsewhere in this symposium. These include infections, hemorrhage, nutrition, pain control, and fracture care, which are considered here only where they illustrate important principles.

The Role of Surgery in Palliation

Surgeons have long been involved in all aspects of cancer care, including prevention, diagnosis, and curative treatment as well as palliation and rehabilitation. Indeed, there are few tumors that never involve surgery in their management and few surgeons who are never involved in the care of a cancer patient. Thus it is

Recent Results in Cancer Research, Vol. 108

helpful to first consider the principles relevant to palliative surgery of all types before the more specific problems that follow, as these principles overlap those of surgery in general.

Patients Are Surgical Patients as Well as Cancer Patients

Patients with cancer having surgery are firstly surgical patients. The most important aim for the surgeon in supportive care of patients is to avoid or minimize the physical and psychological stress that can be associated with any operative procedure. All patients can be apprehensive about an operation. It is not just the hospitalization, anesthetic, and disfigurement that can be a consequence of surgery that are stressful but also the anxiety associated with total reliance on another person for part of the treatment. An awareness of these potential problems can allow the surgeon to plan palliative procedures in a way that minimizes patient stress at each step.

Direct the Surgery at the Consequences of the Tumor

Morbidity in advanced cancer is a consequence of tumor site as much as disease stage. A single primary that erodes a major blood vessel can cause death by hemorrhage even if the tumor is benign. Another patient with distant metastases from malignant testicular teratoma might have the disease controlled without any surgical intervention. Hence, the primary attack by the surgeon palliating advanced cancer should be directed at the symptoms and not necessarily at the malignant processes themselves.

Integrate Surgery into Both Specific Treatment and Supportive Care Programs

Surgery for palliation must be an integrated part of the total treatment program of both specific and supportive therapy for the particular cancer. Specific tumor palliation may result from various modalities. For example, both reduction of tumor bulk by surgery and control by chemotherapy of a tumor causing marrow depresion with consequent anemia or bleeding could improve a patient's quality of life. Careful planning of the surgery to allow optimal drug delivery, which does not interfere with wound healing or recovery of the patient from an operation, is necessary to optimize these specific palliative maneuvers.

Avoid Unreasonable Delay of Palliative Surgery

Palliative surgery should be completed as soon as is practical. There is little to gain by postponing surgery when it is obvious that a particular intervention can benefit the patient. Quality of life is improved by avoiding prolongation of symptoms, and it is also improved by avoiding the anxiety that stems from uncertainty when a patient does not have a clear idea as to what is planned. Thus, if a laparotomy is necessary to determine the extent of tumor before embarking on addition al treatment this should be done as soon as the need for it becomes apparent. Delaying a surgical procedure while additional investigations are done is often particularly stressful and also unreasonably costly.

There are, however, also situations where prudent management without intervention can be the best form of palliation. For example, the patient who has a small bowel obstruction as a result of adhesions from previous surgery or radiotherapy may recover with nasogastric suction and intravenous feeding; an operation in such a patient may not only be hazardous, with its high risk of bowel perforation and difficult wound healing, but also stimulate the tendency to further bowel obstruction from adhesions. Equally, when an established small bowel obstruction is present and it is clear that it will not resolve without surgery, then delay in the surgery is a great disservice to the patient and can compromise the outcome.

Surgical Problems May Have a Benign Cause - Obtain Histological Findings Where Possible

There are particular examples of definitive palliative surgery that illustrate the uncertain intent of the surgery prior to its commencement. Patients with obstructive jaundice and known cancer could have infiltrative metastatic malignancy in the liver causing jaundice, extrahepatic biliary obstruction from lymph nodes or primary tumor, or even a benign cause such as an abscess or cholelithiasis. In such cases an early laparotomy and biopsy wherever possible are often in the patient's best interests. The surgery can palliate successfully by bypassing an extrahepatic obstruction or cure the jaundice if it has a benign cause. Although some investigations are necessary, the surgery should be undertaken as soon as it is clear that no additional diagnostic information can be obtained and that the patient is fit for operation.

Principles of Preoperative Care in Advanced Cancer

Consultations and Explanations

Wherever possible the patient and close friends or relatives must be given a clear understanding of the premise on which the operation is based and of the potential benefits. It is always helpful to discuss this carefully, even when considerable time is necessary, to avoid misunderstandings. Not only the aims of the operation, its potential outcome, and possible complications should be considered, but also the likely course of events if no surgical intervention is undertaken. If the operation planned is based on the sound premise of a likely improvement in quality of life when due consideration is given to the morbidity and potential complications of the procedure, then the explanation is more straightforward. On occasions, the intent of surgery and its potential may not be apparent until after the operation has commenced - for example, if surgery is planned for an obstructing carcinoma of the cecum it may not be apparent until laparotomy is underway whether or not resection is possible. This degree of uncertainty should also be explained. Anxiety is based largely on uncertainty or expected discomfort. The surgeon can carefully direct his discussion and explanations to avoid such potential anxiety.

Preoperative Planning for Immediate and Long-Term Care

The results obtained from palliative surgery may depend largely on the adequacy of preoperative preparation and assessment. Cancer patients can suffer all the major complications of surgery during and after operations and often suffer them more frequently and to a worse degree; so assessment must include not only the tumor type and extent but also the medical state of the patient. In particular, disordered fluid and electrolyte balance, poor wound healing, renal shutdown, and postoperative infections and hemorrhage can be the cause of fatalities. An adequate assessment of the patient's nutritional status and steps to correct it are essential. For major surgery such as bowel resection or nephrectomy, assessment of fluid and electrolyte balance, pulmonary status, cardiovascular function, renal function, and hemostasis is the minimum requirement. Patients with advanced cancer are also often older, thus aggravating these problems. There are many reasons for taking great care.

Many additional people are important to a patient preparing for an operation. A stomal therapist, for example, is a skilled nursing professional who is very well equipped to discuss problems associated with a colostomy. All aspects of colostomy will require consideration at some time, and a stomal therapist usually has the best judgment as to when these should be considered preoperatively and postoperatively for a particular patient. The possible role of additional people is best considered preoperatively for every patient. Details of the role of these people is considered elsewhere.

The postoperative recovery and recuperation environment of the patient should be clearly established before a procedure is undertaken. If the patient is likely to have a long recovery period ahead of him, and only a short stay in hospital with intensive nursing, the ultimate outcome can be compromised by lack of appropriate nursing and supportive care after discharge. It is particularly unfortunate if a patient is allowed to reach such a situation as a result of inadequate early planning.

Principles of Operating for Advanced Cancer

A badly placed incision can compromise what is otherwise a successful operation. An incision in a patient with advanced cancer may heal slowly. Incisions placed where they will give not only good access but also good healing are desirable. Some incisions such as midline lower abdominal incisions are notoriously poor healers and should be avoided. Previous areas of radiotherapy are also best avoided and to achieve this innovative planning and sound judgment may be required.

Other principles important for all operations must be vigorously upheld. The tissues of patients with advanced cancer are very fragile and vascular and may tear or bleed unless handled with care and gentleness during an operation. Hemostasis must be meticulous. Wounds should be sewn up with great care - interrupted sutures are preferred to continuous sutures and suture material that persists for at least 6 weeks is essential.

Each patient must undergo the procedure that is optimal for them. The decision as to whether to attempt a resection or bypass in bowel obstruction, for example, must be made in the light of the particular patient's fitness, age, and the available postoperative care facilities. A noncurative resection for bowel obstruction with an anastomosis and removal of tumor might well be a better palliative procedure in terms of quality of life than a short simple bypass that is likely to cause additional complications or pain by virtue of the continued presence of the tumor. The decision as to whether to resect bowel or not may be complicated by prior radiotherapy. An irradiated bowel does not heal well and incisions through it must be avoided. Decisions as to the precise way in which a particular operation should be conducted in the presence of irradiated tissue must be made with great care and fine judgment.

Other modalities of specific treatment for palliation must have been considered before the operation is commenced as this may suggest the need for additional operative procedures that otherwise would be neglected. For example, metastatic liver disease might be treated better with an intra-arterial catheter placed in the hepatic artery at the time of surgery.

Decisions as to which procedure is undertaken may depend upon a patient's particular wishes, thus underlining the importance of the preoperative consultation and discussion. For example, whether or not a colostomy is done at the time of operation must be consistent with the patient's understanding and wishes.

Postoperative Care in Palliative Surgery

The aim of postoperative care is to optimize recovery by avoiding complications. If it is not possible to avoid complications then we should at least aim to detect them early and treat them vigorously. All the complications of surgery can be particularly troublesome in cancer patients, including hemorrhage; there is often disordered hemostasis, infection, poor wound healing, electrolyte disorders (in particular acid-base imbalance and renal failure), airway obstruction, and problems of prolonged immobilization such as pressure care, bed sores, pulmonary embolus, muscle wasting, and psychological stress from inactivity and confinement. Many of these are potentially fatal, but early diagnosis and aggressive treatment can prevent a minor problem from becoming disaster.

No operation on cancer patients should be undertaken unless it is clear that optimal postoperative care is available. Many potential postoperative complications can be avoided by careful preoperative planning and attention to the detail of the principles discussed previously. Unfortunately, the complication rate following surgery of patients with advanced cancer is high, and it is only with the utmost vigilance that this high rate can be lowered.

Bleeding problems can result from many causes, including tumor involvement of the liver and bone marrow as well as marrow suppression from prior or concurrent cytotoxic therapy or radiation. Bleeding from abnormal tissues around tumors is often venous, low pressure, and easy to control, but concurrent clotting disorders can be a problem with high pressure arterial bleeding and may require transfusion of appropriate blood components, including platelets or fresh plasma.

Many patients having cancer surgery have a preexisting compromised nutritional state and may have difficulty with oral feeding for a period subsequent to their operation. Intravenous nitrition should be considered preoperatively in all cancer patients, and introduced if there is doubt about its need. It is safer for the patient to have a short course of potentially unnecessary hyperalimentation than to reach a difficult situation where it is introduced too late, with wound healing already severely affected and infection, electrolyte disorders, and ultimately renal failure likely to ensue.

Infection in cancer patients following surgery is best treated intensively at the outset until it is clear what the specific antibiotic sensitivities are for particular organisms. If delay occurs in instituting adequate therapy the patient may die because of an inadequate ability to use reserves in other organ systems. The principle of overtreatment at the earliest opportunity is the safest guideline for avoiding complications.

Special Palliative Procedures

Particular complications and problems can arise in cancer patients beyond those discussed elsewhere (such as hemorrhage, infection, and difficulty with wound healing and electrolyte imbalance that occur following operation). Most of these should be managed according to the following principles, already considered:

1. Maintain a heightened awareness of the possibility of the complication arising in all early cancer patients.
2. Diagnose benign causes at the outset by histology where possible.
3. Commence more than adequate treatment early.
4. Tailor the treatment to maximize resolution of the problem and to improve the quality of life with minimum morbidity from the treatment.

The Problem of Cord Compression

Approximately half the patients with cord compression have advanced disease with metastases [1]. Not all require surgery but it is particularly appropriate for those patients who have radioresistant tumors, or if prior radiotherapy precludes its further use.

An awareness of the significance of symptoms such as minor tingling in the fingers or toes or an ipsilateral weakness is necessary, and symptoms should always be actively inquired about on regular review. The tragedy of a patient with permanent paraplegia or incontinence is avoidable if this awareness is present. Although modern radiological imaging techniques can clearly identify the site and distribution of metastatic tumor deposits, prolonged investigations are no substitute for urgent decompression if a level of block and compression has been identified. The principles of preoperative care and postoperative management discussed previously also apply. It is the awareness of the possibility of the problem, however, that is most important in preventing potential difficulties developing into irretrievable disaster. The particular advantage of surgical palliation in this case is that the diagnosis might not be apparent in terms of tumor type, and histological evidence will be obtained. If radiation therapy is used for tumor control, careful monitoring of the patient will be required in case surgical decompression needs to be added if the condition worsens. The relative merits of alternative therapies remain uncertain [2, 3] and controlled trials are required.

Brain Metastases

Patients with melanoma, breast cancer, and lung cancer may have the complication of cerebral metastasis and overall some 20% of patients might be affected [4]. This is a life-threatening situation, and on occasions (particularly with melanoma patients) when the metastasis is solitary, surgery might be an appropriate intervention as a life-saving step [5]. Surgical resection might be followed with advantage by radiotherapy if the tumor is radiosensitive [6]. Many patients, however, will be treated by nonoperative modalities.

Metastases to Other Viscera

The potential of palliative surgery for other visceral meastases is largely dependent on the availability or not of additional systemic cytotoxic chemotherapy with sufficient efficacy to be used in conjunction. Although isolated metastases can be removed as a palliative step (and occasionally a curative one), the morbidity and potential hazards of the operation frequently outweigh the possible gain. It is in tumors such as metastatic testicular teratoma, where cisplatinum-containing cytotoxic regimens have been so useful, that palliative surgery of metastases in viscera such as the lungs has proven particularly valuable. Consideration needs to be given to the tumor type and its chemosensitivity, the site and number of metastases, physical status and health of the patient in terms of ability to withstand the planned operation, and the available facilities for postoperative patient care. Failure to consider each of these components before embarking on surgery can result in untreatable complications and loss of life.

The Palliative Role of Bulk Reduction

Bulk reduction has long been employed in certain tumors, particularly ovarian carcinomas, as a palliative procedure which is believed to improve the duration and quality of life. Hard evidence that it prolongs survival is difficult to find, although bulk reduction appears to have been used successfully in improving the outcome of patients with Burkitt's lymphoma. The principle followed has been that surgical resection of bulk disease, even if incomplete in terms of total tumor removal, may allow more efficient control of residual disease. It follows that effective systemic treatment modalities must be available to control the residual disease to justify the bulk reduction. Although it has been demonstrated that the amount of tumour bulk remaining after surgery does correlate with survival, this does not mean that the survival is better because of the lesser disease - it is still plausible that the patient with better survival was better able to contain their tumor and was going to have a better survival whether the tumor bulk was reduced or not.

Surgery as Specific Palliative Treatment

Some tumors, for example malignant melanoma, are relatively resistant to chemotherapy and radiotherapy and are best treated definitively by surgery whether or not the intent is palliative or curative. Many patients with melanoma at various sites have had cure or long survival achieved by surgical excision - particularly with deposits around the inguinal region. Many others have short survival despite surgery, and the absence of other specific treatments is no justification for poorly planned surgery. It is still essential to balance potential gains against potential morbidity in each individual patient.

Future Directions

Adherence to the principles considered can allow palliative surgery to be used optimally. Beyond this most advances will come from the non-operative supportive care measures. New scientific data from other disciplines will improve preoperative assessment and patient preparation for surgery - particularly with management of infections and nutritional support. Progress in the quality of postoperative care might allow more extensive surgery to be undertaken where it is clearly to the patient's benefit.

I would expect more specific progress to come in two areas. First, surgery has more to offer when it is combined with definitive systemic therapy. Increasingly, we will see what is now "palliative surgery" used with curative intent - perhaps where a mechanical problem has arisen - because curative specific systemic therapy is available. Such surgery will at times be adjuvant to the other specific therapy.

The second area for progress will come from controlled trials of the use of surgery as a palliative procedure in cancer patients with proper attention to quality of life. For example, evaluation of bulk reduction, bypass versus resection, the timing of surgery, the type and extent of investigations, infection control, and wound healing can be undertaken in well-designed trials. The measurement of quality of life should be a key component of such trials.

The principles discussed here are important. If they are challenged by new ideas and appropriate randomized trials then both the patients and their treating surgeons will benefit.

References

1. Bhalla SK (1970) Metastatic disease of the spine. Clin Orthop 73: 52-60
2. Gilbert et al. (1978) Epidural spinal cord compression from metastatic tumour: diagnosis and treatment. Ann Neurol 3: 40
3. Young et al. (1980) Treatment of spinal epidural metastases: randomised prospective comparison of laminectomy and radiation therapy. J Neurosurg 53: 741
4. Posner JB (1977) Management of central nervous system metastases. Semin Oncol 4: 81
5. Winston KR, Walsh JW, Fischer EG (1980) Results of operative treatment of intracranial metastatic tumours. Cancer 45: 2639-2645
6. Galicich JH, Sundaresan N, Thaler HT (1980) Surgical treatment of single brain metastases. J Neurosurg 53: 63-67

Palliative and Supportive Surgery for Gastrointestinal Cancer

U. Metzger, W. Weder, D. Mona, and F. Largiadèr

Departement Chirurgie, Universitätsspital, 8091 Zürich, Switzerland

Gastrointestinal cancer is a common medical problem in Western countries. One-third of the 16000 annual cancer deaths in Switzerland are attributed to gastrointestinal cancer [1]. This means that 1 in 12 inhabitants of this country will eventually die of such a tumor. Due to the limited efficacy of alternative treatment modalities (radiotherapy, chemotherapy), surgery plays the major role in the treatment of gastrointestinal tract cancer. Early stage tumors can usually be cured by surgical resection. However, in population-based studies, these prognostically favorable cases are extremely rare. Only 93 UICC stage I cases (0.7%) were registered at the Birmingham Cancer Registry among 13175 patients with gastric carcinoma from the West Midland area during the period 1960–1969 [2]. Eighty percent of the population in this study had metastatic UICC stage IV disease far beyond any chance of cure. Similar low resectability rates are being found in esophageal cancer, hepatobiliary carcinoma, and pancreatic cancer. Fortunately, in the most common gastrointestinal malignancy, colorectal carcinoma, resectability is much higher, 70%–75%, and half of these patients will be cured by radical resection [3]. Considering the long-term results for all other gastrointestinal carcinomas, even so-called curative resections must in fact be considered palliative procedures. What are the role and potential of surgery for palliation in gastrointestinal cancer?

The Palliative and Supportive Role of Surgery

The main goals of palliative surgery are:

1. Restoration of regular alimentary passage
2. Relief of tumor-related symptoms (pain, bleeding, hormonal symptoms)
3. Prevention of tumor-related complications (bleeding, obstruction, perforation)

These aims can be accomplished by palliative resection and – in part – through bypass procedures. Additional surgical measures include debulking of chemosensitive or hormone-producing tumors and staging procedures for gastrointestinal lymphomas. Finally, supportive treatment is feasible through the surgical place-

Recent Results in Cancer Research, Vol. 108

ment of various internal stents, the insertion of feeding tubes, the insertion of intra-arterial, intraportal, or intraperitoneal catheters for regional chemotherapy, and the placement of interstitial implants for radiation therapy. At every laparotomy, a thorough intraoperative diagnostic workup should be performed to allow adequate planning of subsequent combined modality therapy.

The ultimate goal of all these surgical interventions is the amelioration or maintenance of the patient's quality of life with or without prolongation of survival.

Palliative Resection

Blunt transhiatal dissection of the esophagus for lower third lesions and thoracoabdominal resection for tumors of the middle and upper thirds are indicated if an R_0 (no residual disease) or an R_1 (microscopic residual disease) resection can be achieved by this procedure. Reconstruction is carried out either by a gastric pull-through or by colonic interposition with an end-to-end anastomosis, preferably in the cervical area. For all other cases, bypass procedures or the placement of internal tubes (Celestin, Häring) with or without radiation therapy should be considered.

In the absence of bulky tumor or advanced metastatic dissemination, palliative resection of gastric carcinoma is usually indicated. In most instances, subtotal gastrectomy will be sufficient for this purpose, though sometimes palliative total gastrectomy might be necessary to achieve negative margins. Reconstruction of the alimentary passage is by Roux-en-Y esophago- or gastrojejunostomy.

Palliative resection of pancreatic, primary liver, and bile duct cancer is rarely indicated because of rapid regrowth following incomplete resection. On the other hand, small bowel and large bowel carcinoma should always be resected in order to prevent emergency situations.

Reviewing 1000 major cancer interventions performed at our institution over a 3-year period, more than half of the 631 operations for gastrointestinal neoplasms were already considered palliative at the time of surgery. In elective interventions, operative mortality was 5%, whereas in emergency situations it rose to 20%–40% [4]. Such situations should be avoided whenever possible, taking into account patient's age, tumor biology, and expected survival without treatment.

Palliative resection is also clearly indicated for symptomatic hormone-producing tumors, e.g., carcinoid tumors, where removal of bulky liver deposits reduces urine 5-HIAA excretion and relieves the carcinoid syndrome (flush, diarrhea). More recently, we also removed liver metastases of chemosensitive tumors (ovarian cancer, sarcoma), facilitating subsequent chemotherapy. These liver resections are increasingly being performed in this decade because of significant reduction of surgical morbidity and mortality. Among 30 major liver resections, hospital mortality in our institution was 6.6%, which is comparable to the 5%–6% reported in the surgical literature [5, 6].

In the case of gastrointestinal lymphoma, the primary lesion should be resected with healthy margins to allow safe anastomosis, together with regional lymph nodes. Staging procedures to determine the extent of intra-abdominal spread must be performed. This includes sampling of intra-abdominal and periaortic nodes, a liver biopsy, and often a splenectomy.

Bypass Procedures

Bypass procedures are directed toward relief of obstructive symptoms in the case of locally nonresectable cancer. Because primary tumor is left in place, bypass procedures are of minor palliative value. Tumor-related symptoms like pain and bleeding are not influenced and the formation of blind intestinal loops sometimes creates additional nutritional problems. Again, tumors of the small and large intestine should be removed irrespective of the actual tumor stage. The most common bypass operation is gastroenterostomy for obstructing inoperable tumors of the duodenal area. With the introduction of endoscopically placed esophageal tubes and percutaneously or endoscopically placed endoprostheses for bile duct obstruction, the number of bypass procedures in these anatomical areas has significantly decreased during the last decade. Surgical morbidity and mortality for bypass procedures are almost identical to those for palliative resections and should therefore never be the reason for not performing tumor removal.

Other Supportive Surgical Techniques

Other nonresectional procedures include the surgical placement of catheters through various routes for regional chemotherapy, allowing a higher drug concentration at the target organ. Due to the predominant arterial blood supply of liver tumors and to hepatic extraction of several cytostatics, intra-arterial chemotherapy for primary and secondary liver cancer is increasingly being used. Fully implantable drug delivery systems with portable or implantable pumps allow continuous infusion chemotherapy on an outpatient basis. Higher local drug concentration leads to better response and hepatic extraction minimizes systemic toxicity, thus increasing patients' quality of life. During the last 3½ years we have treated 19 patients with liver metastases of colorectal origin with intra-arterial chemotherapy (5-fluorouracil 1 g/m^2 per 24 h; dose escalated to 2.5 g per 24 h by continuous infusion for 5 days followed by a single mitomycin C dose of 10 mg/m^2 administered by 2 h infusion). The cycles were repeated every 6-8 weeks. Of 14 fully evaluable patients with a total of 124 chemotherapy cycles, seven experienced mild nausea and two had moderate local pain and mucositis. Catheter-related complications comprised seven occlusions (five reversible, two irreversible) and one dislocation. One complete remission (normal CEA, negative CT scan) lasting for 6 months and seven partial remissions were seen. Median survival has not yet been reached at 16 months; maximal survival is 36 months. Treatment was fairly well tolerated and only one patient refused continuation of treatment. Death was always attributed to rapid extrahepatic progression; none of the patients had liver failure.

Intraperitoneal chemotherapy should be considered for patients with peritoneal carcinomatosis with or without malignant ascites. Limited experience showed good tolerance of 2 g 5-fluorouracil given as a weekly intraperitoneal infusion with 100 ml physiological saline. Rapid disappearance of malignant ascites was noted in a young patient with disseminated mucinous carcinoma of the appendix.

Because regional chemotherapeutic approaches are still considered experimental, they should be restricted to prospective controlled clinical trials.

Intractable malignant ascites can also be alleviated by the insertion of peritoneovenous catheters (Denver Shunt, LeVeen Shunt). Initial experience in six patients with ascites and cancer not responsive to systemic therapy showed good palliation and a median patency duration of 6 months. We recommend complete paracentesis at the time of surgical placement of the peritoneovenous catheter to avoid fluid overload and shower of protein products. In addition, we use peroperative heparinization and subsequent anticoagulation to prevent disseminated intravascular coagulation. The following are not considered good candidates for peritoneovenous shunt for palliation of malignant ascites: patients with high ascitic fluid protein content (>4.5 g/liter), with a large number of malignant cells ($>10^6$/ml), with loculated ascites, with peritoneal mesothelioma, or with prior severe renal or cardiac disease [7, 8].

Feeding tubes are inserted to provide continuous enteral nutrition in the case of obstructing upper gastrointestinal tumors. Esophageal tubes (Celestin, Häring) allow oral intake and swallowing of liquids and semisolids and can be placed under local anesthesia through flexible endoscopes. Gastrostomy tubes can now be inserted without laparotomy by percutaneous placement of a small balloon catheter into the inflated and illuminated stomach under direct visual gastroscopic control (Vestweber KH, personal communication).

We have used a modified technique of needle catheter jejunostomy for enteral feeding immediately following cancer surgery to allow adequate nutritional support in the early postoperative period following major resection for upper digestive tract neoplasms. There has been no catheter-related morbidity or mortality, and, if needed, enteral artificial feeding with low residue whole diet solution could be applied over a prolonged period without increasing morbidity [9]. Enteral nutrition following cancer surgery is safe, more effective, physiological, and less expensive compared to the parenteral route.

A few centers are testing the value of intraoperative radiation therapy for pancreatic, gastric, and pelvic tumors. The placement of interstitial implants is also being used for residual or nonresectable tumors at laparotomy. At every laparotomy, the surgeon should perform adequate staging for calculation of prognosis and planning of subsequent combined modality treatment.

Conclusions

The vast majority of surgical interventions for gastrointestinal cancer are palliative procedures either by intent or as a result of the ultimate course of the disease. Due to the very limited efficacy of other treatment modalities, surgery offers the best palliation for a selected group of patients. The primary aim of surgery is the restoration of regular alimentary passage and the relief of tumor-related symptoms. Modern surgery is expanding its capacity for palliation through various innovative approaches to alleviate symptoms of the disease and side-effects of treatment and to prevent emergency situations.

Looking to the future, more effective cytotoxic drugs are urgently needed as well as sophisticated radiation procedures, e.g., intraoperative radiation, brachytherapy, and high-energy heavy particle beam sources, to be integrated into combined modality strategies.

References

1. Gubéran E (1980) Tendances de la mortalité en Suisse, 3. Tumeurs: 1921-1978. Schweiz Med Wochenschr 110 [Suppl 11]: 1-18
2. Fielding JWL, Roginski C, Ellis DJ, Jones BG, Powell J, Waterhouse JA, Brooks VS (1984) Clinicopathological staging of gastric cancer. Br J Surg 71: 677-680
3. Clarke DN, Jones PF, Needham CD (1980) Outcome in colorectal carcinoma: seven-year study of a population. Br Med J 280: 431-435
4. Brugger JJ, Metzger U, Largiadèr F (1985) Karzinomchirurgie heute: Analyse der Komplikationsrate und der Letalität bei 1000 konsekutiven Fällen. Schweiz Rundschau Med (Praxis) 74: 145-148
5. Adson MA, Van Heerden JA (1980) Major hepatic resection for metastatic colorectal cancer. Ann Surg 191: 576-580
6. Fortner JG, Maclean BJ, Kim DK, Howland WS, Turnbull AD, Goldiner P (1981) The seventies evolution in liver surgery for cancer. Cancer 47: 2162-2166
7. Quazi R, Savlov ED (1982) Peritoneovenous shunt for palliation of malignant ascites. Cancer 49: 600-602
8. Souter RG, Wells C, Tarin D, Kettlewell MGW (1985) Surgical and pathologic complications associated with peritoneovenous shunts in management of malignant ascites. Cancer 55: 1973-1978
9. Mona D, Metzger U, Geroulanos S, Uhlschmid G (1983) A modified technique of needle catheter jejunostomy for enteral artificial feeding following cancer surgery. J Exp Clin Cancer Res 3: 299-302

Surgical Supportive Care in Pediatric Oncology

J. Plaschkes

Kinderklinik, Inselspital, Universität Bern, 3010 Bern, Switzerland

It is not easy to define supportive care precisely and to draw a clear distinction between aspects relating to it and others relating to actual treatment. It is also difficult to deal with the subject systematically, so that selected examples are provided to illustrate some of the topics.

From a pragmatic point of view there are essentially two different types of consideration for the surgeon. On the one hand there are the *purely technical ones*, and on the other the more *general ones*. Both are equally important in providing support to the child with cancer and to his whole family in the extremely difficult situation they have to face [1].

General Aspects

Continuity of Care

The complicated and often painful measures and procedures in treating malignancies can only be sustained if the patient has a reasonable measure of confidence in the doctor. One of the important ways of maintaining this confidence is to ensure continuity of care throughout. For the surgeon this means essentially that all procedures (biopsy, operation, etc.) and their explanations should be carried out by the same person. The hierarchical structure of surgical departments and the demands of teaching render this difficult, but it makes a significant contribution to the success or failure of the whole venture and should be given due priority over other considerations.

Postoperative Support

In children it is frequently necessary to use restrictive measures such as bed rest and immobilization to protect the operative results. One should make a special effort each time to determine whether all the measures are absolutely essential. With

Recent Results in Cancer Research, Vol. 108

a modicum of thought and more flexibility it is possible to reduce these measures to a minimum or at least to make them more tolerable. Ingenuity is the key to success here.

Technical Aspects

Quality of Life

Many of the apparently purely technical aspects of surgery can in fact help to improve quality of life in the widest sense.

Venous Access for Treatment and Nutrition

In all meetings on supportive care pride of place is given to this subject. The indications, advantages, and risks of the various implantable devices or open-ended catheters have been exhaustively discussed [2]. For this reason, and not because they are unimportant, they will not be discussed further.

Some of the difficulties and pitfalls we have encountered recently using the implantable Port-a-Gath system in selected patients will be mentioned here. As a rule we try and introduce the central catheter via the subclavian vein by a Seldinger-type puncture technique. The "peel away sheath" system has caused some difficulties due to the relative thinness of the sheath and buckling if the introduction needs too much force. We now use a more rigid sheath which does not peel away and find this better. In the selected children we have encountered more difficulties in introducing the catheter than expected and have thought that venous anomalies might be the problem. A recent case in which an angiogram was performed because of such difficulties revealed a thrombosis of the left innominate vein (Fig. 1). As seen from the collateral circulation, it would have been dangerous to place another catheter on the right side in this situation because thrombosis of this side would have blocked all venous return from the head.

The message is that in patients who have already had numerous intravenous treatments or previous central catheters (the selection criteria in our patients), such unexpected blockages may be more common than has been realized. With the modern safer digital angiographic techniques there may be a place for more routine angiograms in such patients.

Protection of Organs from Radiation

A number of surgical maneuvers are useful for protecting various organs in the field of radiation. The gonads are the main ones requiring protection. Ovaries can be fixed medially or laterally by well established techniques used extensively in Hodgin's disease [3]. It has been shown that fertility can be maintained with these techniques and it does not seem necessary to put the ovaries back in their normal position at the end of treatment [4]. The testes can be placed in the thigh if the

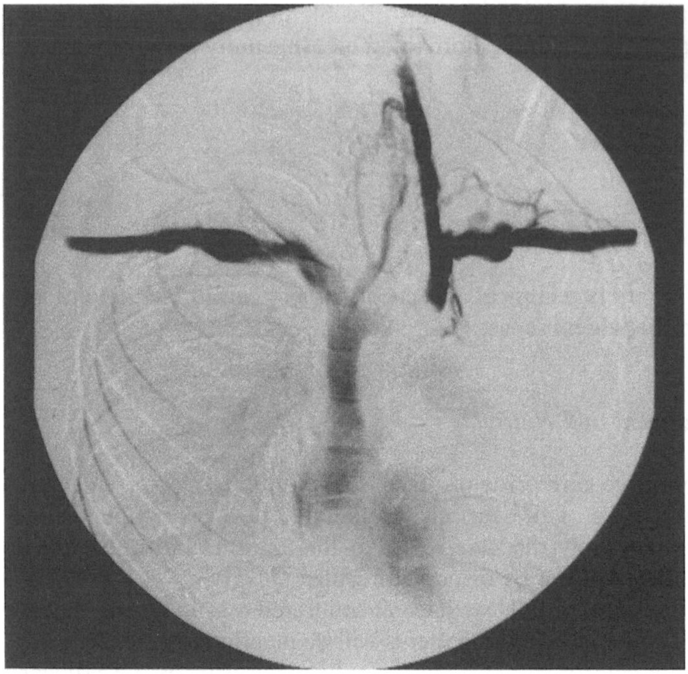

Fig. 1. Obstructive thrombosis of left innominate vein

scrotum has to be irradiated. In this situation it is obviously necessary to return the testes to the scrotum. This is made much easier if the cord is wrapped in a Silastic sheath at the first operation, a technique we have used a number of times.

It is also possible to displace the lungs or intestine to avoid direct radiation. Various nets of nonabsorbable or absorbable material have been used for this purpose. One of the best techniques is to use inflatable Silastic bags, often employed in plastic surgery as tissue expanders [5].

Treatment of Complications

A not infrequent complication of chemotherapy is extravasation of drugs which cause skin and tissue necrosis. Immediate surgical evacuation is the best treatment. This type of necrosis can be prevented by a simple incision made as soon as possible; the result of such an incision is usually excellent.

Function- and Organ-Preserving Surgery

One cannot discuss support and quality of life without mentioning some of the more conservative, functional organ-preserving operations that are now possible, particularly in the solid tumors of childhood which frequently respond to chemo-

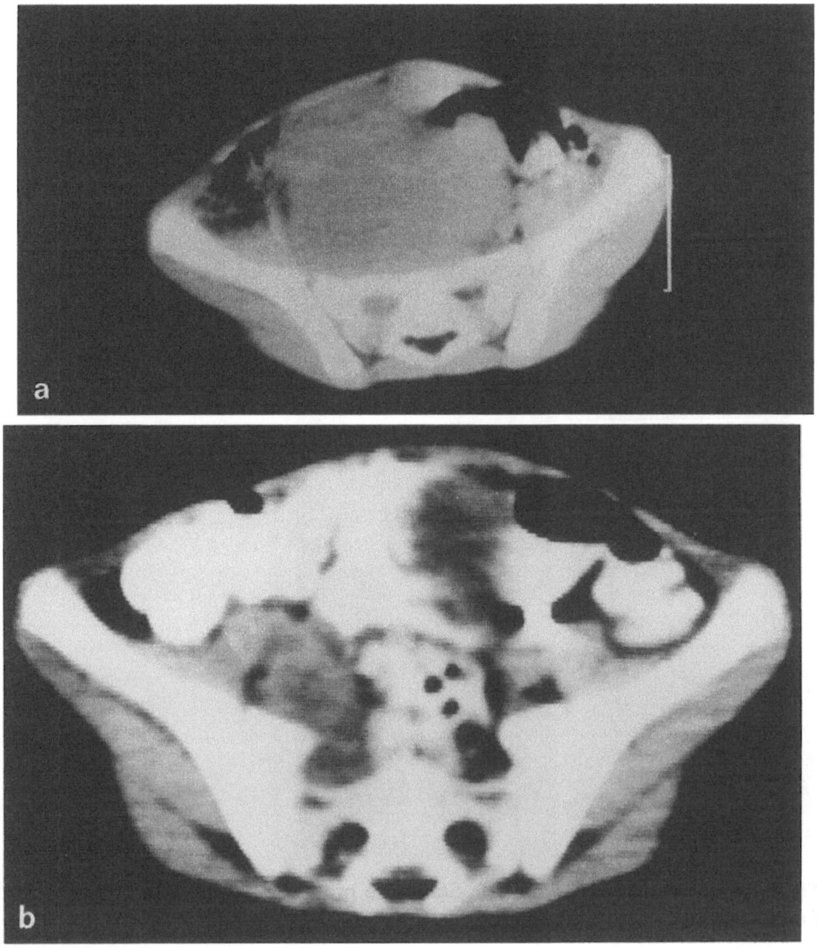

Fig. 2. **a** Large pelvic tumor before chemotherapy CT-scan. **b** Regression of tumor after chemotherapy CT-scan

therapy much more dramatically than those seen in adults. Two groups of tumors are particularly suitable for this type of surgery, where nowadays preoperative chemotherapy is the rule rather than the exception. These are the *rhabdomyosarcomas of the pelvic region and urogenital tract* [6] and *bone tumors of the extremities* [7, 8, 9].

A large pelvic rhabdomyosarcoma treated with preoperative chemotherapy can become much smaller and more localized and can be excised without sacrificing the bladder or other organs (Figs. 2).

Amputation of an extremity for osteosarcoma or Ewing's sarcoma can be avoided with a localized resection and replacement with a custom-made expandable "growing" prosthesis specially designed for children (Fig. 3).

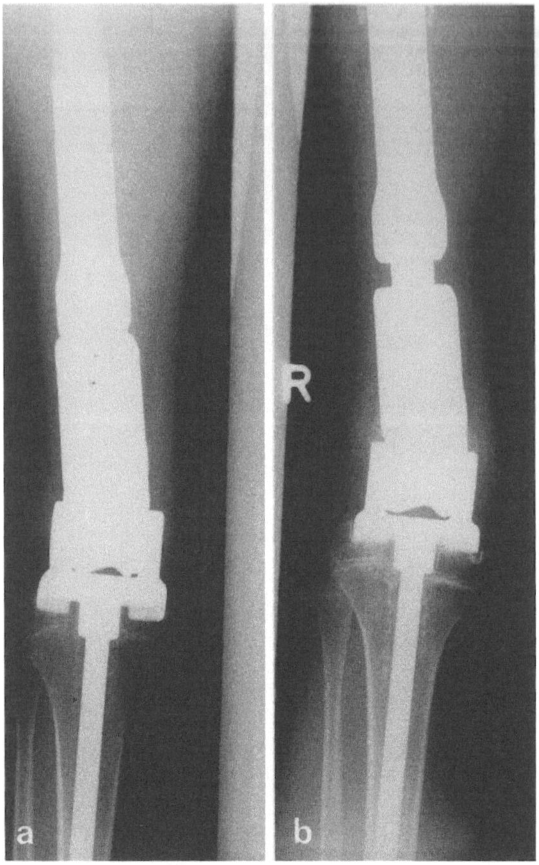

Fig. 3. **a** "Growing" custom-made Stanmore prothesis before extension. **b** Prothesis after first extension

Summary and Conclusion

An attempt has been made to describe some of the more practical surgical concepts and techniques which are used in pediatric surgical oncology. They do not fall into a coherent logical sequence and are not particularly specific to the cancer patient. But they do have one thing in common, namely they can all help to give more support to the child and his family. It should be clear that interaction between the doctor and the patient is also important. The support of one depends to a large extent on the support of the other.

References

1. Plaschkes J (1986) Surgical oncology in children. In: Voute PA, Barrett A, Bloom MJG, Lemerle J, Niedhardt MV (eds) Cancer in children. Clinical management. Springer, Berlin Heidelberg New York Tokyo, pp 46-53
2. Van der Stack F, Bokkerink T, Lippens R, Severijnen R (1986) Totally implantable systems for intravenous drug delivery. Experiences in children with cancer. Z Kinderchir 41: 39-42
3. Nahhas WA, Nisce LZ, D'Angio GJ, Lewis JL (1971) Lateral ovarian displacement. Obstet Gynecol 38: 785-788
4. Horning S, Hope RT, Kaplan HS (1981) Female reproductive potential after treatment for Hodgkin's disease. N Engl J Med 304: 1377-1321
5. Sasaki GH (1985) Tissue expansion, guidelines and case analysis. Dow Corning
6. Hays DM (1985) The surgical approach to sarcomas of children and young adults. Preservation of organs and function. In: D'Angio GJ, Evans AE (eds) Bone tumours and soft tissue sarcomas. Arnold, London, pp 94-104
7. Rao BN, Champion JE, Pratt CB et al. (1985) Limb salvage procedures for children with osteosarcoma. An alternative to amputation. J Pediatr Surg 18: 901-908
8. Scales JT (1983) Bone and joint replacement for the preservation of limbs. Br J Hosp Med 29: 220-232
9. Plaschkes J, Bettex M (1986) Glied- und organerhaltende Operationen bei malignen soliden Tumoren im Kindesalter. Ther Rundschau 49: 824-828

Prognostic Significance of Nutritional Status in Cancer Surgery

P. Schlag, T. Fritz, and T. Hölting

Chirurgische Klinik, Sektion für chirurgische Onkologie, Universität Heidelberg, Im Neuenheimer Feld 110, 6900 Heidelberg, FRG

Malnutrition is a common accompaniment of malignant disease [5, 9]. The presence of nutritional deficiencies in patients for whom surgical therapy is indicated is of clinical importance because a relationship between the existence of such deficiencies and the occurrence of postoperative morbidity and mortality is assumed. Based on this premise the need for perioperative intensive nutritional repletion in malnourished cancer patients was established [1, 2, 10]. Only a few studies demonstrated that preoperative total parenteral nutrition reduced postoperative complication rates in cancer surgery. The available data are inconclusive and might be influenced by patient selection [8, 11, 12]. Further, the retrospective approach in most of the reported studies is questionable [4, 6, 7]. The problems related to these trials mainly concern the identification of the surgical cancer patient in need of supportive nutrition. Various parameters like secretory proteins, delayed hypersensitivity skin test, and skinfold thickness are taken to be of relevance to the nutritional status of the patient [7]. Buzby et al. described a computer-generated regression equation designed to predict the risk of postoperative complications [3]. This parameter is called the *Prognostic Nutritional Index (PNI)*. The PNI includes serum albumin and transferrin concentration, triceps skinfold thickness, and delayed hypersensitivity skin test reactivity. Our objective was to test in a prospective trial the validity of the single nutrition-related factors as well as the whole model in predicting the operative risk in GI tract cancer patients.

Material and Methods

From March 1986 through January 1987 a total of 133 consecutive patients with histologically proven GI tract malignancies who underwent gastrointestinal cancer surgery were included in this study. The different diagnostic groups are depicted in Table 1. Within 24 h of referral to the hospital, patients underwent nutritional assessment including anthropometrics (triceps skinfold thickness), measures of secretory protein status (total serum protein, serum albumin, and serum transferrin), and delayed hypersensitivity skin test (Multitest, Institut Mérieux, Lyon, France). Based on these data the PNI was calculated as reported elsewhere [3, 11]. No par-

Recent Results in Cancer Research, Vol. 108

Table 1. Diagnostic groups

	All patients	Patients with extensive or major operative procedures
Esophageal cancer	14	14
Gastric cancer	33	28
Colon cancer	24	18
Rectal cancer	32	30
Prim. and sec. liver cancer	30	14
Total	133	104

Table 2. Operative treatment groups

Extensive operative procedures	*43*
Esophagectomy	14
Abdominothoracic gastric resection	8
Total gastrectomy	16
Hemihepatectomy	5
Major operative procedures	*61*
Subtotal gastrectomy	4
Hemicolectomy	18
Anterior resection	15
Miles procedures	15
Segmental liver resection	9
Minor operative procedures	*29*

enteral or specific nutrition was administered preoperatively to change the nutritional status of the patients but substitution for electrolytes, hemoglobin, or albumin was obligatory in those with deficient parameters. The different operative procedures performed are shown in Table 2. To exclude other interrelationships only one surgeon (P. S.) was involved, and perioperative treatment was standardized. Antibiotic prophylaxis was administered on the day of the operation in all large procedures. The clinical course of all operated patients was monitored for objective complications until death or discharge from the hospital. Clinical signs of septic complications were continuing fever, leukocytosis, and local signs of inflammation. Wound infections and deep or intra-abdominal abscesses were proved on culture and required pus drainage. Pneumonia was defined as fever and evidence of pulmonary infiltrate on roentgenograms, with a requirement for antibiotic therapy. A tracheal smear was not always taken. Statistical analysis was performed by the Wilcoxon rank sum test, the chi-square test, and the Armitage linear trend test. Significance was set at $P<0.05$.

Results

During the postoperative course, 38 of the 133 patients suffered from postoperative complications. This corresponds to a total morbidity of 29%, including 15%

Table 3. Postoperative morbidity and mortality

Complications	Number	Deaths
Wound infection	12	–
Intraabdominal abscess	6	–
Anastomotic leakage	8	1
Severe pneumonia	7	–
Organ insufficiency	5	1
Total	38/133 (29%)	2/133 (1.5%)

Table 4. Occurrence and severity of complications in relation to age

	Median age	±	SD
No complications	59.9		13.5
Minor complications	61.3		9.7
Major complications	53.7		14.7

Table 5. Complication rate according to operative procedure

	Minor operations	Major or extensive operations
Major complications	1/28	19/104
Major complications	–	18/104
Total	1/28 (4%)	37/104 (36%)

Table 6. Summary of the nutritional parameters

	Mean	±	SD
Albumin (g/liter)	40.1	±	4.8
Transferrin (mg/dl)	275.4	±	111.1
Skinfold (mm)	7.8	±	6.1
Multitest (score)	1.8	±	1.8
PNI (%)	18.1	±	27.3

minor and 14% major complications. The different complications are listed in Table 3. There was no correlation between complication rate and age of the patients (Table 4). As expected, an obvious relationship existed between the extent of the chosen surgical procedure and postoperative morbidity (Table 5).

On the average the different nutritional parameters were within the normal range, though with a high individual variation (Table 6). The PNI of the analyzed patients corresponded to a left-shifted Gaussian curve (Fig. 1). Patients with progressed disease usually had worse nutritional parameters but it has to be kept in mind that in most of these patients less invasive and nonresecting operations were

Table 7. PNI distribution according to operative procedure

	No.	PNI		
		Mean	±	SD
Minor operations	29	32	±	21
Major operations	104	13	±	28

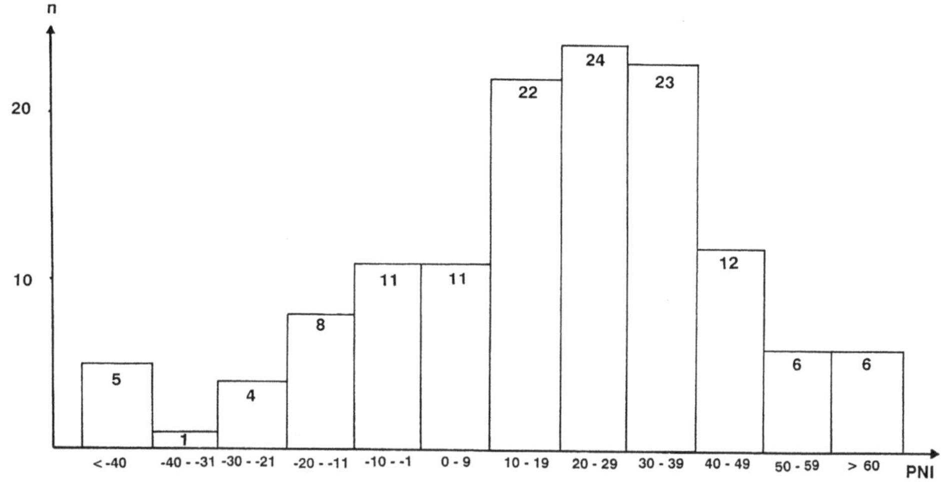

Fig. 1. PNI distribution ($n=133$)

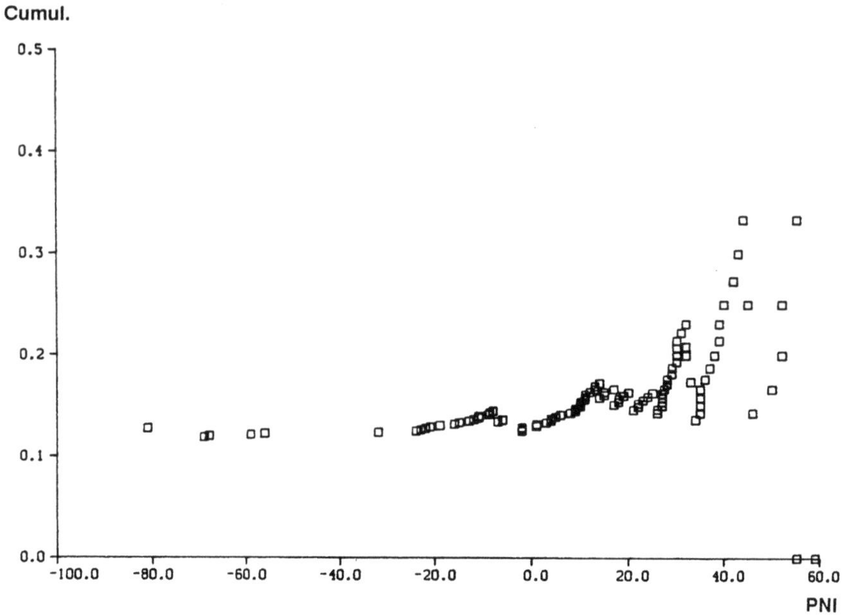

Fig. 2. Cumulative complication rate according to the PNI

performed (Table 7). These two factors are therefore dependent on each other, and the correlation between the rate of postoperative complications and nutritional parameters had to be stratified for the different kinds of operation. The complication rate in the group of minor surgical procedures was only 1 in 28, so that a correlation to patient's nutritional status could not be determined. Thus it was of great interest whether a correlation could be established in the group with major operations, where nearly all the complications were seen. The analysis of the different investigated parameters alone did not show a correlation with the postoperative complication rate. Multifactorial analysis according to the PNI, however, showed another result: While the complication rate in cases with PNI levels less than 40 was constantly low, an increasing number of complications could be seen in patients with PNI levels more than 40 (Fig. 2). Nevertheless, it was again not possible to show a statistically significant relationship because the group of patients with PNI over 40 was too small in our cohort.

Discussion

The postoperative complication rate is influenced by several different parameters [7]. The aim of our analysis was to determine the significance of the nutritional status and whether these factors influence postoperative morbidity and mortality. We therefore tried to keep other influencing factors like the involved surgeon, pre- and postoperative therapy, and primary disease quite constant to permit comparison. This is something which has not been considered sufficiently in recent trials, so that the correlation seen there cannot be regarded as conclusive [4, 6, 8, 11].

Previous studies have shown that nutritional parameter deteriorate with progressive disease, especially when there is metastatic spread [5, 9]. We observed this in our trial, too. Our patients, however, had a much better preoperative condition than those in other trials [3, 11]. Unlike former analyses, we could not show a strong correlation between nutritional parameters and postoperative complication rate. Only among those of severely malnourished patients (as defined according to the PNI) who underwent major surgery was there an increase in postoperative complications. The low complication rate in our patients and the small number of malnourished patients may be the reasons why we could not show a correlation, unlike Buzby et al. [3]. Thus to summarize it was not possible to correlate the preoperative nutritional status and the postoperative complication rate in general but only in patients with severe malnutrition who underwent major surgical procedures. Further, as already stated, in our study we did not generally use preoperative nutrition for malnourished patients but substitution of albumin or hemoglobin deficiency was obligatory. This might also have influenced our results. On the other hand, other underlying factors like the skill and experience of the surgeon and the severity of the operation are more important in predicting the risk of surgery. Our conclusion is that among surgical cancer patients, only in the severely malnourished, who were extremely rare in our patient cohort, might nutritional factors have an important influence on indication for therapy and therapy itself.

References

1. Askanazi J, Weissman CH, Rothkopf M, Starker PM (1987) Perioperative nutritional support. Nutr Int 3: 12-18
2. Brennan MF (1981) Total parenteral nutrition in the cancer patient. N Engl J Med 305: 375-382
3. Buzby GP, Mullen JL, Maathews DC, Hobbs CH, Rosato EF (1980) Prognostic nutritional index in gastrointestinal surgery. Am J Surg 139: 160-167
4. Heatley RV, Williams RHP, Lewis MH (1979) Preoperative intravenous feeding: a controlled trial. Postgrad Med J 55: 541-545
5. Heberer D, Byerly LO, Chlebowski RT (1985) Metabolic abnormalities in the cancer patients. Cancer 55: 225-229
6. Holter AR, Fischer MD (1977) The effects of perioperative hyperalimentation on complications in patients with carcinoma and weight loss. J Surg Res 23: 31-34
7. Meguid MM, Mughal M, Meguid V (1987) Risk benefit analysis of malnutrition and perioperative nutritional support: a review. Nutr Int 3: 25-34
8. Müller JM, Brenner U, Dienst C, Pichlmaier H (1982) Preoperative parenteral feeding in patients with gastrointestinal carcinoma. Lancet 9: 68-71
9. Shizgal HM (1985) Body composition of patients with malnutrition and cancer. Cancer 55: 250-253
10. Silberman H (1983) Preoperative nutrition therapy. West J Med 138: 248-249
11. Smale BF, Mullen JE, Buzby GP, Rosato EF (1981) The efficancy of nutritional assessment and support in cancer surgery. Cancer 47: 2375-2381
12. Thompson BR, Julian TB, Stremple JF (1981) Perioperative total parenteral nutrition in patients with gastrointestinal cancer. J Surg Res 30: 497-500

Surgical Management of Tumor-Related Limb Fractures

B. G. Weber

Orthopädie am Rosenberg, Rorschacher Straße 150, 9006 St. Gallen, Switzerland

Tumor manifestation in the skeleton may be isolated, multifocal, or disseminated, resulting in one or several fractures. If several fractures are present, they may have arisen at different times or simultaneously. Whenever tumor-related fractures occur, the patient suffers pain and loss of limb function. The treatment therefore concentrates on compensating for loss of function and relief of pain.

In fractures related to a benign tumor, the treatment must not merely aim for temporary restoration of function and transitory relief of pain, as, for instance, would be offered by total hip replacement in cases of fracture of the proximal femur caused by fibrous dysplasia. In fractures caused by benign tumors, reconstruction to restore normal anatomy must be the challenge of treatment, given that recurrence of the tumor is unlikely because the tumor mass is resected radically at the time of surgery. The operation consists as a rule in resection of the tumor mass and fixation of the destabilized bone (femur, tibia, humerus, or forearm) by metal plates or medullary nails and by compensation of bone defect with autologous bone grafts harvested from the patient's pelvis.

In fractures related to a malignant tumor, treatment must take into account all aspects of the given case, especially the patient's life expectancy. The better the prognosis, the more the treatment will focus on relief of pain and "prosthetic compensation" of the destabilized bone to enable the patient to ambulate (broken leg) or to use the arm again (broken humerus or forearm). In other words: if life expectancy is good, the treatment should be similar to that for fracture caused by a benign tumor. If life expectancy is limited, the treatment should offer maximum temporary efficiency with minimum burden for the patient, i.e., it should relieve pain immediately and enable the patient to be mobilized again. Quality of life is to be restored for the patient's expected duration of life.

The decision on the appropriate type of fracture treatment depends on the assessment of the patient's general condition. Such an assessment is made in teamwork between the oncologist, the radiologist, and the orthopedic surgeon. The specific problems facing the orthopedic surgeon, who should restore the broken bone and relieve local pain, are still complex once a decision is reached by the team: To fix rigidly a fracture due to malignant alteration of the bone, be it primary (osteosarcoma) or secondary (metastatic), requires special surgical techniques which are

Recent Results in Cancer Research, Vol. 108

not the same as for "normal" fractures. Tumor-altered bone does not have the same mechanical quality as normal broken bone; apart from metallic screws, plates, and nails, additional reinforcement is often required by means of "bone cement," i.e., methyl methacrylate, a material which is used in orthopedic surgery to fix artificial joints in cases of joint resection for degenerative joint disease. Moreover, tumor-altered bone does not have the same healing capacity as normal broken bone. Internal fixations of such fractures must therefore provide longlasting hold. They are more bulky than fixations for normal fractures, and are at risk of fatigue fracture if the bone itself never does unite owing to delayed fracture healing. When the patient lives long enough but the fracture does not unite at all, fatigue fracture of the metallic fixation will occur 1 or 2 years after the operation. Sometimes new internal fixation may become necessary.

With successful treatment of tumor-related fractures, the patient's quality of life, already overshadowed by the underlying disease, is dramatically improved, at least for a certain time (Fig. 1) and in most instances until death. With regard to such improvement in the quality of life, the restoration of the locomotor system is an important element.

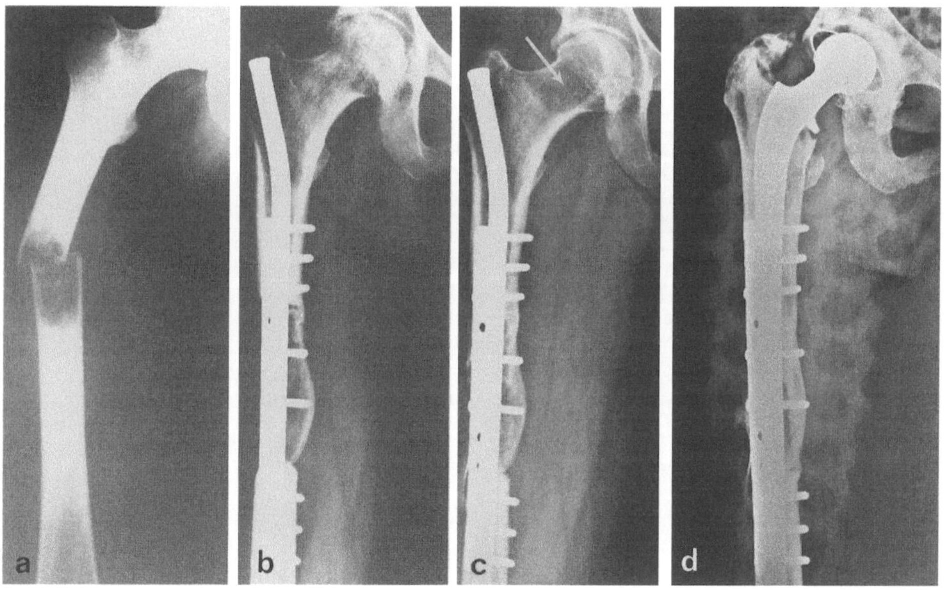

Fig. 1a–d. Tumor-related fracture and treatment. Pat. nr. 3209-3, 114.049, G. E., ♀, 48 years. **a** Metastatic fracture 1 month after nephrectomy for hypernephroma. **b** Tumor resection, internal fixation, and autologous grafting. **c** One year later new metastasis in the femoral neck (↗). **d** Two years after resection of the hip joint, after total hip replacement. The affected limb was free of pain with full function, allowing the lady to perform as a professional classic dancer until she died (4) years after the fracture owing to generalized metastases

Summary

Tumor-related fractures require internal rigid fixation with adapted surgical techniques in accordance with the altered bone quality. Internal fixation results in relief of pain and restoration of function, i. e., in walking capacity in the case of leg fractures and manual action in the case of arm fractures. Restoration of pain-free function in the case of tumor-related fractures is therefore an important part of the treatment of tumor patients.

Surgical Management of Tumor-Related Spinal Instability

F. Magerl and B. Jeanneret

Klinik für Orthopädische Chirurgie, Kantonsspital, 9007 St. Gallen, Switzerland

The majority of malignant tumors affecting the spine are metastases, breast cancer being the most common primary tumor [2, 6, 9]. The patients are usually elderly. Tumor invasion may result in pain, instability, or neurological deficit or all three. The goals of surgery are to provide pain relief, restore spinal stability, and enhance the chance of neurological recovery [1]. Surgery should facilitate nursing care and allow for early mobilization without cumbersome external support. In planning spinal surgery, a team approach which includes pathologists, oncologists, and radiotherapists as well as the surgeon is essential.

The surgical procedure may include decompression, tumor resection, and stabilization. When tumor invasion and/or decompression creates spinal instability, stabilization is mandatory. Surgery may be carried out via an anterior [2, 3, 5, 6, 7], posterior [4, 8, 9], or combined approach [1, 3, 5]. In the cervical spine, anterior techniques are usually employed, while in the thoracic and lumbar spine posterior techniques are preferred, as they are less traumatic. Combined approaches are sometimes indicated, in order to achieve sufficient stability. Bone loss is most often replaced by synthetic material. Metal implants are used for stabilization.

Postoperative management must include chemo- and/or radiotherapy as appropriate for the tumor type [9].

Material

Between 1964 and 1986, 64 patients (30 females and 34 males) with malignant spinal tumors were operated on at the Department for Orthopedic Surgery, Kantonsspital, St. Gallen. Most operations were performed by the senior author (F. M.). The charts of all patients were reviewed.

Results

The average age of the patients was 56 years (range: 24–82 years); the age distribution is shown in Fig. 1. Cancer of the breast was the most commonly encoun-

Recent Results in Cancer Research, Vol. 108

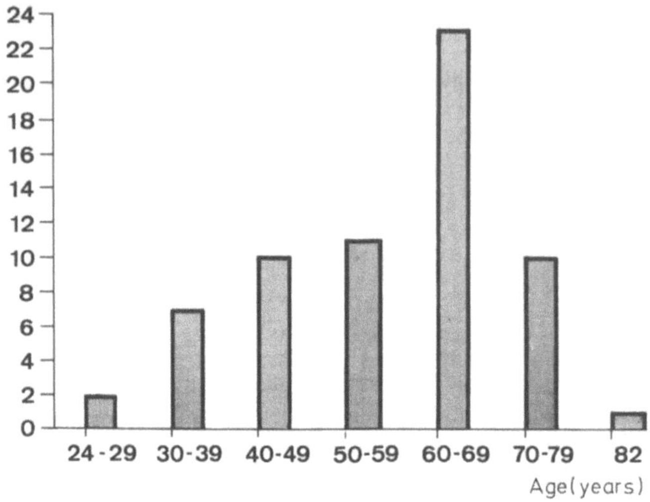

Fig. 1. Age distribution of the 64 patients

Table 1. Primary sites of the tumors

Carcinomas	No.	Other tumors	No.
Breast	19	Lymphoma	2
Renal	6	Plasmacytoma	7
Lung	5	Chordoma	3
Prostate	4	Chondrosarcoma	2
Thyroid	3	Others	3
Others	6		
Unknown	4		

tered tumor, followed by plasmacytomas and renal and lung tumors (Table 1). The distribution of the affected spinal level is shown in Fig. 2; the upper half of the cervical spine was very frequently affected. In 24 cases, the tumor involved more than one vertebra.

Six patients had previously been treated elsewhere by laminectomy; 26 had had chemo- and/or radiotherapy.

Indication for surgery was a neurological deficit in 45 patients. Nine had a radicular paresis, 30 an incomplete cord lesion, and six a complete cord lesion. Instability was present in 62 patients. All patients had pain. Walking was impaired in eight patients and impossible in 16 preoperatively.

Eighty-two operative procedures were performed in the 64 patients. Laminectomy without stabilization was performed in eight cases, a posterior stabilization with plates, wires, autologous bone graft, or methyl methacrylate in four, and a combination of both in ten. In 22 patients, anterior decompression and stabilization were accomplished by using autologous bone graft, methyl methacrylate, or

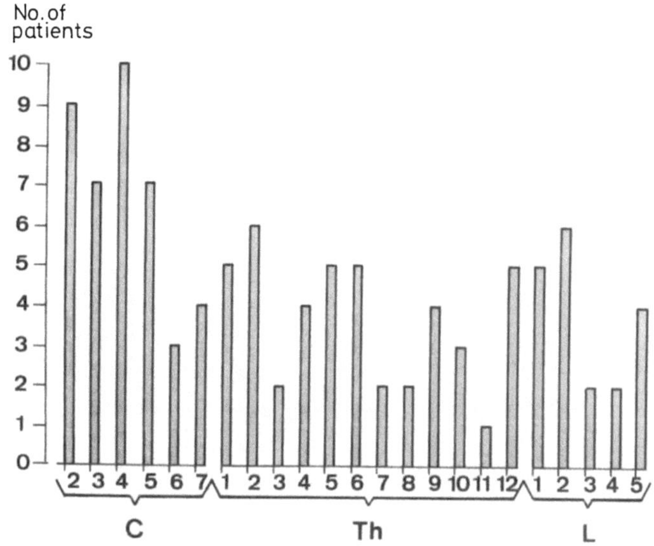

Fig. 2. Tumor distribution, C2-L5

hydroxyapatite with or without additional metal implants. In 13 patients anterior decompression and stabilization were performed, followed by a posterior stabilization (Figs. 3, 4). A posterior total vertebrectomy with stabilization was performed in seven patients (Fig. 5). Five patients received an occipitocervical composite fusion (Fig. 6).

Following surgery, the neurological status improved to normal in three patients, improved subtotally in 24, remained unchanged in 16, and deteriorated in two. Of the 24 patients with preoperative walking difficulties, seven improved to normal, 16 remained unchanged, and one was worse. Two nonambulators regained walking ability after the intervention; neither of them had a complete cord lesion preoperatively. All patients experienced substantial relief of pain.

Eight complications occurred in eight patients (two infections, two pulmonary embolisms, one myocardial infarction, one hematoma, and two cases of neurological deterioration), four of them resulting in death (one infection, two pulmonary embolisms, one myocardial infarction). The deaths occurred between the second week and the second month postoperatively. Only one death, namely the infection, could be attributed to the surgery itself.

Fifty-five patients succumbed to their disease with an average survival time of 15 months postoperatively. Seven patients remain alive with an average follow-up of 6 years (range: 3 months to 10 years). Two patients were lost to follow-up. A survivorship analysis is presented in Fig. 7. As the curve indicates, one-third of the patients lived longer than 1 year. The patients with plasmacytomas (mean survival time: 23 months) and cancer of the prostate (mean survival time: 26 months) had the best prognosis, while patients with carcinomas of the lung had the worst (mean survival time: 3 months). Patients with breast cancer had a mean survival time of 12 months.

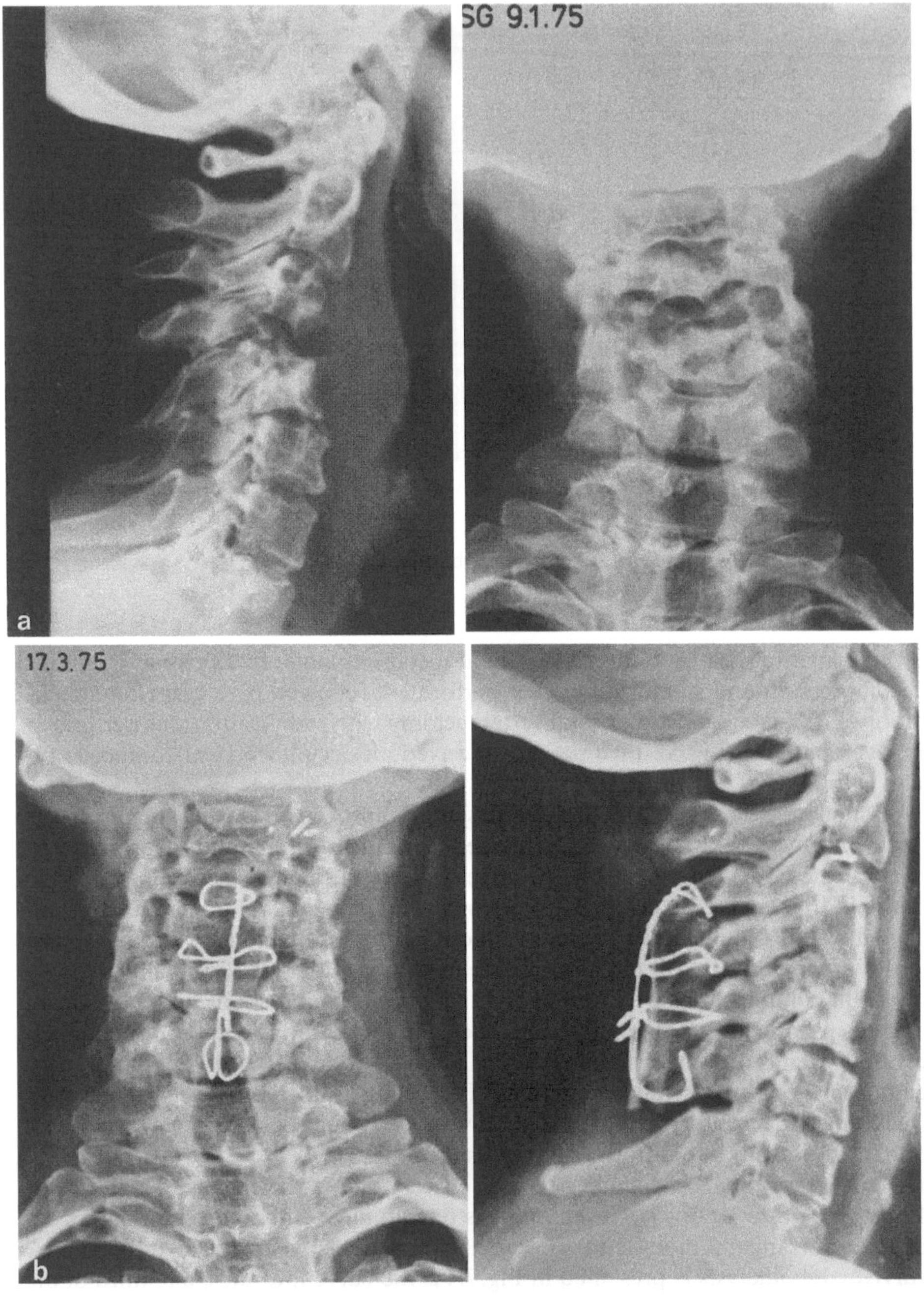

Fig. 3. In this 51-year-old woman with destruction of two cervical vertebrae caused by a rhabdomyosarcoma (**a**), combined anterior and posterior decompression and stabilization were employed (**b**). Autologous bone graft was used for the fusion, together with a posterior wire fixation. The fusion held and the root paresis resolved. The patient lived an additional 3 years without local recurrence

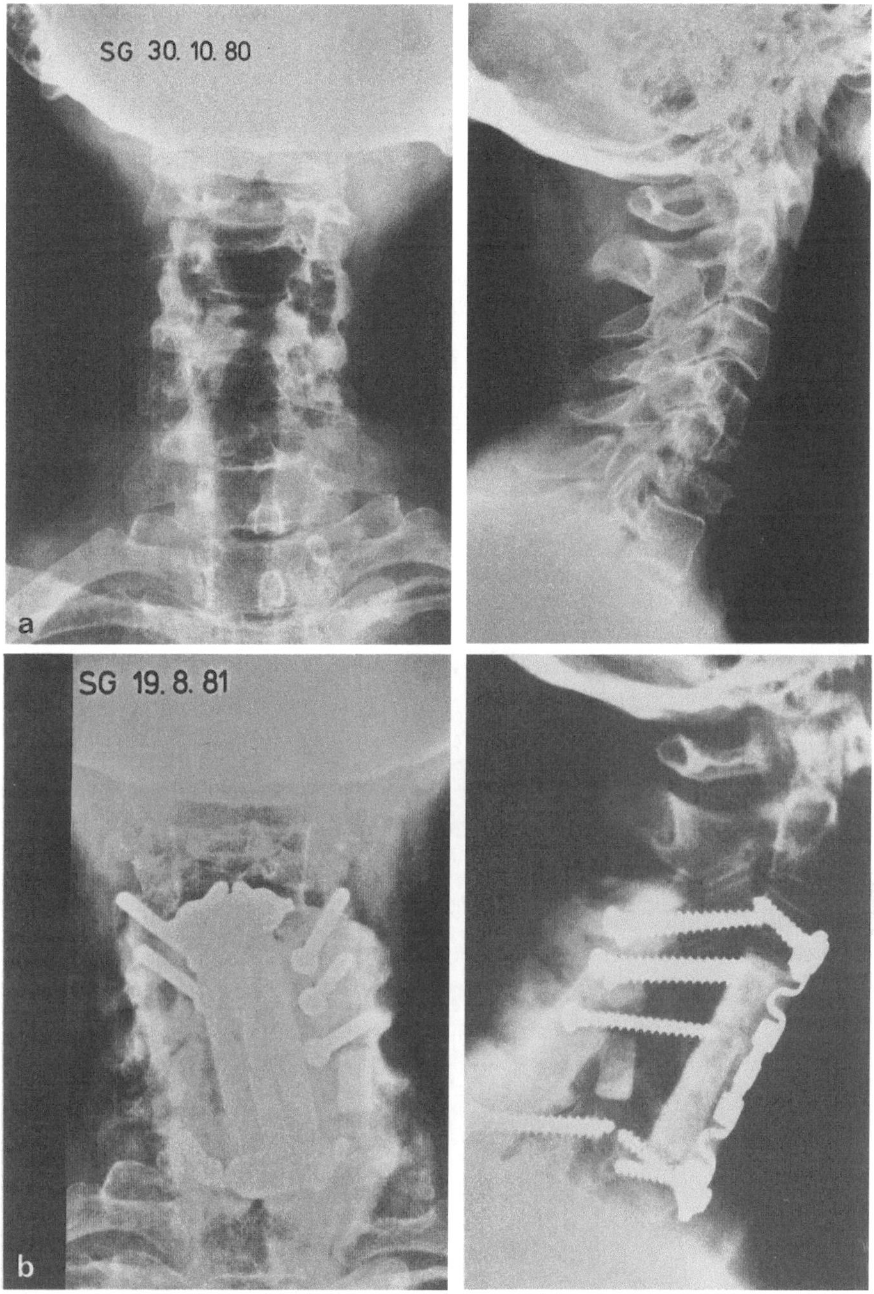

Fig. 4. A 44-year-old woman with anterior and posterior destruction of three cervical vertebrae and painful root paresis due to breast cancer (**a**). Anterior stabilization was achieved by an hydroxyapatite block and plate fixation. Posterior fixation was performed with methyl methacrylate anchored to facet screws (**b**)

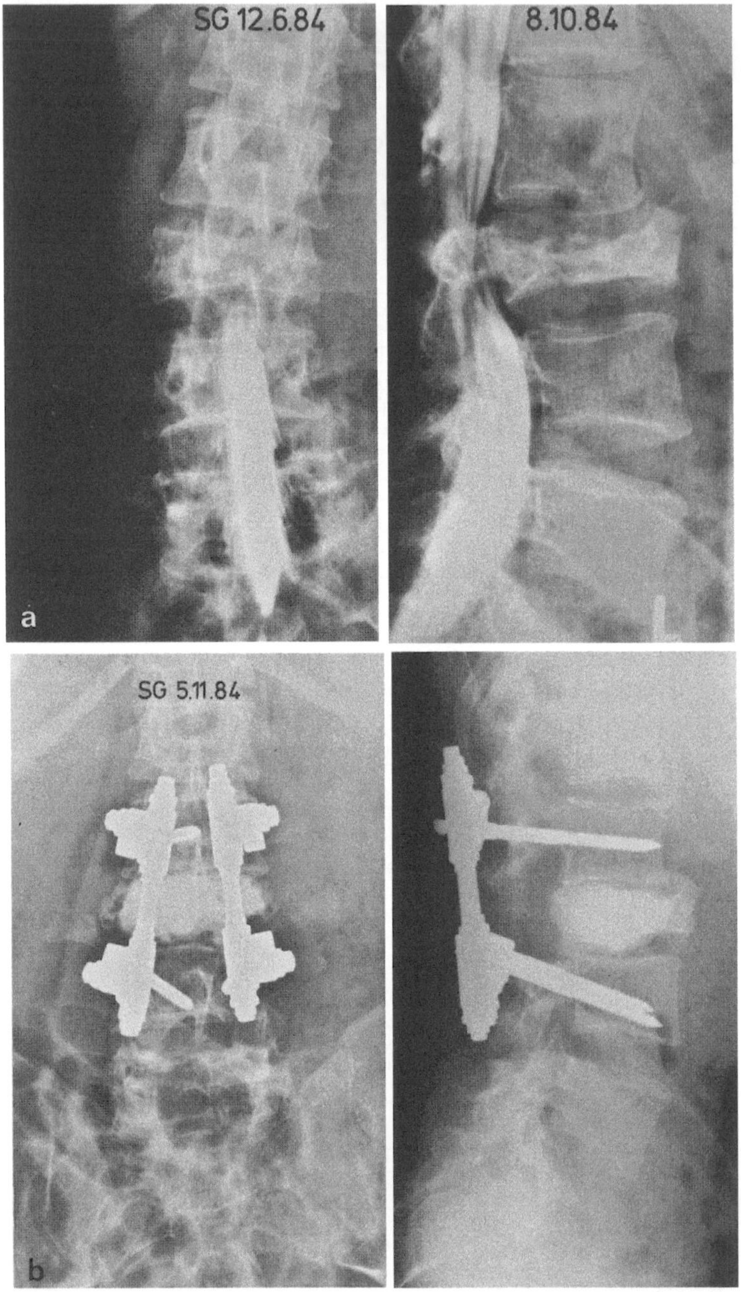

Fig. 5. A 37-year-old male with an incomplete cauda equina lesion due to metastatic lung carcinoma at L3 (**a**). A total vertebrectomy was performed from dorsally: the posterior vertebral elements were exposed and removed by a standard midline approach, the soft tissues retracted, and the vertebral body resected in piecemeal fashion. Following this, the resulting space between the adjacent vertebral bodies was filled with methyl methacrylate. Stabilization was completed by an internal fixator (**b**)

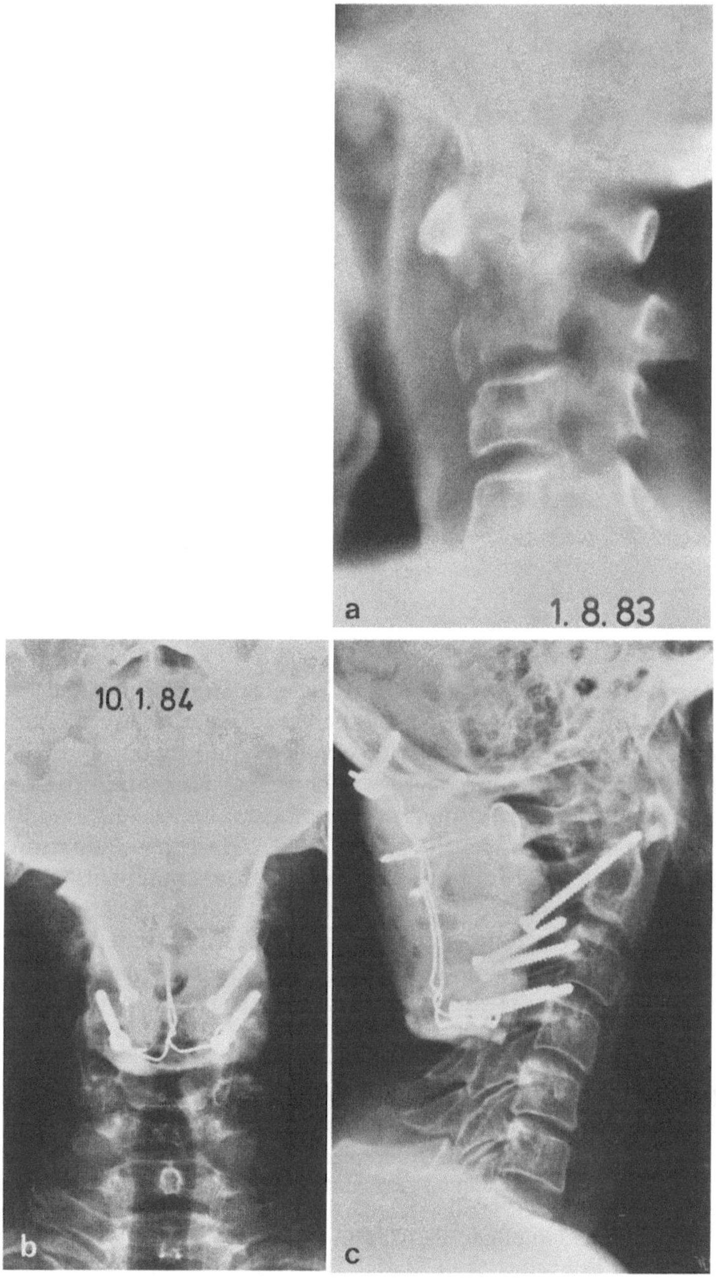

Fig. 6. A 60-year-old male with severe pain caused by destruction of C2 due to metastatic prostate carcinoma (**a**). Composite posterior fusion from the occiput to C4 with methyl methacrylate restored spinal stability (**b, c**). Complete pain relief allowed the patient to resume his work for 1 year

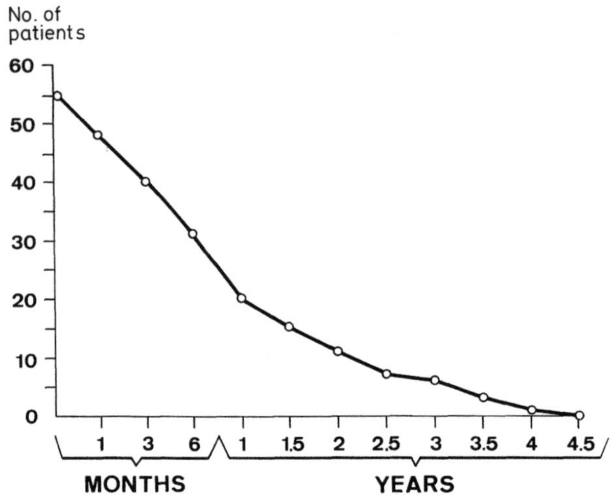

Fig. 7. Survival rate according to length of time after operation (55 patients). This figure concepts only patients who died before follow-up. At that time, 7 patients were still alive

Discussion

The survival time of our patients reflects the benefit of surgery combined with the contribution of chemo- and radiotherapy in cases where the tumor was amenable to this treatment. We feel that the quality of the remaining lifetime can be substantially improved by proper surgery; however, this is hard to quantitate in a retrospective study. Improvement of neurological deficit (e.g., regaining the ability to walk) certainly improves the quality of life. However, patients in whom neurological deficit does not improve also benefit from spinal surgery since it contributes substantially to pain reduction and facilitates nursing care.

At the present time, sufficient decompression and stabilization are practically always achievable by modern surgical techniques. Therefore, this surgery plays an important role in the supportive treatment of cancer patients.

References

1. DeWald RL, Bridwell KH, Prodromas C, Rodts MF (1985) Reconstructive spinal surgery as palliation for metastatic malignancies of the spine. Spine 10: 21–26
2. Fidler MW (1985) Pathological fractures of the cervical spine: palliative surgical treatment. J Bone Joint Surg [Br] 67: 352–357
3. Johnson LR, Leatherman KD, Holt RT (1983) Anterior decompression of the spinal cord for neurological deficit. Spine 8: 396–405
4. Jomin M, Lesoin F, Rousseaux M, Villette L, Autricque A (1985) Abord direct des métastases rachidiennes dorso-lombaires par voie postéro-latérale. J Chir (Paris) 122: 573–575
5. Kostuik JP (1983) Anterior spinal cord decompression for lesions of the thoracic and lumbar spine, techniques, new methods of internal fixations, results. Spine 8: 512–531
6. Onimus M, Schraub S, Bertin D, Bosset JF, Guidet M (1985) Le traitement du cancer secondaire du rachis. Rev Chir Orthop 71: 473–482

7. Polster J, Brinckmann P (1977) Ein Wirbelkörperimplantat zur Verwendung bei Palliativoperationen an der Wirbelsäule. Z Orthop 115: 118-122
8. Roy-Camille R, Saillant G, Bisserié M, Judet T, Hautefort E, Mamoudy P (1981) Résection vertébrale totale dans la chirurgie tumorale au niveau du rachis dorsal par voie postérieure pure. Rev Chir Orthop 67: 421-430
9. Roy-Camille R, Saillant G, Lapresle P, Mazel C, Mariambourg G (1985) Traitement chirurgical des métastases du rachis par stabilisation à l'aide de plaques postérieures vissées dans les pédicules vertébraux. Rev Chir Orthop 71: 483-492

Indications for and Results of Nutritional Therapy in Cancer Patients

G. Ollenschläger, K. Konkol, and B. Mödder

Medizinische Universitätsklinik II, Poliklinik, Joseph-Stelzmann-Straße 9, 5000 Köln 41, FRG

Malnutrition is one of the typical consequences of tumor burden and tumor therapy. Its first clinical manifestations are weight loss in adults and failure to gain weight in children. The etiology of cancer patients' malnutrition is multifactorial, and, as yet, incompletely understood.

Different factors may induce or maintain catabolism in the tumor-bearing organism, e.g., anorexia, dysphagia, oral and gastrointestinal lesions, due to tumor infiltration or antineoplastic therapy, vomiting, diarrhea, malassimilation, and hypermetabolism (Table 1). Anorexia is regarded to be the main problem. The spontaneous oral intake of nutrients is often inadequate during the progress of the disease, either in terms of sufficient supply or relative to increased protein and energy demand.

The mediators leading to early satiety or aversion to specific meals, tastes, or smell or to eating as a whole are not exactly known. In recent years, endorphins as well as imbalances of neutral amino acids with special regard to the central nervous serotoninergic and dopaminergic system have been discussed as factors which may modify appetite [12, 21].

Beside tumor-induced anorexia, one can differentiate between therapy-induced and psychogenic anorexia. Appetite may be influenced by mental stress,

Table 1. Etiology of cachexia

Inadequate Substrate		
Intake	Loss	Metabolism
Starvation	Vomiting	Hypermetabolism
Anorexia	Diarrhea	Catabolism
Pain	Malassimilation	Liver insufficiency
Oral lesions	Protein-losing gastroenteropathies	Inherited enzymatic defects
Dysphagia	Nephrotic syndrome	
GI obstruction	Consuming diseases	
Neurological/psychiatric syndroms	Drainages/dialysis	

Recent Results in Cancer Research, Vol. 108

from which tumor patients very often suffer. In these situations, e.g., fear of outcome or side-effects of tumor therapy, most of the patients are not able to eat sufficiently [5, 14, 20].

Tumor therapy is a relevant inducer of anorexia. During the perioperative period the patients are not allowed or are unable to eat adequately. Postoperative complications may delay the beginning of spontaneous oral intake. Depending on the type of surgical intervention, nutrient absorption may be reduced (Table 2).

Radiation therapy, especially of the oral cavity, the head and neck region, and the small bowel, may lead to reduced oral intake as a consequence of anorexia, mucositis, dysphagia, or abdominal pain [20, 26] (Table 3).

In most cases oncological chemotherapy leads to anorexia, nausea, or vomiting, and it quite often induces mucositis (Table 4). The decrease in spontaneous oral intake is of great relevance for those patients who are treated with chemother-

Table 2. Effects of radical resection leading to malnutrition

Resected organs	Effects
Oral cavity, pharynx	Dependence on tube feeding
Esophagus	Vagotomy:
	gastric stasis
	fat malabsorption
Stomach	Dumping syndrome
	Anorexia
	Fat malabsorption
	Generalized malabsorption
	Blind loop syndrome
Small intestine	Fat to generalized malabsorption
Pancreas	Fat malabsorption
	Insulin deficiency
Colon	Water and electrolyte loss

Table 3. Localized effects of radiotherapy leading to malnutrition

Region	Effects
Central nervous system	Nausea
	Vomiting
Head and neck	Loss of taste
	Loss of smell
	Anorexia
	Mucositis
	Dysphagia
Thorax	Dysphagia
Abdomen/pelvis	Nausea
	Vomiting
	Anorexia
	Enteritis
	Diarrhea

Table 4. Localized effects of oncological chemotherapy leading to malnutrition

Region	Effects
Central nervous system	Nausea Vomiting Loss of smell and taste Anorexia
Oral cavity, pharynx	Alterations of taste Mucositis Dysphagia
Esophagus	Dysphagia
Stomach	Gastritis Vomiting
Small intestine	Enteritis Malabsorption Diarrhea
Liver	Impaired protein synthesis
Whole body	Catabolism

apeutic agents for a long time, e.g., because of acute leukemia. The oral intake may decrease to about 20% of the daily RDA, and patients often lose about 10% of their usual body weight within 2 weeks (see Fig. 1). Because of this, reconstitution of the damaged organs may be delayed, and quality of life is significantly impaired (Fig. 2).

Chemotherapeutic agents, as well as radiotherapy of the oral cavity and also the influences of the tumor itself, can cause alterations in taste sensation. DeWys noted that one-third of his patients had an elevation of the recognition threshold for sweet; one-sixth had lowering of the threshold for sour and salt sensations [5]. During cytostatic treatment, taste sensations change from day to day, depending on the type of specific and supportive therapy (e.g., antibiotics) [8].

In addition to anorexia, alimentary canal obstruction localized to the oropharynx, esophagus, or stomach frequently results in decreased intake [5, 7]. Nausea, vomiting, abdominal pain, and disordered intestinal peristalsis can be associated both with tumors of the GI tract and the antineoplastic therapy. Ineffective assimilation of nutrients may be caused by tumor infiltration, blind loops, or chemo- and radiotherapy. Malnutrition itself results in intestinal mucosal atrophy and further compromise of the bowel's absorptive functions [34].

The degree of malnutrition seen in cancer patients is often thought to be greater than that which can be explained solely on the basis of decreased nutrient intake [5]. It has been a constant controversy whether elevated energy expenditure is one of the main factors underlying the weight loss seen in cancer patients. Lundholm and co-workers have been able to show that the resting energy expenditure of weight-losing cancer patients is significantly higher than that of weight-losing noncancer patients (about 580 vs. 450 kcal/mole potassium [15]). Several organs or tissues may be involved in this phenomenon.

Whereas the turnover rate and protein synthesis rate of muscle are depressed in the tumor-bearing host [5, 15], visceral organs as well as the immunoreactive cells are regarded as the main factors underlying the increased energy turnover.

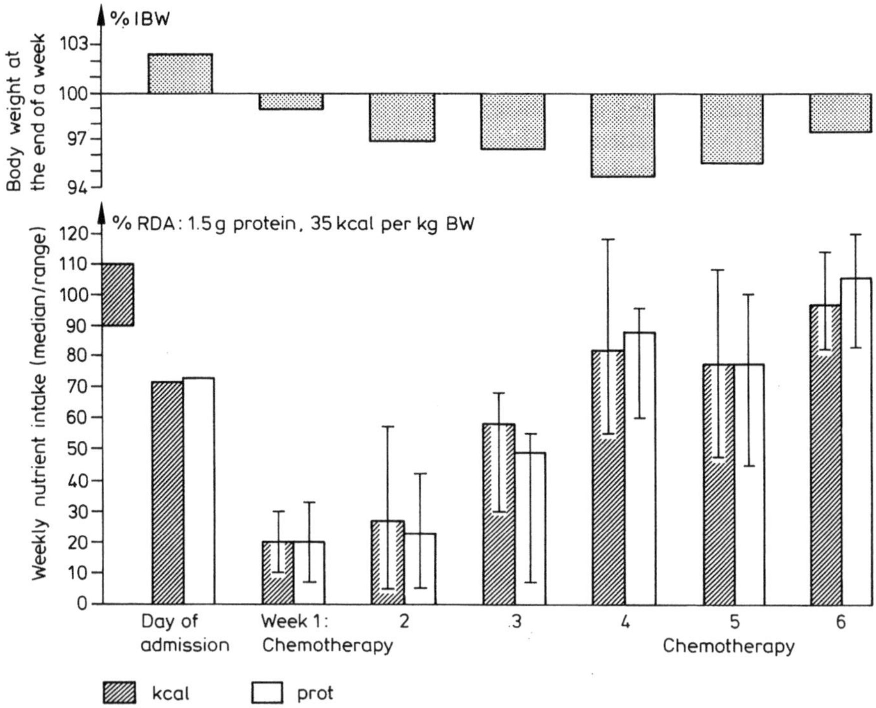

Fig. 1. Weight change and nutrient intake of a female patient during induction therapy for acute myelogenous leukemia (LAM-6 protocol). *Above:* Body weight at the day of admission and at the end of each week (% ideal body weight = *IBW* = (1-100)-[(1-152) × 0.4] where *l* = length/cm. *Below:* Intake of energy (kcal/*hatched*) and protein (g/*circles*) per week (median, range) (in % of offered daily nutrients = 1.5 g protein, 35 kcal per kg IBW and day)

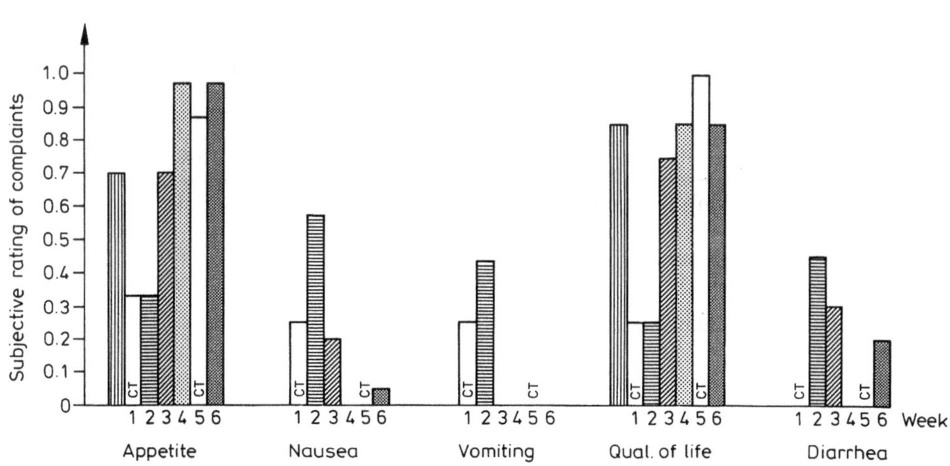

Fig. 2. Changes in appetite, subjective complaints, and quality of life of the patient from Fig. 1 - each column represents the mean number of complaints in that week. *CT*, chemotherapy

For example, increased hepatic protein synthesis and RES function and the cell proliferation or the inadequate metabolism of the tumor may contribute to the elevated energy consumption.

With respect to the metabolism of the nutrient substrates, glucose turnover is increased in cancer patients. This may explain about 50% or more of the elevated energy expenditure, leading to a weight loss of about 0.5-1 kg per month [15]. The glucose uptake of muscle is disturbed - due to insulin resistance in the peripheral organs - wheres liver, immunoactive cells, and tumor may have an increased glucose uptake [9, 15, 24, 33]. Experimental and clinical data have suggested an increased whole body oxidation of lipids in cancer patient [1, 6, 7, 15, 24]. Amino acid flux is increased dependent upon the increased hepatic protein synthesis. During inadequate spontaneous oral intake, skeletal muscles are wasted due to depressed protein synthesis rather than increased breakdown. When the tumor host is supported by nutrients, protein synthesis will be initiated independent of the route of feeding [1, 15].

In conclusion, tumor cachexia is primarily due to insufficient oral intake, caused by anorexia. Beside this a number of tumor patients have an elevated resing and total energy expenditure which is not decreased during starvation. This situation is different from the metabolism in starved nontumor patients. Its aim is to provide life-supporting protein synthesis and the immune system with precursors and energy [6, 15].

Indications for Nutritional Therapy

Patients with malignancy with or without antineoplastic therapy have a high risk of becoming malnourished. DeWys et al. [4] found that, depending on the tumor type, 12%-67% of 3047 cancer patients had a significant weight loss in the 6 months prior to chemotherapy (Table 5). Our own results showed that 68% of a

Table 5. Frequency of weight loss in cancer patients. (DeWys et al. [4])

Tumor type	No.	Weight loss over 6 months		
		>5%	5%-10%	>10%
Favorable non-Hodgkin's lymphoma	290	18	8	10
Breast	289	14	8	6
Acute myelogenous leukemia	129	12	8	4
Sarcoma	189	18	11	7
Unfavorable non-Hodgkin's lymphoma	311	28	13	15
Colon	307	28	14	14
Prostate	78	28	18	10
Lung, small cell	436	34	20	14
Lung, non-small cell	590	36	21	15
Pancreas (over 2 months)	111	54	28	26
Nonmeasurable gastric	179	62	32	30
Measurable gastric	138	67	29	38

Table 6. Indications for intensified nutritional therapy

A. Apparent malnutrition
- Actual body weight <90% IBW
- Weight loss >10% over 6 months or 5% within 1 months
- Serum albumin <3.5 g/100 ml
B. Imminent malnutrition
- Inadequate spontaneous oral intake (<60% predicted nutrient requirements for more than 1 week)
- Intensive antineoplastic therapy planned
- Sepsis

heterogeneous group of outpatients with cancer lost more than 5% of their usual body weight during the 6 months prior to the date of diagnosis, compared to 21% of nontumor patients [19]. Analysis of the absolute actual body weight yielded no valid information enabling us to discriminate between tumor and nontumor patients. Eighty-five percent of the tumor patients had a body weight more than 90% of ideal body weight. Oncological patients with apparent or imminent malnutrition (see Table 6) should be contacted by a nutrition specialist (nutrition team or registered dietitian) when hospitalized for more than 1 week. Especially for those patients who receive antineoplastic therapy with a high risk of reduced oral intake, an individual nutrition program should be introduced some days before the beginning of the specific therapy.

There are several tumor types, therapeutic interventions, and clinical situations in which malnutrition has to be anticipated quite often:

Tumor Types with a High Incidence of Malnutrition

According to the data of DeWys et al. [4], patients with pancreatic or gastric cancer have the highest incidence of malnutrition (Table 5); however, highly malignant lymphomas and colon, prostate, and lung carcinomas are also associated with significant weight loss. In addition, tumors of the central nervous system, the head and neck region, and the esophagus often lead to severe malnutrition because of anorexia or dysphagia.

Antineoplastic Strategies with a High Risk of Malnutrition

Surgery

In addition to the perioperative catabolism, radical resections within the oral cavity, the head-neck area, and the GI tract are typical precursors of malnutrition (Table 2). In a pilot study on the quality of life of gastrectomized patients, Raab et al. [27] were able to show that 37% of the patients were malnourished before operation, while the percentage was 70% 2 weeks and 81% 1 year after operation. Intestinal malabsorption is of minor relevance for this development. Rather the decreased oral intake is the prime reason for malnutrition and stems from the symptoms of the dumping syndrome or abdominal pain.

From the correlation of malnutrition and postoperative complications, Meguid and Meguid deduced three risk groups of tumor patients [16]: *Group 1,* the high-risk patients, are those with tumors of the esophagus, liver, gallbladder, or pancreas, with intra-abdominal retroperitoneal sarcoma, or with abdominal carcinomatosis. Intensive nutritional therapy should be started immediately postoperatively. In malnourished patients, a preoperative nutritional period of about 7–10 days [18] may be useful. *Group 2* comprises well-nourished patients younger than 40 years, regardless of their primary carcinoma. *Group 3* includes patients with tumors of lymphoproliferative or genitourinary/gynecological origin without malnutrition. These patients need to be carefully observed (e.g., daily weight control). Patients in groups 2 and 3 should be treated by intensive nutrition if there are complications or the period of inadequate oral intake lasts longer than 10 days.

Radiotherapy

Radiation therapy predominantly of the oral cavity or the pharynx constitutes an indication for intensive nutrition because of the anorexia, mucositis, and dysphagia that result (Table 3). Especially enteral nutrition via a tube is very helpful in maintaining the nutritional status. When the small bowel is radiated, abdominal pain and diarrhea will occur. In animals, feeding via total parenteral nutrition was able to prevent radiation enteritis, whereas usual feeding induced diarrhea and weight loss [20, 26].

Oncological Chemotherapy

Most cytostatic substances cause nausea, vomiting, anorexia, and often mucositis (Table 4). In addition, protein synthesis - and as a consequence anabolism of nutrient substrates - may be diminished during chemotherapy, as well as GI absorption [10, 20]. In part, toxicity of antineoplastic agents increases during malnutrition [17]. The chemotherapy-induced malnutrition, which is primarily dependent upon decreased oral intake (Fig. 1), will be relevant for the outcome of the patient if the spontaneous oral intake is less than 60% of the recommended substrate intake over a period of more than 1 week. This means diminished quality of life and prolonged phases of infection [29].

Most stressful for the nutritional status of cancer patients are combined strategies of radio- and chemotherapy, e.g. in the treatment of acute leukemia by bone marrow transplantation [31, 35]. Without the support of artificial nutrition, the side-effects of high-dose chemotherapy and total body irradiation on the nutritional status are intolerable.

Strategies of Nutritional Therapy

There are different ways of feeding the tumor patient, namely orally or enterally (via a nasoenteral tube, percutaneous endoscopic gastrostomy, or fine-needle catheter jejunostomy) [19, 22, 30].

When these routes or a combination of them are not tolerated by the patient or cause clinical problems, partial or total parenteral nutrition becomes necessary if the spontaneous oral intake is inadequate.

Oral Nutrition

As long as possible, i. e., as long as the nutrient intake is adequate for the clinical situation, the cancer patient should eat orally. The basis for a longstanding acceptance of oral nutrition - even during anorexia and while a higher amount of nutrients than usual may be necessary (see Table 7) - is the offer of meals of choice during hospitalization. Especially alterations of taste and smell reduce the oral intake significantly. These side-effects of antineoplastic therapy must be overcome variations of flavor and seasoning, which may change from day to day. Frequently anorexia is combined with aversion to meat. It is known that a lot of tumor patients refuse beef and pork first, and poultry and fish later. The high protein demand of the tumor patient (Table 7) can be met for a longer time with the help of egg and milk protein.

Early satiety is a typical consequence of anorexia. Patients may tolerate the recommended daily nutrient supply better when six to eight small meals are offered instead of the usual three big ones. Liquid formula diet with a high amount of protein and calories can be offered between meals. The different flavors of these formula diets are necessary to keep pace with the changes in taste of the tumor patient [8, 19]. It is also possible to mix the usual diet with formula diet of neutral flavor for enrichment with protein and calories.

During antineoplastic therapy which induces nausea, emesis, and mucositis, neutral tasting meals should be offered to the patient. Spiced food will intensify mucositis-associated pain and dysphagia. Beside this, chemotherapy-related anorexia and vomiting are known to result primarily from a learned aversion [5, 20, 21]: the incidence and intensity of anorexia and vomiting are triggered by those qualities of taste and smell which were experienced when suffering the side-effects of antineoplastic therapy [21]. The main problem with oral nutrition in cancer pat-

Table 7. Intensified oral nutrition for cancer patients

- Nutrition education program
- Documentation of daily body weight and food intake
- During hospitalization: meals of choice, including formula diet
- Daily offer:
  a) Patients without malnutrition or metabolic stress 1.3-1.5 g protein, 30-35 kcal per kg IBW
  b) Patients with malnutrition or metabolic stress 1.5-2 g protein, 35-45 kcal per kg IBW

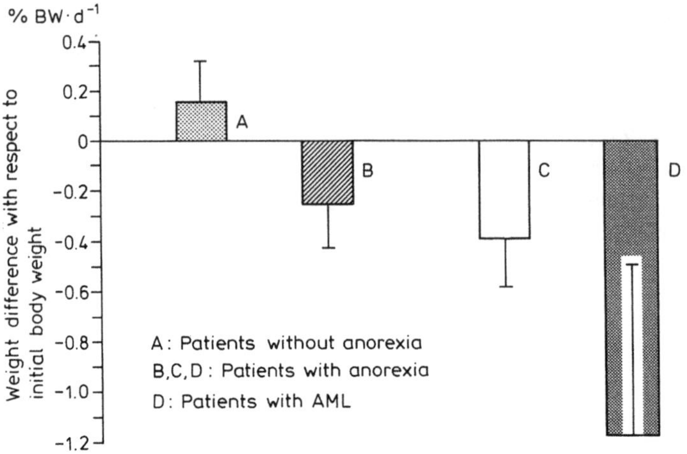

Fig. 3. Daily weight changes in patients during induction therapy for high-grade non-Hodgkin's lymphoma (NHL) and acute myelogenous leukemia (AML). Group A (NHL + AML) - intensive oral nutrition: daily intake of 2 g protein, 50 kcal per kg IBW. Group B (NHL+AML): daily intake of 1 g, 30 kcal. Group C NHL - free diet. Group D AML - free diet

ients with anorexia is the relatively low tolerance to ingestion of higher amounts of protein and energy. However, with the help of nutrition educational provided by a dietitian on a daily basis, it is possible to maintain the nutritional status of highly motivated patients even during phases of cytostatic treatment (see Fig. 3). Patients who accepted a daily intake of 2 g protein, 50 kcal per kg ideal body weight (IBW), i.e., double the usual recommended daily supply, maintained their body weight, whereas patients on usual intake (1 g, 30 kcal per kg IBW per day) lost weight continuously during chemotherapy.

If the daily amount of nutrient cannot be achieved by the oral route alone, partial or total artificial nutrition becomes necessary. The institution and duration of artificial nutrition depend on the degree of malnutrition and metabolic stress, the clinical situation (e.g., whether fever is present), and the expected duration of inadequate oral intake. Especially for patients with nontreatable, end-stage tumor burden, quality of life must be the main indicator of whether artificial nutrition is necessary.

Enteral Nutrition (Tube Feeding)

Tube feeding has become an alternative to parenteral nutrition since the development of ultrafine, very flexible tubes, which can be used for weeks and months without significant local irritation. Nearly all types of cancer patient can be fed by enteral tubes if there is no danger of ileus, vomiting, or aspiration. In patients undergoing cytostatic treatment the risk of nausea and vomiting may be intensified by a nasally applied tube. Dislocation of the tube - and as a consequence aspiration - might be a catastrophe for an immunocompromised patient. That is why in our hospital antineoplastic therapy with a high incidence of vomiting is a contraindication for nasogastric or duodenal tubes. Except for this restriction, tube feeding is a very helpful method of nutritional therapy, especially for patients with anorexia and dysphagia. Main indications are tumors of the oral cavity, the head-neck area, and the esophagus.

If the patient does not tolerate the nasal access, and artificial nutrition will be necessary for more than 4 weeks, percutaneous endoscopic gastrostomy (PEG) (Vestweber [30, pp 42–51]) is an alternative technique for enteral access. Indications are primarily tumors of the head and neck region and the esophagus. PEG is also being used more and more, without relevant complications, for nontreatable end-stage tumor patients whose nutrition needs to be delivered via artificial access [13].

Solutions of protein (milk, soya protein, casein), maltodextrin, fat, and essential elements are the nutrient substrates for tube feeding if gastric (or sometimes duodenal) feeding is used. The optimal composition of formula diets for oral and tube feeding has been intensively discussed elsewhere [3, 28, 30].

For jejunal feeding and also duodenal feeding in patients undergoing aggressive antineoplastic therapy, hydrolysates of protein and polysaccharides, namely oligopeptides, amino acids, and oligosaccharides, are used in combination with essential fatty acids, medium chain triglycerides, and essential elements. This is of special advantage for those tumor patients in whom malabsorption (due to malnutrition, infiltration, or specific therapy) is apparent [20, 24, 26, 34].

Enteral nutrition is nowadays available as home-enteral nutrition. Pharmaceutical companies offer effective distribution systems to supply the patients with nutrition solutions and application material [30].

Parenteral Nutrition

In the 1970s parenteral nutrition was the only effective means of artificial feeding, and most metabolic and clinical studies on nutritional therapy in the cancer patient have been performed on the basis of parenteral nutrition [1, 6, 15, 25]. As a consequence of increasing use of enteral nutrition, parenteral access has become more and more restricted to those patients who refuse enteral tubes or in whom enteral tubes may be too dangerous. Especially during oncological chemotherapy, parenteral nutrition is used either as partial (in combination with oral feeding) or total parenteral nutrition (TPN). Situations in which enteral access should be avoided are vomiting, thrombocytopenia, and ileus.

Partial parenteral nutrition can be given in the following way: 800 kcal will be supplied in 1250 ml, containing 500 ml amino acid solution 5%, 500 ml glucose solution 10%, and 250 ml lipid emulsion 20%. The solution, with an osmolarity of about 500 mosmol/liter, can be infused via peripheral veins over 8 h, e.g., overnight. TPN has to be infused through a central line, because of the high osmolarity of carbohydrate solutions. Over 24 h 4000 kcal can be given as a maximum, with 1500 ml amino acid solution 10%, 1500 ml glucose solution 40%, and 500 ml lipid emulsion 20%. If the patient has to be treated longer than 1 week, vitamins and trace elements must be added [23].

In our opinion, there is almost no indication for home parenteral nutrition in the tumor patient, because home enteral nutrition can avoid the problems of handling, especially of asepsis, which is the basis for safe parenteral therapy.

Results of Nutritional Therapy in the Cancer Patient

Multiple studies have been done in a prospective randomized manner, as reviewed by Brennan and co-workers [1, 25]. If one combines all the studies on surgical tumor patients, it is possible to demonstrate statistically significant decreases in complications associated with TPN, but there is no statistical difference in mortality [25]. Also as an adjunct to radiotherapy and - with one exception - to oncological chemotherapy, intensive nutrition has no influence on survival, whereas the nutritional status can be improved regardless of the route of access [19].

Yamada et al. [36] randomized 34 stage 3 and 4 gastric cancer patients who received adjuvant chemotherapy (5-fluorouracil) postoperatively for as long as possible, either to 2000 kcal TPN for 18 days postsurgery + free oral intake, or to free oral intake. The disease-free interval until recurrence was 452 ± 289 days in the TPN group and 229 ± 174 days in the non-TPN group. Patients in the TPN group were able to take more than double the 5-fluorouracil dose than the non-TPN group (total administered: 159 ± 96 g vs. 69 ± 73 g). The 3-year survival rate of the TPN patients was 54% vs. 0% among the non-TPN patients. The authors concluded that intensive postoperative nutritional therapy induces increased tolerance to 5-fluorouracil due to improved nutrition and increased cell-mediated immunity. There are also other results which underline the dependence of cell-mediated immunity on the nutritional status in patients with gstrointestinal cancer [2]. A further speculative interpretation of these results is that a tumor may become more susceptible to chemotherapy if there is an adequate substrate supply to the host during chemotherapy [24, 32].

With respect to tumor growth, there are some indices of its stimulation by forced feeding in experimental animals [6]. However, no definitive studies are available regarding the effect of nutritional support on tumor growth in cancer patients. Experimental data on rat sarcomas suggest that starvation of the tumor-bearing host metabolically favors the tumor over the host [9].

In conclusion, intensive nutritional therapy of the tumor patient is able to correct existing specific nutritional deficits, to diminish and reverse weight loss, to prevent further malnutrition, and to increase the quality of life (Table 8) - without evidence of inappropriate increased tumor growth - if it is combined with antineoplastic therapy. There are some studies on increase of cell-mediated immunotolerance and improved tolerance to surgical and cytostatic interventions owing to

Table 8. Aims of intensive nutritional therapy in tumor patients

- Treating existing nutritional deficits
- Preventing nutritional depletion
- Meeting the needs for nutrients during the metabolic stress of antineoplastic therapy
- Improving the patient's quality of life

intensive nutritional therapy. Thus, although it is frequently questioned whether intensive nutritional therapy for a limited time during tumor reduction therapy can influence an inexorable pathological process, initiated years before therapy, the truly appropriate question is whether nutritional therapy can permit effective cancer treatment (relative to survival) in a chronically debilitated or metabolically stressed patient [16]. Among patients whose tumors are progressive and no longer treatable, artificially administered nutrition has to be restricted to those whose quality of life will increase in spite of the disadvantages of an artificial feeding access.

References

1. Brennan MF, Ekman L (1984) Metabolic consequences of nutritional support of the cancer patient. Cancer 54: 2627-2634
2. Burke M, Hesp R, Kark AE (1983) The effect of undernutrition and disease site and stage on cell-mediated immunity in gastrointestinal cancer. Clin Oncol 9: 203-211
3. Dempsey DT, Mullen JL (1985) Macronutrient requirements in the malnourished cancer patient. How much of what and why? Cancer 55: 290-294
4. DeWys WD, Begg C, Lavin PT et al. (1980) Prognostic effect of weight loss prior to chemotherapy in cancer patients. Am J Med 69: 491-497
5. DeWys WD (1982) Pathopyhsiology of cancer cachexia: current understanding and areas for future research. Cancer Res [Suppl] 42: 721s-726s
6. Ekman L, Lindmark L, Lundholm KG (1985) Nutritional manipulation of cancer patients. In: Bozzetti F, Dionigi R (eds) Nutrition in cancer and trauma sepsis. Karger, Basel, pp 68-77
7. Fearon KCH, Plumb JA, Calman KC (1986) Nutritional consequences of cancer in man. Clin Nutr 5: 81-89
8. Gallagher P, Tweedle DE (1983) Taste threshold and acceptability of commercial diets in cancer patients. JPEN 7: 361-363
9. Goodgame JT, Lowry SF, Reilly JJ, Jones DC, Brennan MF (1979) Nutritional manipulations and tumor growth. Am J Clin Nutr 32: 2277-2284
10. Herrmann VM, Garnick MB, Moore FD, Wilmore DW (1981) Effect of cytotoxic agents on protein kinetics in patients with metastatic cancer. Surgery 90: 381-387
11. Heim ME, Leweling H, Edler L, Queißer W (1985) Adjuvant parenteral nutrition in patients with colorectal cancer receiving polychemotherapy: a randomized clinical trial. Tumor Diagn Ther 6: 129-133
12. Holm E, Schimpf F, Schlickeiser GG, Söhner W, Staedt U, Striebel JP (1987) Aminosäurenstoffwechsel bei Tumorkrankheiten. Aktuel Onkol 35: 25-54
13. Keymling M, Wörner W, Lübke HJ, Weithofer G, Bloch R (1983) Ambulante pumpenassistierte kontinuierliche Sondenernährung bei Patienten mit metastasierendem Karzinom. Klin Ernährung 12: 145-156
14. Kokal WA (1985) The impact of antitumor therapy on nutrition. Cancer 55: 273-278
15. Lundholm KG (1985) Energy and substrate metabolism in the cancer-bearing host. In: Bozzetti F, Dionigi R (eds) Nutrition in cancer and trauma sepsis. Karger, Basel, pp 78-89
16. Meguid MM, Meguid V (1985) Preoperative identification of the surgical cancer patient in need of postoperative supportive total parenteral nutrition. Cancer 55: 258-262
17. Mihranian MH, Wang YM, Daly JM (1984) Effects of nutritional depletion and repletion on plasma methotrexate pharmacokinetics. Cancer 54: 2268-2271
18. Müller JM, Brenner U, Dienst C et al. (1982) Preoperative parenteral feeding in patients with gastrointestinal carcinoma. Lancet 2: 68-71

19. Ollenschläger G, Sander F (1985) Indikationen und Ergebnisse der enteralen Ernährung in der Onkologie. Z Gastroenterol [Suppl] 23: 64-76
20. Ollenschläger G (1986) Einfluß aggressiver Tumortherapie auf die Nährstoffverwertung und den Ernährungszustand. Infusionstherapie 13: 70-77
21. Ollenschläger G, Jansen S, Fischer H, Mödder B (1987) Zur Pathogenese und klinischen Bedeutung der Anorexie onkologischer Patienten. Aktuel Onkol 35: 12-24
22. Ollenschläger G (1987) Indikationen und Methoden der klinischen Ernährung bei onkologischen Patienten. Klin Ernährung 25: 177-188
23. Ollenschläger G, Fischer H, Mödder B (1987) Stoffwechselkomplikationen bei langdauernder parenteraler Ernährung. Med Klinik 82: 619-623, 666-669
24. Ollenschläger G, Jansen S (1988) Besonderheiten der Substratverwertung bei onkologischen Patienten. Infusionstherapie (in press)
25. Paidas CN, Jeevanandam M, Brennan MF (1985) Nutritional support of the cancer patient. In: Bozzetti F, Dionigi R (eds) Nutrition in cancer and trauma sepsis. Karger, Basel, pp 90-110
26. Pezner R, Archambeau JO (1985) Critical evaluation of the role of nutritional support for radiation therapy patients. Cancer 55: 263-267
27. Raab M, van Maercke P, Stützer H (1987) Lebensqualität nach Gastrektomie - Vergleich der Magenersatzmethoden nach Longmire und Roux. (in preparation)
28. Roth E, Ollenschläger G, Hackl JM (1985) Grundlagen und Technik der Infusionstherapie und klinischen Ernährung. Reissigl H (ed) Handbuch der Infusionstherapie und klinischen Ernährung, Vol 2. Karger, Basel
29. Ruffmann R, Schlick E, Tartaris T, Chirigos MA (1986) Proteinmangel, Körperabwehr und natürliche Anti-Tumor-Immunität. Infusionstherapie 13: 106-112
30. Sailer D, Kolb S, Neff H (1986) Künstliche Ernährung zu Hause. In: Bässler KH, Grünert A, Kleinberger G, Reissigl H (eds) Infusionstherapie und klinische Ernährung, vol 14. Karger, Basel
31. Szeluga DJ, Stuart RK, Brookmeyer R, Utermohlen V, Santos GW (1985) Energy requirements of parenterally fed bone marrow transplant recipients. JPEN 9: 139-143
32. Torosian MH, Tsou KC, Daly JM, Mullen JL, Stein TP, Miller EE, Buzby GP (1984) Alteration of tumor cell kinetics by pulse total parenteral nutrition. Potential therapeutic implications. Cancer 53: 1409-1415
33. Van Eys (1985) Nutrition and cancer: physiological interrelationships. Ann Rev Nutr 5: 435-461
34. Weiner R, Matkowitz R, Hartig W, Conradi G, Laue R (1979) Enterale Resorption und Tumorkachexie. Z Ges Inn Med 34: 57-61
35. Weisdorf S, Hofland C, Sharp HL et al. (1984) Total parenteral nutrition in bone marrow transplantation: a clinical evaluation. J Pediatr Gastroenterol Nutr 3: 95-100
36. Yamada N, Koyama H, Hioki K, Yamada T, Yamamoto M (1983) Effect of postoperative total parenteral nutrition (TPN) as an adjunct to gastrectomy for advanced gastric carcinoma. Br J Surg 70: 267-274

Parenteral Nutrition in Tumor Patients

J. M. Müller, P. Thul, M. Halber, and P. Huber

Chirurgische Universitätsklinik, Joseph-Stelzmann-Straße 9, 5000 Köln 41, FRG

The role of parenteral nutrition (PN) in the operative management of cancer patients has been well recognized for the past 10–15 years; a great number of surgeons believe it to be the most effective method of improving the nutritional status of cancer patients perioperatively. We can not absolutely agree with them, since PN is also a potentially hazardous and expensive therapy. One must therefore evaluate its risks and its benefits before recommending its use in daily practise. In this context we have to answer the following questions.

1. Which additional complications result from PN in the operative treatment of cancer patients?
2. Can preoperative PN induce anabolism and preserve or improve the nutritional status of cancer patients with in an acceptable period of time?
3. Does preoperative PN reduce the postoperative complication rate in major surgery?
4. Is PN superior to infusion of water and electrolytes in the postoperative period, regarding the final outcome of an operation as the crucial criterion of effectiveness?

Complications of PN

Parenteral nutrition adds little to the perioperative complication rate. Complications related to the insertion of the central venous catheter must be excluded because most of the patients or procedures in which PN is indicated need a central venous line for intra- and postoperative monitoring. In our experience a central venous catheter is placed in a superior manner when electively performed for PN than when performed just prior to operation. In two prospective randomized trials we observed one subclavian vein thrombosis and five catheter-related episodes of sepsis. The sepsis rate per 1000 days preoperative PN was 2.4 cases. Rises in the transaminases and alkaline phosphatase were the only metabolic complications that occurred in our patients. None of the above-mentioned complications increased the risk of the operation.

Recent Results in Cancer Research, Vol. 108

Table 1. Parameters before and after 7 days' preoperative PN. (Rasmussen et al. [3])

	Before ($n=10$)	After ($n=10$)
Weight (kg)	57.6 ± 2.1	59.0 ± 2.7
Albumin (μmol/liter)	474 ± 27	461 ± 12
Transferrin (μmol/liter)	52 ± 1.2	49 ± 2.3
IgG (μmol/liter)	60.0 ± 2.7	61.0 ± 3.4
Cutan test (mm)	6 ± 0	20 ± 2

Metabolic Effect of Preoperative Parenteral Nutrition

Regarding the nutritional effect of preoperative PN, all studies agree that a positive nitrogen balance and an increase in body weight can be achieved even in extremely malnourished patients. Assessment of body composition by in vivo neutron activation analysis or other methods has shown that most of the weight gain is due to an increase in body water. This finding has to be kept in mind when trying to interpret the different results of measurement of protein concentrations before and after preoperative PN.

In several studies, as in that by Rasmussen et al. [3], the concentrations of plasma proteins or immunoglobulins (Table 1) stayed constant after 7 days of preoperative PN despite or because of a water retention of 1.4 liters. The only result in favor of preoperative PN in this study was a significant increase in T cell activity as measured by intracutaneous application of seven different antigens.

In our two trials of preoperative PN one group of patients (group I) received the regular hospital diet and two other groups 1.5 g amino acids per kg body weight per day and 45 kcal per kg body weight per day in the form of a glucose (group II) or lipid (group III) regime for 10 days. The mean weight gain between admission and surgery was 2.3 kg in group II and 1.8 kg in group III. The controls lost 0.9 kg during the same period. In patients who received the normal hospital diet, total protein, prealbumin, and retinol binding protein fell significantly between the day of admission and the day of operation. In group II, which received the glucose regimen, the concentrations of prealbumin, transferrin, IgG, IgM, retinol binding protein, and C3a increased significantly. Those patients who had received the lipid regimen showed distinctive increases only in transferrin, IgM, and C3a levels.

In both preoperative PN groups we observed an increase in the central venous pressure. This was probably due to an expansion of the intravascular fluid compartment. We therefore corrected the protein concentration on the day of operation according to the changes in the hematocrit between the day of admission and the day of operation. After this correction, the difference in concentration of all proteins between the day of admission and the day of operation decreased in group I and increased in groups II and III.

In considering the effect of preoperative PN on nutritional status we should not forget what happens to patients with a devastating illness such as cancer who receive no nutritional support during the preoperative period. Pinchcofsky and

Table 2. Increasing malnutrition during hospitalization. (Pinchcofsky et al. [2])

	Admission	Reassessment	*P*
Kwashiorkor patients ($n=192$)			
Albumin	2.6 ± 0.05	2.2 ± 0.02	<0.05
Lymphocyte count	850 ±21	653 ±16	<0.05
Ideal body weight (%)	129 ± 1.1	113 ± 1.4	<0.05
Marasmus patients ($n=61$)			
Albumin	3.65± 0.02	3.4± 0.01	<0.05
Lymphocyte count	1994 ±23	1332 ±20	<0.05
Ideal body weight (%)	67.8 ± 0.8	63.6± 1.4	<0.05

Kaminski [2] found increased malnutrition during hospitalization (Table 2). When the nutritional status of malnourished patients was reassessed after 3 weeks of hospitalization the concentration of albumin, the total lymphocyte count, and the percentage of ideal body weight had dropped significantly. Patients who had received hospital diet in our trial for an average of 8.5 days before surgery showed a similar phenomenon. The decrease in several plasma proteins was more pronounced in well nourished than in malnourished patients, probably because the latter were better adapted to the reduced intake due to certain diagnostic procedures which required an empty gastrointestinal tract. When we compared the protein, immunoglobulin, and complement levels on the day of operation between patients on a regular hospital diet and patients who received 10 days' preoperative PN the concentrations of total protein, prealbumin, retinol binding protein, transferrin, IgG, IgM, and C3a were found to be significantly higher in group II, which received the glucose regimen, than in group I, and the concentrations of transferrin, IgM, and C3a were markedly higher in group III, which received the lipid regimen, than in group I.

Clinical Effect of Preoperative Parenteral Nutrition

Several randomized and nonrandomized trials have been carried out to demonstrate the beneficial effect of preoperative PN especially in cancer patients. We selected four of them because the duration of preoperative PN, the amount of nutrients given, and the number of patients who entered the trial were sufficient to draw a conclusion.

In 1979 Heatley and Williams [1] reported the results of a randomized trial in which 74 patients (Table 3) with a preoperative diagnosis of gastric or esophageal cancer received either a 3000 calorie oral diet or the same oral diet plus 7-10 days of preoperative PN in the form of 1.5 g amino acids and 40 kcal per kg. The only benefit observed in the preoperative PN group was a significant reduction in postoperative wound infections (Table 4). The interpretation of these data is confounded by the fact that malnutrition was not a criterion of stratification or entrance into the study. In addition, the preoperative diagnosis proved incorrect in 14 patients. Seven patients in each group either had a benign lesion or no pathology was demonstrated at the time of surgical exploration.

Table 3. Clinical details of patients admitted to Heatley and Williams' randomized trial [1]

	Treated group	Control group
No.	38	36
Age (years)	65.6	66.4
Male: female ratio	26:12	20:16
Pathology at operation		
Negative laparotomy	2	2
Benign pathology	5	5
Operable cancer	19	22
Inoperable cancer	12	7

Table 4. Complications and deaths in Heatley and Williams' randomized trial [1]

	Treated group ($n=38$)	Control group ($n=36$)	*P*
Wound infection	3	11	<0.05
Anastomotic leakage	2	3	n.s.
Death	6	8	n.s.

In 1981 Smale et al. [4] analyzed the postoperative course of 159 patients who had undergone a major intra-abdominal, intrathoracic, or head and neck operation for palliation or cure of malignancy. The course of 54 patients who had received 6 or more days of preoperative PN providing 35 kcal and 1.5 g amino acids per day was compared to that of 105 patients who had received no preoperative PN. The effect of preoperative PN was correlated with nutritional status on admission by stratifying the patients retrospectively according to their prognostic nutritional index. In patients (Fig. 1) who were poorly nourished and had a PNI of more than 40%, preoperative PN was associated with a 2.1-fold reduction in all postoperative complications, a 2.9-fold reduction in major sepsis, and a 2.7-fold reduction in mortality.

In our first trial of preoperative PN, cancer patients were stratified according to the site of the primary tumor and nutritional status. As already mentioned, they were randomly assigned to three groups. Group I served as a control. Group II received preoperative PN for 10 days in the form of a glucose regimen and Group III, PPN for 10 days in the form of a lipid regimen. The three groups (Table 5) were comparable in terms of age, sex distribution, tumor site, stage of tumor at surgery, nutritional status, preoperative risk factor, and type and duration of surgical procedure. The smaller number of patients in group III is explained by a premature termination of the trial in this group. A planned evaluation after two-thirds of the patients had entered the trial revealed a significantly higher mortality in group III than in group II. The reason for this result is unclear. We presently have few data suggesting that the high load of fat given to these patients may have led at least to a partial blockade of some macrophage and granulocytic function.

The rates of wound infection, pneumonia, major complications affecting the site of operation, and mortality were generally lower in group II than in the con-

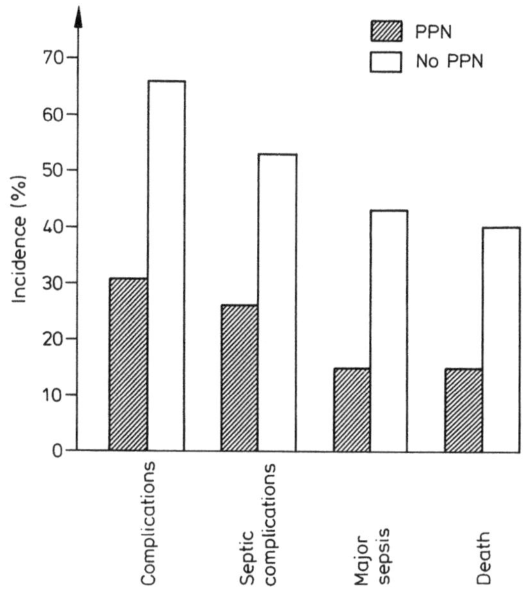

Fig. 1. Comparison of morbidity and mortality in malnourished (PNI 40) cancer patients with and without preoperative PN *(PPN)*. (Smale et al. [4])

Table 5. Patient characteristics of the three groups in the first trial of preoperative PN

	Group		
	I (control)	II (PPN: AA, G)	III (PPN: AA, G, F)
N°. of patients	59	66	46
Mean age ± SD (yr)	59.4 ± 12.6	58.9 ± 11.5	58.6 ± 10.4
Sex ratio (M/F)	34/25	42/24	29/17
Tumor site			
	%	%	%
Esophagus	6 (10.2)	8 (12.1)	5 (10.8)
Stomach	28 (47.5)	30 (45.5)	24 (52.1)
Colon	11 (18.6)	12 (18.2)	8 (17.4)
Rectum	11 (18.6)	10 (15.2)	6 (13.0)
Pancreas	3 (5.1)	6 (9.1)	3 (6.5)
Tumor stage			
I	11 (18.6)	6 (9.1)	3 (6.5)
II	9 (15.3)	13 (19.1)	10 (21.7)
III	28 (47.5)	33 (50.0)	22 (47.8)
IV	11 (18.6)	14 (21.2)	11 (23.9)
Type of operation			
Curative procedures	45 (76.3)	45 (68.2)	30 (65.2)
Palliative procedures	14 (23.7)	21 (31.8)	16 (34.8)
Mean duration of the operation ± SD (min)	235 ± 95	229 ± 80	215 ± 84

AA, amino acids; *F*, lipid emulsion; *G*, glucose.

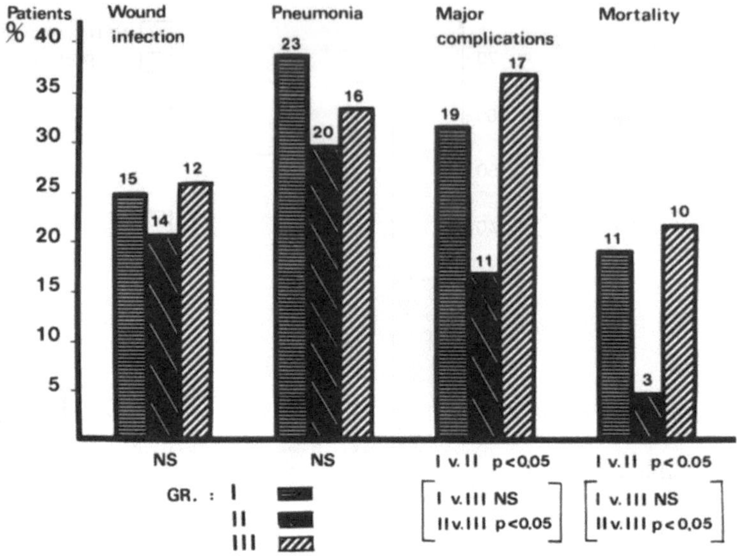

Fig. 2. Postoperative complications in the three groups in the first trial of preoperative PN

trol group (Fig. 2). The differences were significant only for major complications and mortality. It is statistically incorrect to compare group III with the other two groups because of the insufficient number of patients who entered the trial. The postoperative complication rate in group III was not very different from that in group I, but especially regarding major complications and mortality it was higher than in group II.

All deaths occurred between the 3rd and the 14th postoperative day and were caused either by a major complication affecting the site of operation or by bronchopneumonia. None of the patients died of rapidly progressing cancer.

To limit the indication for preoperative PN for high risk patients, we divided the groups according to tumor stage, tumor location, and nutritional status and compared the subgroups. We expected that malnourished patients would show the most benefit from preoperative nutritional support. This was not the case. The greatest difference in mortality between the control group and the second group was found for carcinomas of the upper gastrointestinal tract. We believe that the probable cause of these findings in this subgroup is the high incidence of malnutrition as well as the need to undergo a major operation. The difference in mortality between the control group and group II was more than 20%.

We thought that the easiest way to validate the first study would be to observe patients with carcinoma of the upper GI tract only. This study was carried out in the same way as the first one. In each group 55 patients with carcinoma of the stomach and esophagus were entered in the trial. Group I served as controls and group II received 10 days of preoperative PN. The patient characteristics in the two groups were comparable (Table 6). We again found lower rates of wound infection, pneumonia, major complications at the site of operation, and mortality in the preoperative PN group. The difference between the groups was statistically

Table 6. Patient characteristics in the two groups in the study of preoperative PN in patients with carcinoma of the upper GI tract only

	Group	
	I	II
N°. of patients	55	58
Mean age ± SD (yr)	57.4±11.6	58.2±11.5
Sex ratio (M/F)	31/24	38/20
Tumor site		
Esophagus	10	12
Stomach	45	46
Tumor stage		
I	7	3
II	6	12
III	31	33
IV	11	10
Type of operation		
Resection	42	43
Palliative	13	15
Mean duration of the operation ± SD (Min)	236.6±50.1	231.6±64.6

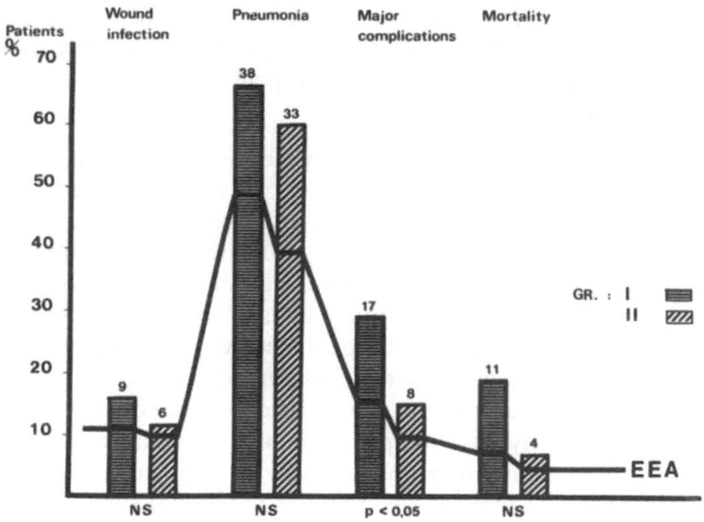

Fig. 3. Postoperative complications in the two groups in the study of preoperative PN in patients with carcinoma the upper GI tract only

significant for major complications only (Fig. 3). This result was astonishing because from the first study we had expected a significant difference for all four types of complication. One explanation for these unexpected findings might be an alteration of our surgical technique, which took place during the period of the second trial. An EEA stapler was used for esophageal-jejunal anastomosis after gastrectomy and a blunt dissection of the esophagus was carried out instead of a transthoracic resection. Comparing the patients in both groups who were operated according to the new techniques, we found that the difference for wound infection was only 5%, for pneumonia 4%, and for major complications and mortality 6%. These numbers are still in favor of preoperative PN, but with such a small therapeutic difference one would need more than 500 patients in each group to prove in a prospective randomized trial that preoperative PN reduces the postoperative complication rate significantly.

Postoperative Parenteral Nutrition

There is general agreement that postoperative PN reduces the metabolic consequences of an operative trauma. Several studies have reported an improvement in nitrogen balance, protein fractions, and immunocompetence with postoperative PN as compared to water and electrolyte therapy only. Unfortunately there is not a single prospective randomized trial which was able to prove that for whatever type of cancer surgery postoperative PN is superior to water and electrolyte infusion in terms of the postoperative complication rate. On the basis of our own clinical experience and the results of various uncontrolled studies, the following conclusions may be drawn. If the postoperative morbidity and mortality are the primary criteria for judging the therapeutic effectiveness of postoperative PN in cancer surgery:

1. The necessity of every form of postoperative PN must be called into question with regard to operations which do not involve the gastrointestinal tract. I personally think that PN is unnecessary in these patients.
2. Postoperative PN does not have an advantage compared to water and electrolyte therapy after surgery for gastrointestinal cancer, if the patient was not malnourished preoperatively and if he is allowed to start oral intake within 5 days after surgery. In our clinic patients receive postoperative PN routinely only after esophagectomy, gastrectomy, and pancreatectomy.
3. In malnourished patients PN should be started preoperatively and continued postoperatively until the patient is able to eat adequately. Due to the fact that after gastrectomy or esophagectomy patients not seldom develop malnutrition within 2 or 3 months we continue nutritional support via an intraoperatively placed needle jejunostomy for several weeks in selected cases. A prospective comparative trial is planned to evaluate this approach.

References

1. Heatley RV, Williams RHP (1979) Preoperative intravenous feeding - a controlled trial. Postgrad Med J 55: 541
2. Pinchcofsky GD, Kaminski MV (1985) Increasing malnutrition during hospitalization: documentation by a nutritional screening program. J Am Coll Nutr 4: 471
3. Rasmussen A, Segel E, Trier Aagaard M, Hessov I (1985) The effect of preoperative nutrition on the immune system. Clin Nutr 4: 175
4. Smale BF, Mullen JL, Buzby GP, Rosato EF (1981) The efficacy of nutritional assessment and support in cancer surgery. Cancer 10: 2375

Nutritional Management of the Ambulatory Patient

J. H. Hartlapp

Medizinische Klinik, Rheinische Friedrich-Wilhelms-Universität, Venusberg, Sigmund-Freud-Straße 25, 5300 Bonn, FRG

Cancer has a recognized negative influence on the nutritional condition of the patient, which may be worsened by the effects of chemotherapeutic treatment [15]. As a result, patients suffer significant degrees of malnutrition, associated with a number of untoward clinical effects [2, 13].

Nutritional Status of the Cancer Patient

The most common effects are weight loss, associated reduction of body fat, depletion of protein, progressive weakness resulting in prolonged bed rest, and skin breakdown. Endocrine changes produce secondary nutrient depletion and apathy. Furthermore, patients suffer from electrolyte fluid imbalance, depressed immune mechanisms accompanied by impaired phagocytosis of the granulocytes and by decreased macrophage mobilization, and retarded wound healing. In addition, malnutrition leads to a delay in the diagnostic and therapeutic program. Increased morbidity and mortality have been reported [10].

The management of patients showing evidence of these clinical effects often consists in a compensating hyperalimentation [11]. However, the importance of considering the patient's nutritional status at the time of diagnosis has been emphasized; at this early moment, malnutrition can be more easily prevented or corrected. The objective should be to integrate nutritional support into the therapeutic approach. For the ambulatory cancer patient undergoing chemotherapy, preventing malnutrition becomes a focus of particular concern [14].

Guidelines for Enteral Nutrition, Especially in Ambulatory Patients

The first and most striking step in the nutritional program is the instruction of the patient and his relatives. When the patient is being informed about the side-effects of chemotherapy, the physician has to underline the need to maintain an adequate nutritional status by ingesting an optimal diet voluntarily. The major concern is to make the patient aware of his health and to make him understand the reasons for

Recent Results in Cancer Research, Vol. 108

an optimal nutritional therapy. Cancer patients should become as compliant as patients suffering from diabetes and following a dietary regimen.

Nutrition as a supportive therapy consists in a program tailored to the patient's individual needs and life-style while considering the nutritional status. Oral feeding should be the preferred method of nutritional support for as long as possible [5]. With regard to individual taste, appetite, and ability to eat, the patient should be encouraged to ingest mainly normal food. Provision of adequate nutrition is particularly important since numerous different essential nutrients have to be considered and provided in appropriate quantities to prevent deficiencies during a caloric-sufficient diet [3, 10]. If loss of weight is observed, patients have to be given a nutritional drinkable supplement. Oral feeding may be unsatisfactory due to pain on chewing and swallowing; for these patients, formula diets guarantee adequate nutrition over a long period.

Tube feeding via nasogastric, nasoduodenojujenal, or percutaneous-endogastric intubation according to the individual situation is still exceptional in ambulatory treatment. It is not known whether parenteral nutrition improves survival [1]. Apart from individual or small series of case reports, only a few studies have been conducted and the results have always been reported as exceptionally good [6, 7, 9, 12].

The maintenance of an adequate nutritional status can be easily followed by recording the body weight at regular intervals. On these occasions, the patient can also be motivated anew and encouraged to follow a balanced diet.

Patients and relatives should be taught that few voluminous meals are less appropriate than frequent small meals. This kind of nutrition is easier to digest and from the physiological point of view more effective. An aversion can be prevented by varying foods. A nicely prepared meal and a decorative layout may enhance the joy of eating. According to the individual taste, an appetizing composition and small quantities of alcoholic beverages before or during the meals may stimulate the appetite. Communal eating also raises and holds the appetite and furthermore creates a pleasant atmosphere and intensifies the joy of life.

Regulation of Oral Feeding Under Cytostatic Treatment

During the days of cytostatic treatment, the food intake is additionally decreased by the side-effects of the drugs. Loss of appetite, nausea, and vomiting can be prevented, at least partially, by antiemetics. On the day before treatment, the fluid intake should be intentionally augmented; on the evening before starting the cytostatic course, the patient can be given a mild sedative, possibly combined with an antiemetic. On the morning of the first day of treatment the patient should have a small breakfast and has to take an antiemetic. Paying regard to the individually observed side-effects, the patient should be advised to eat smaller meals than usual. Sufficient fluid intake has to be ensured, if necessary with antiemetic protection. Beginning with the first day after therapy, the patient should try to return to his normal eating practice. The administration of antiemetics 15-30 min before the meal may help.

Possibilities for Improving Nutrition

When the therapeutic program is first presented, patients and relatives should be informed about all devisable possibilities for improving nutrition. Light and digestible diets with between meal snacks may prevent lack of appetite and early satiety. Many patients complain that foods have lost their taste. Increased seasoning and experimenting with a variety of flavors (including flavoring extracts) and aromas may be appropriate. Patients who develop a dislike for beef and especially pork mostly continue to accept fish and poultry. If an aversion to all foods containing animal proteins should subsist, adequate protein intake may still be maintained with dairy products, eggs, legumes, and peanuts. Ice creams, milk shakes, puddings, custards, and commercial supplements can be rendered more appealing by fresh fruits. In general, between meal snacks improve the daily protein and calorie intake.

Diet should be modified in consistency according to the patient's individual needs. Nowadays, meals are easily prepared with mixers, achieving bland, soft, or liquid textures. Coffee, tea, or water can be ameliorated by adding fruit juices or other high caloric beverages such as milk or cream. Patients with stomatitis should be given foods and beverages at room temperature or even cold. Likewise, patients should be encouraged to eat what they desire - even unusual requests for foods should be fulfilled. Many patients prefer breakfast-type meals in the evening; therefore, this kind of meal should be made available at any time of the day.

Tube feeding is indicated for patients with developing or manifest malnutrition. Oral feeding is also contraindicated when there is pain on swallowing and impaired swallowing mechanisms. Patients with partial or total obstruction may be fed via intubation through various insertions [8]. Commercially available tubes are of small caliber, soft plastic material and have proved to be well tolerated. Nevertheless, there remains the cosmetic impairment caused by tubes inserted through the nose. When obstruction occurs in the esophagus or the stomach, a percutaneous-gastric or duodenojejunal tube is generally used. For ambulatory patients without digestive or absorptive disorders, formula diets can be given. Feedings should be applied in small initial doses, gradually increasing to optimum amounts, to avoid sensation of repletion, meteorism, and diarrhea and to enhance patient compliance [4].

Conclusion

In conclusion, a dietary concept should be included early in cancer therapy for the ambulatory patient to prevent malnutrition and to correct any existing nutritional deficiences. The quality of life is thereby improved and therapy is facilitated and might be rendered more effective. We have data to suggest that inclusion of nutritional therapy in the treatment of cancer patients is justified. It is true that controlled clinical trials in large series of patients are still lacking, but we are nevertheless paying increased attention to this elementary sort of therapy, which contributes to the patient's sense of well-being and improves the quality of life for a longer time.

References

1. Copeland EM, Daly JM, Ota DM (1979) Nutrition, cancer and intravenous hyperalimentation. Cancer 43: 2108-2116
2. Daly JM (1986) Malnutrition and metabolic abnormalities in cancer patients. Infusionstherapie 13: 66-68
3. Dickerson JWT (1983) Nutrition of the cancer patient. Adv Nutr Res 5: 105-131
4. Dobbie RP, Butterick OD (1977) Continuous pump/tube enteric hyperalimentation - use in esophageal disease. JPEN 1: 100-104
5. Hartlapp JH, Illiger HJ, Wolter H (1984) Aspekte der praktischen Onkologie. Onkologie 7: 23-27
6. Issels BF, Valdivieso M, Zaren HA (1968) Protection against chemotherapy toxicity by i.v. hyperalimentation. Cancer Treat Rep 62: 1139-1143
7. Joyeux H, Dubois JB, Solassol C, Pujol H (1982) Cyclic intermittent parenteral nutrition (CIPN): a first adjuvant therapy in radio-chemotherapeutic combination for advanced ovarian tumors (AOT). Proc 13th Int Cancer Congress (abstract) 648: 3705
8. Newmark SR, Simpson MS, Beskitt MP, Black J, Sublett D (1981) Home tube feeding for long-term nutritional support. JPEN 5: 76-78
9. Shamberger RC, Brennan MF, Goodgame JT, Lowrey SS, Maher MM, Pizzo PA (1981) Effect of total parenteral nutrition (TPN) on metabolic parameters of patients undergoing ablative chemotherapy. Proc Am Ass Cancer Res Am Soc Clin Oncol (abstract) 22: 420
10. Shils ME (1979) Nutritional therapy of the cancer patient: guidelines for enteral and parenteral feeding. Curr Probl Cancer 4: 66-76
11. Silberman H (1980) Hyperalimentation in patients with cancer. Surg Gynecol Obstetr 150: 755-757
12. Valdivieso M, Bodey GP, Benjamin RS, Barkley HT, Freemann MB, Ertel M, Smith TL, Montain DF (1981) Role of intravenous hyperalimentation as an adjunct to intensive chemotherapy for small cell bronchogenic carcinoma. Cancer Treat Rep 65: 145-150
13. Waterhouse C (1963) Nutritional disorders in neoplastic diseases. J Chron Dis 16: 637-644
14. De Wys WD (1980) Nutritional care of the cancer patient. JAMA 244: 374-376
15. De Wys WD, Begg C, Lavin PT et al. (1980) Prognostic effect of weight loss prior to chemotherapy in cancer patients. Am J Med 69: 491-497

Nutritional Management of the Childhood Cancer Patient

M. R. Rossi and C. Uderzo

Clinica Pediatrica dell'Università di Milano Centro di Ematologia Pediatrica,
Ospedale di Monza, Via Donizetti 106, 20052 Monza, Italy

Owing to the progress made in recent years, childhood cancers are now generally treatable. This progress is particularly evident in the treatment of lymphoblastic leukemia, lymphomas, and Wilms' tumor; in fact most of these patients remain in remission for such long periods that they may reasonably be considered cured. Much effort has been made to improve support treatment for these patients with the aim of ensuring the best chance of therapeutic success; two examples of this are the notable advances achieved in the treatment of infections and in transfusional regimens. The importance of the nutritional status of cancer patients in obtaining the best possible treatment results has also been stressed in recent years, and numerous studies have been performed in different centers with the aim of clarifying the mechanisms of the protein-energy malnutrition (PEM) that often occurs in these patients. As a result, useful and sophisticated techniques have been developed to investigate nutritional status, and the use of techniques such as total parenteral nutrition (TPN) has been rationalized and widened. TPN has been shown to be fundamental in some patient categories at high risk, such as recipients of bone marrow transplants and subjects with gastrointestinal cancers.

It is well known that patients with neoplastic disease are at risk of developing a negative energy metabolism for numerous reasons, including energy expediture for tumor growth and the negative effects of chemotherapy (nausea, vomiting, anorexia, mucositis, change in taste). Furthermore, chemo- and radiotherapy inhibit proliferation of the intestinal mucosa, thus causing malabsorption, and induce myelosuppression. As a result all cancer patients, be they children or adults, are subject to weight loss, malnutrition, and increased susceptibility to infections with a further worsening of their catabolic condition. It has now been realized that this problem must be approached in different ways in children and adults.

The first evident difference is that the child is a growing organism and for this reason has particular calorie and protein requirements. Pediatric research in the past 15 years has thrown light on these requirements from both the physiological and the physiopathological standpoint. This has led to rationalization in the approach to the nutrition of both healthy children and those with diseases affecting nutritional status (malabsorption syndromes, intolerance, infections, etc.), including cancer. The second difference is that the psychological aspects of nutrition in

Recent Results in Cancer Research, Vol. 108

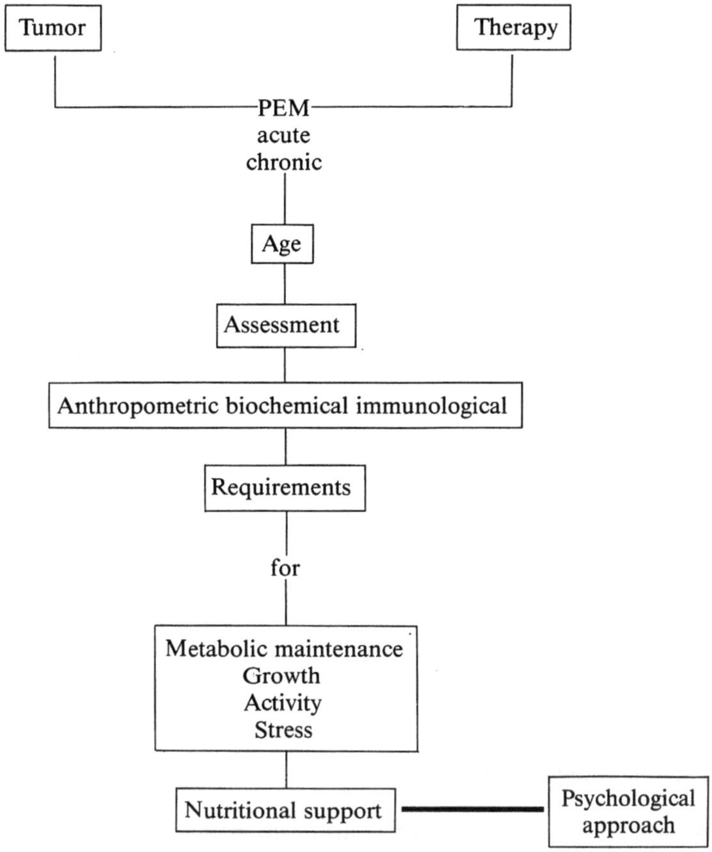

Fig. 1. Approach to nutrition in pediatric cancer

children require much attention, especially in children with tumors. In particular the child's relationship with its parents must be considered, since nutrition cannot be separated from the parental relationship, especially as far as the mother is concerned. These two aspects are particularly important in the small child, and even more so in the infant up to the age of 2 years.

These considerations show the vital role played by a pediatric approach to the nutritional problem in the child with cancer (Fig. 1) and how normal growth of the child is an important objective in view of the possibility of long disease-free survival.

Nutritional Assessment

The nutritional status of each child with cancer should be evaluated, especially if the tumor is a rapidly growing and invasive one or if it involves the alimentary tract. Furthermore, a nutritional assessment should be made of all children who have to undergo radiotherapy (especially to the head, neck, esophagus, and abdomen), major surgery, or intensive chemotherapy. This assessment consists of:

- History
- Physical examination
- Anthropometry
- Biochemical evaluation
- Immunological evaluation

History

Two aspects should be considered: firstly, the type of tumor, the duration of treatment and its possible side-effects (nausea, vomiting, stomatitis, diarrhea, anorexia), and the probability of developing severe infections; secondly, the nutritional history of the patient, anthropometric data from birth until diagnosis of the cancer, idiosyncrasies or intolerances, and dietary habits with due consideration to psychosocial factors (family origin, economic conditions, etc.). The second aspect is important since it shows the quality of growth of the child when healthy and avoids under- and overstimation of the conditions at onset of the disease; in fact a dynamic evaluation of the variations with respect to the preceding period is important rather than a detailed theoretical calculation made at the diagnosis of cancer.

Physical Examination

A physical examination forms part of the patient evaluation at onset of the disease and should include a check for any signs of malnutrition and dehydration (skin, eyes, hair, mucous membranes, etc.). Physical examination should obviously constitute part of the medical program for the duration of the disease, especially if chronic PEM can be expected. Any objective signs suggesting malnutrition must be confirmed by biochemical data since cancer treatment may cause lesions similar to those of PEM.

Anthropometry

Anthropometric measurements must be made periodically, taking into account the patient's age and utilizing the tables of percentiles referring to the population to which the child belongs. The aim is to evaluate any loss of mass of the organism not only at onset of the disease but also at any particular time during treatment. The measurements are repeated periodically in order to check the quality of growth of the child during the disease. As already stated, one of the aims of nutritional treatment of these children is to ensure correct growth, and weight, height, and cranial circumference measurements in particular constitute a series of reliable parameters of growth. Other anthropometric measurements (fatfolds, mid-upper arm circumference, etc.) are possibly of less importance as regards growth of the child; they are nevertheless useful elements for a dynamic evaluation of the ratio between lean and fat body mass although they may be difficult to evaluate in children, especially very young ones, and yield results that are not very reliable. It is worthwhile underlining that anthropometric measurements (excluding height) must be made in conditions of optimal hydration to avoid underestimates (in the case of dehydration) and overestimates (in the case of imbibition).

Biochemical Evaluation

Efforts have been made to rationalize this approach in the attempt to find sensitive and reliable parameters of nutritional status. In evaluating these parameters it must be borne in mind that many factors may interfere with the results, such as infections, drugs administered, and circadian rhythms. Furthermore, these tests are often expensive and require a large amount of blood in addition to that needed for routine tests. Thus they should be kept to a minimum.

Serum albumin (<3 g/dl) and transferrin (<150 mg/dl) are possibly the best specific indicators of protein nutritional status; to these may be added prealbumin (<20 mg/dl), which is a sensitive and early indicator of protein deficiency and which, because of its short half-life, is modified more rapidly than the other two substances, permitting frequent monitoring. Urinary creatinine may be useful since its level of excretion is considered an approximate index of lean body mass; however, in the case of young children, urine collection may not be simple. Some elements, in particular zinc, are deficient in the presence of a decreased alimentary intake and may thus be useful as a nutritional index.

The hematological features and immunological indicators do not have an absolute value and their reliability in patients undergoing chemotherapy with steroids and/or cytotoxic drugs is poor.

Nutritional Requirements

The nutritional requirements constitute a very important aspect of nutrition in the treatment of children with cancer. In fact a patient of a few months or years presents calorie and protein requirements per kilogram body weight very different from those of older children or adults. Table 1 shows the requirements that have been established for healthy children up to 1 year of age (a period in which growth is particularly rapid), to which should be added the requirements relating to the type of tumor and degree of stress.

Three factors must be considered in determining the calorie and protein requirements of a child with cancer:

- Requirements for maintenance of organic functions
- Requirements for growth
- Requirements for the conditions of stress (tumor, infections, etc.)

The maintenance calorie and protein requirements can be derived from indications in the literature; they are about 140 mg/kg of protein daily and 1270 kcal/m^2

Table 1. Average protein and energy requirements in infants. (Modified from Beaton 1985)

Age (months)	Protein (g/kg/day)	Energy (kcal/kg/day)
0-1		124
1-2	2.25	116
2-3	1.82	109
3-4	1.47	103
4-5	1.34	99
5-6	1.30	96.5
6-7		95
7-8	1.25	94.5
8-9		95
9-10		99
10-11	1.15	100
11-12		104.5

daily. The proteins for growth constitute about 25% of the requirement; from the caloric point of view, considering that each gram of growth requires from 0.45 to 1.2 kcal, and with a theoretical daily growth of 0.9 g/kg per day as the objective, the need is from 0.4 to 1.1 kcal/kg. To this must be added the activity requirements that are calculated as about 50% of the basal metabolic requirements. The state of stress due to the tumor or to particular conditions (such as intercurrent infections) requires a further increase that is naturally very variable but has been roughly evaluated as 20% of the basal metabolic need.

These figures are obviously only points of reference, and adjustments can be made based on an evaluation of the nutritional status of each patient and on the requirements relating to the state of health, treatment, and type of tumor.

Nutritional Techniques

Starting from the principle that the normal nutritional intake of a healthy child is insufficient to meet the requirements of a child with cancer, and bearing in mind the difficulties in oral hyperalimentation (also because of the presence of anorexia, mucositis, change in taste, etc.), there are basically two techniques that are widely used: enteral nutrition and total or partial parenteral nutrition.

Much has been written on the technique of TPN, due particularly to studies performed on newborns who were the first pediatric patients to undergo this procedure. It is worth emphasizing the improvement obtained in the treatment of children with cancer due to the introduction of silicon catheters with a subcutaneous tunnel (Hickman or Broviac types). Furthermore, advances in the quality of infused nutritional solutions continuously improve the approach to the problem.

Since the percentage of these cases with severely impaired nutritional status is not very high, depending on the type of tumor and particular conditions of risk (Table 2), enteral nutrition with elementary or semielementary products with low osmolarity is in our opinion very promising. With the aim of avoiding problems of

Table 2. Frequency of various types of childhood neoplasm and associated risk of protein-energy malnutrition. (Modified from Rickard et al. [4])

Type of neoplasm	% of total childhood neoplasms	Incidence of PEM at diagnosis
Acute leukemia	30.2	6%
Lymphocytic	25.7	
Non-Lymphocytic	4.5	
Lymphomas	13.6	
Hodgkin's	4.3	?
Non-Hodgkin	9.3	10–15%
CNS tumors	18.6	?
Neuroblastoma	7.7	47%
Retinoblastoma	2.6	?
Soft-tissue sarcoma	6.5	?
Wilms' tumor	6.1	31%
Bone sarcomas	4.6	
Osteosarcoma	2.3	12.5%
Ewing's	2.3	67%
Liver tumor	1.2	?
All others	8.9	?

malnutrition in children with acute leukemia, we administered a semielementary diet using a silicon nasal-gastric tube. The preliminary study included 21 children aged between 58 days and 12 years (median 5 years) with leukemia at onset or in relapse, and a control group of 15 children comparable for age, leukemia, and treatment who received the usual hospital diet. The semielementary nutrient used was Alfare (Nestlè, Vevey, Switzerland), in increasing concentrations from 8% to 25% if well tolerated. Since the energy value was 480 kcal/100 g of powder, the higher concentrations permitted hyperalimentation. The product was administered for 7–50 days (median 28 days). The weight increase obtained was 7.7 ± 5.5(SD) g/day whereas in the control group there was a weight loss in all except one child. All the patients except for two with protein-losing enteropathy maintained a normal albumin value; thyroxine-binding prealbumin (TBPA) and retinol-binding protein (RBP) were under normal values at the start of the study but showed an increase at subsequent check-ups, in some cases even to standard values. The only notable side-effect was transient diarrhea in some patients. The study was thus considered positive, and now we use this diet for patients with poor but not severe malnutrition in whom side-effects due to chemotherapy, such as mucositis and anorexia, can be expected.

Conclusions

A malnourished child manifests inadequate growth, greater susceptibility to infections, deterioration of psychological condition, and possibly, if very young, retarded cerebral development. When a child with cancer presents these risks, adequate nutritional intake must be the immediate response. A child in a good nutritional condition will tolerate treatment better and be more stable psychologically; moreover prognosis may be improved since it will be possible to give the full cancer treatment. In the meantime correct development of the whole organism will have been ensured.

References

1. Van Eys J (1986) The pathophysiology of undernutrition in the child with cancer. Cancer 58: 1874-1880
2. Rickard KA, Loghmani ES, Grosfeld JL et al. (1985) Short- and long-term effectiveness of enteral and parenteral nutrition in reversing or preventing protein-energy malnutrition in advanced neuroblastoma. Cancer 56: 2881-2897
3. Kokal WA (1985) The impact of antitumor therapy on nutrition. Cancer 55: 273-278
4. Rickard KA, Baehner RL, Coates TD et al. (1982) Supportive nutritional intervention in pediatric cancer. Cancer Res 42: 766-773
5. Donaldson SS (1982) Effects of therapy on nutritional status of the pediatric cancer patient. Cancer Res 42: 729-736
6. Van Eys J (1977) Nutritional therapy in children with cancer. Cancer Res 37: 2457-2461

Malnutrition and the Role of Nutritional Support for Radiation Therapy Patients

H.-J. Thiel, R. Fietkau, and R. Sauer

Klinik und Poliklinik für Strahlentherapie, Universitätsstraße 27, 8520 Erlangen, FRG

General Aspects of Radiogenic Nutritional Disturbances

The effect of radiotherapy, like that of chemotherapy, cannot be exclusively restricted to the malignant cell populations; neither modality can be prevented from adversely affecting the surrounding normal tissue and from giving rise to specific nutritional problems (Table 1). The nutritional disorders caused by irradiation depend on:

1. The type of irradiation
2. The dose, fractionation, and duration of radiotherapy
3. The localization of the tumor or of the region irradiated
4. The volume irradiated
5. The combination with other therapy modalities (23)

Dose, Fractionation, and Duration of Treatment

Acute radiation reactions are usually of limited duration and therefore affect the nutritional status less adversely than chronic radiation sequelae. Therefore it is of particular importance for the clinician to make due allowance for the tolerance dose of the various organs at risk in planning the radiation dose and the pattern of fractionation as well as in selecting the target volume [23, 62].

High individual doses as part of a hypofractionation program increase the late effects of irradiation and should no longer be applied. The same holds true for the still widely observed bad habit of irradiating only one field daily for reasons of economy in the case of parallel opposing field arrangements. This is because a very high individual dose is applied to the soft tissues close to the surface, which leads to the so-called edge effect, i.e., to severe fibrosis of intervening structures [30].

Recent Results in Cancer Research, Vol. 108

Table 1. Localized effects of radiotherapy leading to nutritional alterations. (Modified from Donaldson and Lenon [23])

Region	Acute effects	Chronic effects
CNS	Nausea Vomiting	
Head and neck	Mucositis Sore mouth and throat Dysphagia Odynophagia Dry mouth (xerostomia) Loss of taste (hypo-/ageusia) Dysgeusia Loss of smell (hypo-/anosmia) Dysosmia Anorexia	Xerostomia Loss of taste Dental caries Ulcer Osteoradionecrosis Trismus
Thorax	Dysphagia	Fibrosis Stenosis Perforation Fistula
Abdomen and pelvis	Anorexia Nausea Vomiting Diarrhea Acute enteritis Acute colitis Choleretic enteropathy	Diarrhea Maldigestion Malabsorption Chronic enteritis Chronic colitis Ulcer Stricture Obstruction Diarrhea Perforation Fistula

Location of the Tumor or of the Region Irradiated

The severity and incidence of weight loss and malnutrition are primarily determined by the location of the tumor or the body region irradiated. The two phenomena develop mainly in patients in whom sections of the gastrointestinal tract are irradiated [13, 14, 20, 21, 23, 25, 37, 44, 47–50, 63, 73–75]. The side-effects (Table 1) of irradiation pertinent to malnutrition are:

1. *Inadequate oral food intake,* caused by mucositis, xerostomia, alterations in the sensations of smell and taste, odynophagia, and dysphagia if the oral cavity, oropharynx, and esophagus are irradiated.
2. *Anorexia, nausea, and vomiting* if as a result of the irradiation of the salivary glands the saliva becomes viscid and finally dries up or if large portions of the thorax or abdomen lie in the field of irradiation.
3. *Defective digestion, malabsorption, and diarrhea* whenever large portions of the small intestine and colon are irradiated.

Table 2. Weight loss experienced by irradiated patients. (Modified from Pezner and Archambeau [53])

Irradiated region	Patients	% patients with weight loss during XRT	Average weight loss (kg)	% patients with weight loss >10% of body weight
Head and neck [23]	122	93	3.7	9
Head and neck [13]	74	94	-	-
Head and neck [70]	36	50	4.0	10
Larynx and hypopharynx [14]	110	-	3.1	3
Larynx stage I+II [53]				
XRT field <7×7 cm	26	19	1.5	0
XRT field >7×7 cm	9	67	5.3	22
Abdomen [23]	67	88	3.4	13
Pelvis [53]	40	38	2.4	0

Owing to these side-effects, patients are no longer able to eat, they no longer like to eat, or they are no longer in a position to absorb the nutritive substances administered.

The Volume Irradiated

The second important factor determining both the incidence and severity of malnutrition is the volume of the gastrointestinal tract irradiated (Table 2). Thus in 35 patients with a laryngeal carcinoma, stage I or II, a mean weight loss of 1.5 kg was observed only in 19% of cases with 7×7 cm fields, whereas with fields in excess of 7×7 cm 67% of the patients suffered a mean weight loss of 5.3 kg. In the small field group no patient lost more than 10% of his initial body weight as compared with 22% in the large field group [53].

Among the 40 patients who were subjected to irradiation of the pelvis [53], only 38% lost 2.4 kg on average; by contrast 88% of 67 patients who underwent irradiation of the abdomen [23] lost 3.4 kg on average. A weight loss above 10% of the initial body weight was seen in 13% of the abdominally irradiated patients, whereas such a loss did not occur in any of the patients subjected solely to pelvic irradiation.

Combined Radiation Therapy/Chemotherapy

Only a very limited number of data are available on the impact of a combined modality therapy on nutritional status, although especially combined chemotherapy/radiotherapy has been seen to interfere most strongly with rapidly proliferating cell populations, such as those involving the skin, the mucosa, and epithelium of the gastrointestinal tract [23, 54–56]. How serious the side-effects and complications of such combination therapy can be was demonstrated by an investigation undertaken at the Gustave-Roussy Institute, where 44 children were subjected to aggressive abdominal irradiation and simultaneous polychemotherapy directed against different types of tumor: Fifty-five percent of the children suffered a loss of weight. In 70% acute radiation enteritis with nausea, vomiting, and diarrhea was observed. For this reason is was necessary for 30% of them to receive intravenous infusions. Within a maximum of 2 months following completion of therapy, 36% of the long-term survivors developed chronic radiation enteritis with acute vomiting, diarrhea, and symptoms of small-bowel obstruction. All the children with severe acute enteritis received chemotherapy/radiotherapy simultaneously; 60% received actinomycin D. Eighty percent of the children with chronic enteritis were given simultaneous chemotherapy/radiotherapy; all of them received actinomycin D.

Table 3. Possible problems with treatment of head and neck cancer patients. (Modified from Dwyer [27])

Surgery	Chewing and swallowing difficulties
	Alteration in smell
	Loss of taste
Radiation	Mucositis (sore mouth and throat)
	Dysphagia
	Anorexia, nausea, and vomiting
	Xerostomia (dry mouth)
	Loss of taste (mouth blindness)
	Taste changes (dysgeusia)
	Dental caries
	Weight loss
Chemotherapy	Stomatitis
	Anorexia, nausea, and vomiting
	Candidiasis
	Conditioned food aversions
	Psychogenic emesis
Untreated patient	Alcohol, tobacco
	Insufficient oral intake
	No dietetic experience
	Bad fitting dentures, edentulous
	Difficulty in speaking, chewing, and swallowing
	Obstruction of the alimentary tract
	Infection and ulceration of soft tissues and bone of jaw
	Metastasis to other parts of body
Life style, nutrition, and cancer risk	Heavy drinker
	Excessive smoker
	Poor oral hygiene
	Insufficient dental care
	Bad fitting dentures
	Occupation: - longlasting chronic irritation of oral mucosa
	- repeated or chronic trauma

Special Topographical Problems of Radiotherapy and Their Impact on Nutritional Status

Head and Neck

In patients with tumors involving the head and neck region, the following factors affect the nutritional status:

1. Personality of the tumor patient
2. Subjective and objective tumor findings
3. The side-effects of the treatment [1, 23, 27, 37, 48-50, 53, 71-75]

Most of these patients are obstinate excessive smokers and drinkers with bad eating habits, poor oral hygiene, and a very bad dental status because of inadequate dental care (Table 3).

Owing to the tumor-induced obstruction of the oropharynx (Figs. 1, 2), the frequently extensive anatomically and functionally crippling operation, and the aggressive chemotherapy/radiotherapy required, mastication and swallowing are impaired to such an extent that the patients are only able to take in semisolid or liquid meals rich in carbohydrates and eventually cease to eat at all. As these patients cannot be induced to give up their vices during the radiotherapy, they are seriously afflicted by the acute side-effects of radiation. These are:

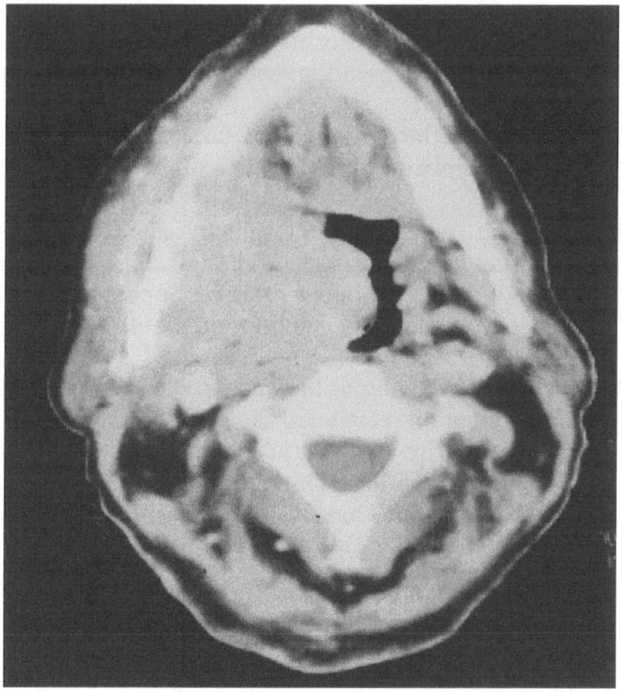

Fig. 1. Gross oropharyngeal cancer, stage T_4N_3, with almost complete obstruction of pharynx

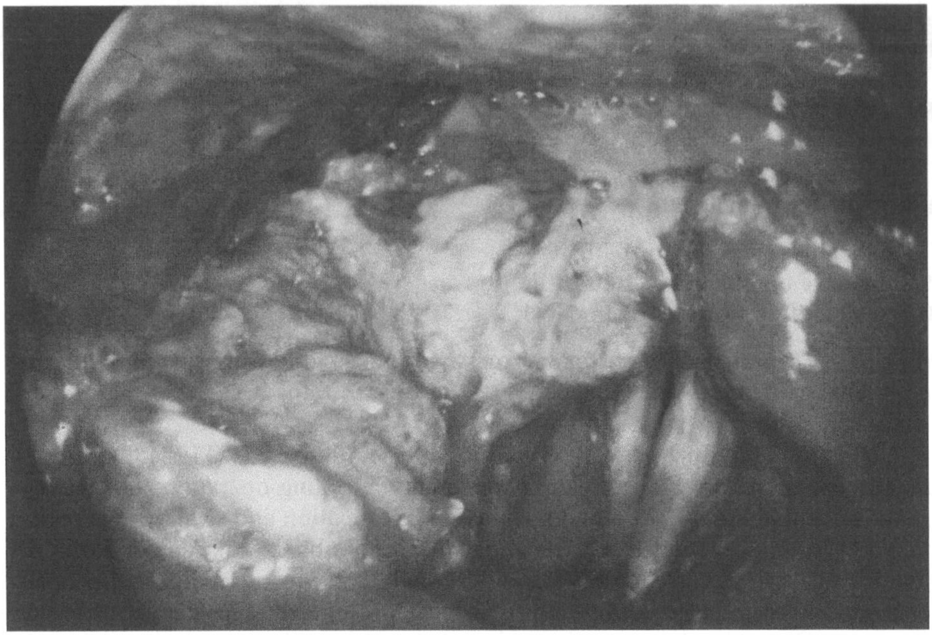

Fig. 2. Direct endoscopic view of bulky hypopharyngeal carcinoma

1. Radiation-induced mucositis with edema and erythema of the mucosa, formation of fibrinous pseudomembranes, and finally superficial ulcerations and hemorrhages [71].
2. Alterations in the sensations of taste and smell, such as hypogeusia, ageusia, dysgeusia, hyposmia, and anosmia (Table 4) [7, 13-15, 16, 19, 21, 23, 27, 33, 37, 48-50, 53, 75].
3. Dry mouth. When the large salivary glands are subjected to radiotherapy, the salivary volume decreases and the saliva quality is altered: the clear and watery solution is converted into a viscid semiopaque mass (Table 4). As a result, mastication and swallowing of solid food are no longer possible [1, 13, 21, 23, 27, 29, 37, 40, 48-50, 53, 71, 75, 77, 78, 80].
4. Dental caries. Owing to the qualitative and quantitative alteration of the saliva and the radiation reaction of the surrounding mucosa, the self-cleaning function of the oral cavity is impaired. The composition of the oral bacterial flora is altered, allowing cariogenic microorganisms to develop and to find an excellent substrate in the tenacious material; finally the tooth becomes easy prey to bacterial destruction (Fig. 3) [21, 23, 27, 30, 37, 39, 43, 57, 72].

The *chronic radiation sequelae* observed are: mucosal ulcerations, hemorrhages, trismus caused by increasing fibrosis of the masticatory musculature, and osteoradionecrosis of the mandible [21, 23, 28, 30, 46].

All these acute and chronic side-effects of radiotherapy are likely to lead to devastating nutritional deficits (Table 5). Donaldson and Lenon [23] studied 122 patients with squamous cell carcinomas of the oral cavity, the oropharynx, and the

Table 4. Long-term effects of radiotherapy (1–7 years after XRT) on taste and salivary function in man. (Modified from Mossman et al. [50])

Subjective complaints			Taste function tests				Saliva function tests	
Xerostomia	Hypo-/dysgeusia	Anorexia	NaCl	Sucrose	HCl	Urea	Flow rate (ml/min)	Protein secretion rate (mg/min)
Before XRT			Detection threshold (mM/liter) ↑					
2/18 (11%)	3/18 (17%)	3/18 (17%)	6/13 (46%)	3/13 (23%)	5/13 (38%)	7/13 (54%)	↓ 12/12 (100%)	↓ 11/11 (100%)
During and after XRT			Recognition threshold (mM/liter) ↑					
12/18 (67%)	12/18 (67%)	9/18 (50%)	7/13 (54%)	4/13 (31%)	7/13 (54%)	8/13 (61%)	0 7/12 (58%)	0 7/11 (64%)
1–7 years after XRT			Taste intensity responsiveness ↓					
15/22 (68%)	11/22 (50%)	7/18 (39%)	salt and bitter >> sweet and sour					

Conclusions:
1. Curative doses of radiotherapy may result in long-term changes in salivary and taste function: 69% had measurable taste loss; every patient who had radiotherapy including the parotid glands had measurable salivary dysfunction.
2. The maximum tolerance doses resulting in a 50% complication rate 5 years after treatment (TD 50/5) are estimated to be 40–65 Gy for xerostomia and 50–65 Gy for taste loss.

hypopharynx who were subjected to radiotherapy over 6–8 weeks with curative intent at Stanford University Medical Center. Ninety-three percent of patients had an average weight loss of 3.7 kg during the treatment; 8.7% lost more than 10% of their initial weight. Sixty-four percent of patients were already undernourished and had a body weight of less than 70 kg before the treatment was started. Our own studies demonstrated that 50% of all ENT patients suffered a weight loss of 4 kg during a radiotherapeutic course despite intensive nutritional support [73, 74].

Thorax

Irradiation of tumors involving the lungs, the mediastinum, or the esophagus leads to esophagitis and thus to dysphagia. The tissue of the trachea and of the bronchial tree is less sensitive.

Late effects that have a considerable impact on the nutritional status are fibrosis of the esophagus with stenosis and obstruction, ulceration, perforation, and formation of fistulae.

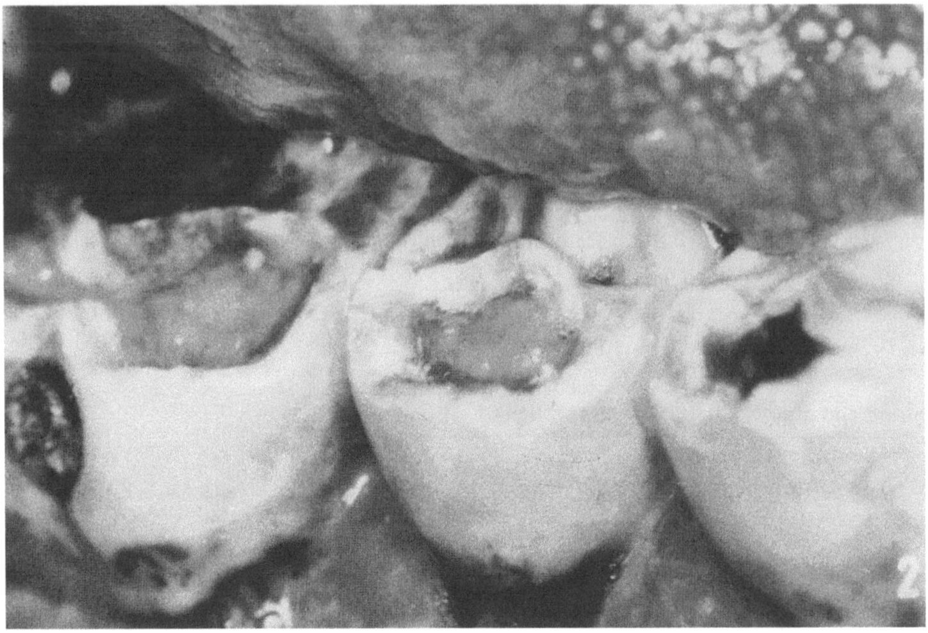

Fig. 3. Patient after irradiation: poor dental hygiene caused loss of dentin; thus the tooth enamel is laid open

Table 5. Nutritional problems of radiotherapy of head and neck cancer patients. (Chencharick and Mossman [13])

Subjective nutritional assessment			Objective nutritional assessment			
			Body weight		24-h dietary recall	
	Before XRT	During XRT	Before XRT	After XRT	Early (1 week)	Late (6 weeks)
Oral complications	25%	>80%	94%	86%	Significant caloric	
Mouth dryness	25%[a]	80%	5 kg $\downarrow$	5.9 kg $\downarrow$	deficiencies (kcal)	
Fluid intake	40%	60%			1746	1698
Abnormal taste function	14%[b]	84%			2400	2400
Foods taste bad	15%	80%			(RDA)	(RDA)
Add sugar	2%	30%			More carbohydrates	
Add salt	15%	15%			172 g	205 g
Dysphagia	40%	70%			More sugar	
Loss of appetite	20%	60%			50 g	84 g

Conclusions:
1. Head and neck cancer patients have subjectively oral and nutritional problems and objectively nutritional deficits prior to radiotherapy which are either exacerbated or sustained during therapy.
2. Nutritional evaluations should be made a routine, integral part of therapy for every cancer patient.

[a] Salivary function tests: all normal.
[b] Measurement of taste function: >90% abnormal.

Abdomen and Pelvis

The stomach appears to tolerate radiation remarkably well. Asymptomatic radiation gastritis accompanied by hyperemia, edema, microscopic hemorrhages, and exudation are likely to develop after approximately 2 weeks of irradiation. Low doses of radiation to the stomach only cause nonspecific anorexia and nausea, while high doses by contrast lead to ulcer formation with epigastric pain, bleeding, vomiting, and progressive weight loss [32, 60, 61, 65].

Irradiation of the *small and large bowel* may be accompanied by the triad of nausea, vomiting, and diarrhea as symptoms of *acute radiation enteritis*. Morphologically irradiation is associated with alterations of the small bowel epithelium with a shortening of villi, alterations in cell kinetics, especially reduction of mitoses, decreased enzymatic activities, and vascular changes [51, 76, 81]. Small-bowel injury leads to variable degrees of malabsorption of fat, carbohydrates, and proteins as well as to a loss of water and electrolytes [4, 23, 36, 44, 58, 59, 68-70]. Moreover, numerous enzymes, including disaccharidase and peptidase, have been shown to decrease in the mucosa [36, 70].

A major reason for steatorrhea diarrhea is the so-called cholerhetic enteropathy [2, 3, 4, 34, 68], i.e., malabsorption of bile salts by the small bowel which gives rise to malabsorption of fat. In addition, the bile salts in the colon inhibit water absorption and stimulate the peristaltic movements of the colon, resulting in a loss of water and electrolytes.

Chronic radiation enteritis [22, 41, 61, 71] is clinically characterized by symptoms of chronic diarrhea or intermittent intestinal obstruction, mucosal ulcerations, perforation, and formation of fistulae. Morphologically it is marked by fibrosis of the small bowel, submucosal telangiectasis, vascular thrombosis, and hyalinization. Typically, there is a progressive loss of water, electrolytes, proteins, carbohydrates, fats, and vitamins. An operative intervention may eventually become necessary.

Nutritional problems related to *chronic radiation colitis* result from diarrhea, tenesmus, and blood loss [61].

Therapeutic Measures for the Improvement of the Nutritional Status

For all patients expected to present nutritional problems in response to radiotherapy, and especially for all ENT patients, the nutritional status is defined by means of a standardized scheme before the treatment is started (Table 6). This schedule comprises anthropometric, biochemical, and immunological parameters which define body and muscle dimensions, fat depots, the status of the function proteins, and that of the cell-mediated immunity [5, 6, 56, 57].

In the nutritional management and nutritional therapy, the dietitian plays a particularly important role. Her tasks can be broken down into three phases (Table 7) [1, 23, 27, 37, 73, 75]:

1. Identification of the problem
2. Interventional measures before and during therapy

Table 6. Nutritional assessment. (Modified from Blackburn et al. [6])

Body mass	BW = body weight	
	BrW = Broca weight	Height (cm) − 100 = BrW (kg)
	WT/HT = Weight for Height Index	(Actual weight/ideal body weight) × 100
	IBW = Ideal body weight	M: IBW = BrW − 0.2(BrW − 52) F: IBW = BrW − 0.4(BrW − 52)
Fat stores (body fat mass)	TSF = Triceps skinfold	M: 12.5 mm F: 16.55 mm
Lean body mass (skeletal muscle protein)	AC = Arm circumference	M: 293 mm F: 285 mm
	AMC = Arm muscle circumference	AMC = AC − (TSF × 3.14) (mm) M: 253 mm F: 232 mm
	CHI = Creatinine Height Index	CHI = (C in 24-h urine/IC) × 100 (%)
	IC = Ideal Creatinine	M: IC = IBW × 23 (mg) F: IC = IBW × 18 (mg)
Visceral proteins	Albumin	35 g/liter
	Prealbumin	180 mg/liter
	Cholinesterase	M: 3300 U/liter, F: 2500 U/liter
	Transferrin	2 g/liter
	Retinol binding protein	30 mg/liter
	Total iron binding capacity	2.4–4 mg/liter
Immune function	Total lymphocyte count	1800/μl
	Lymphocyte transformation assay	
	Delayed hypersensitivity skin testing: SK/SD, mumps, Candida, Multitest Merieux	
	Immunoglobulins	

3. Aftercare of the patients and reviewing of records to assess the therapeutic results

The nutritional therapy must be adapted to the type and extent of malnutrition. As 75% of the tumor patients show medium-to-severe malnutrition of the mixed type, an increased supply of both high energy food and biologically valuable proteins is indicated. The function of the gastrointestinal tract is the determining factor for the optimal feeding of nutrients. The daily demand of calories and proteins depends on both the type and the objective of therapy. As a rule, the daily intake of calories should amount to 2500–3000 kcal and the daily albumin intake to 1.5–2 g albumin/kg nominal weight.

An indication for concomitant nutritional therapy is given:

1. If the oral intake of calories and proteins has dropped below 80% of the standard values prior to the initiation of radiotherapy
2. If the patient has lost more than 10% of his normal body weight

Table 7. Nutritional assessment and support during cancer treatment on an outpatient basis. (Modified from Dwyer [27])

Phase 1: Problem identification

1. *Screening criteria* for patients at risk with respect to jeopardized nutritional status
   - Weight for height
   - Declines in weight
   - Patient's report of appetite, food intake, and problems with eating
   - Analysis of the type of therapy
2. *Further dietetic assessment* of all patients at risk
   - 24-hour recalls of food intake (dietary histories) or food records kept for several days (food intake diaries)
   - History: nausea, taste changes, dryness in the mouth
   - Profile of the patient's likes and dislikes (food preferences)
3. *Detailed nutritional assessment*
   - History data (medical, dietetic, social)
   - Anthropometric
   - Biochemical
   - Clinical
   - Psychological
4. *Formulation of the nutritional care plan*
   - Anticipatory guidance and intervention on a broad front of potential patient problems in the food and eating sphere (side-effects of therapy)

Phase 2: Intervention measures

1. Therapeutic consultation with a nutritionist
2. Special nutritional advice for a specific problem
3. General nutritional advice of the anticipatory type
4. Special help in obtaining food assistance
5. Help with food management
6. General health education

Phase 3: Follow-up and record reviews

- to assess the success of therapies
- to readjust nutritional care plans and protocols

3. If the serum albumin level has dropped below 3.5 g/dl
4. If stomatitis is present or if the function of the gastrointestinal tract has been impaired by any other disorder
5. If during the radiotherapeutic course the patient suffers a weight loss of 0.5 kg/10 Gy, i.e., 0.5 kg/week or more.

Concomitant nutritional management and therapy should be given according to a multistep plan based on the initial diagnostic findings and allowing for the expected increase in the patient's nutritional problems with the duration of the radiotherapeutic treatment (Table 8) [1, 27, 37, 73, 74].

For the food intake basically two routes can be selected: the enteral and parenteral route (Tables 9, 10). The food should be given via the physiological oral and enteral routes for as long as possible. However, the necessity of feeding largely iso-osmolar solutions creates a volume problem for the intake of calories. Most patients fail to take in orally more than 1000 kcal/day and only 2500–3000 kcal with strictly enteral administration. In the case of higher caloric quantities, the patient's

Table 8. Step plan for dietetic counseling and managing of patients

Step 1: Dietetic counseling
Normal oral nutrition
Diet modifications
Mechanical soft diet
Blended diet
Patient motivation
Step 2: Forced oral nutrition
High caloric and high protein supplementary feedings
Fortified milk
High protein eggnog
High protein milkshake
Commercial formula diets
Step 3: Forced enteral nutrition
Tube feeding (nasogastric, nasoduodenojejunal)
Regular tube feedings
Noncommercial ("homemade")
Commercial ("industrial made")
Nutrient defined diet (formula diet)
Oligopeptide diet
Chemically defined diet (elemental diet)
Lactose free tube feedings
Restricted residue diet
Fine needle - catheter - jejunostomy (FNCJ)
Percutaneous endoscopically guided gastrostomy (PEG)
"Home enteral nutrition"
Step 4: Parenteral nutrition (intravenous hyperalimentation)
Partial parenteral nutrition
Total parenteral nutrition
"Home parenteral nutrition"

cooperation diminishes as a result of the volume and time expended on the food intake: a feeling of fullness, overfeeding, and aversion to the taste of food are the consequences. However, due to the use of nutrient pumps it has become possible for the patient to be fed continuously outside his home and during the night.

Many patients find it difficult to accept a nasogastric indwelling feeding tube [74]. They feel uneasy when it is introduced and can hardly bring themselves to tolerate it. They are loathe to go around with it in public. A better alternative is offered by percutaneous endoscopic gastrostomy (PEG), where the feeding catheter is placed directly in the stomach of the locally anesthetized patient by way of a guide wire under endoscopic control (Fig. 4). However, acceptance of this approach by the patient is poor prior to radiotherapy, despite the efforts made to motivate him. It is only owing to the mounting distress caused by the increasing weight loss and the acute reactions to irradiation that he yields. We hope that by performing PEG simultaneously with surgery, patient acceptance can be increased. Presently, we establish an indication for PEG only on an empirical clinical basis in the following instances:

Table 9. How to treat?

Enteral	1. Oral	Drinking-cup Straw
	2. Gastric fistula	Nasogastric tube Kader fistula PEG = percutaneous endoscopically guided gastrostomy (Gauderer, Keymling)
	3. Jejunal fistula	Nasojejunal tube Witzel fistula FNCJ = Fine needle catheter jejunostomy (Delany, Troidl)
Parenteral	1. Peripheral vein	Partial or total
	2. Central vein	Partial or total Broviac catheter Hickman catheter
	3. Central vein with subcutaneous "port"	Port-A-Cath system Infuse-A-Port system
In hospital		
At home	1. Home enteral nutrition (HEN) 2. Home parenteral nutrition (HPN)	

Table 10. What to eat? (Troidl [77])

	Homemade diet high molecular	Formula diet high molecular	Elemental diet low molecular
Composition	Protein Fat Carbohydrates Salts, vitamins Residues	Protein Fat Poly-, oligosaccharides Salts, vitamins Minimal residues	Amino acids, peptides Essential fatty acids Oligo-, monosaccharides Salts, vitamins No residues
Covering of nutrition requirements	incomplete	→	complete
Resorption	partial	→	total
Gastrointestinal tract	loaded	→	unloaded
Preparation	complex	→	simple
Taste	good	→	bad
Psychological situation	good	→	bad
Side-effects	minimal	→	present
Costs	minimal	→	high

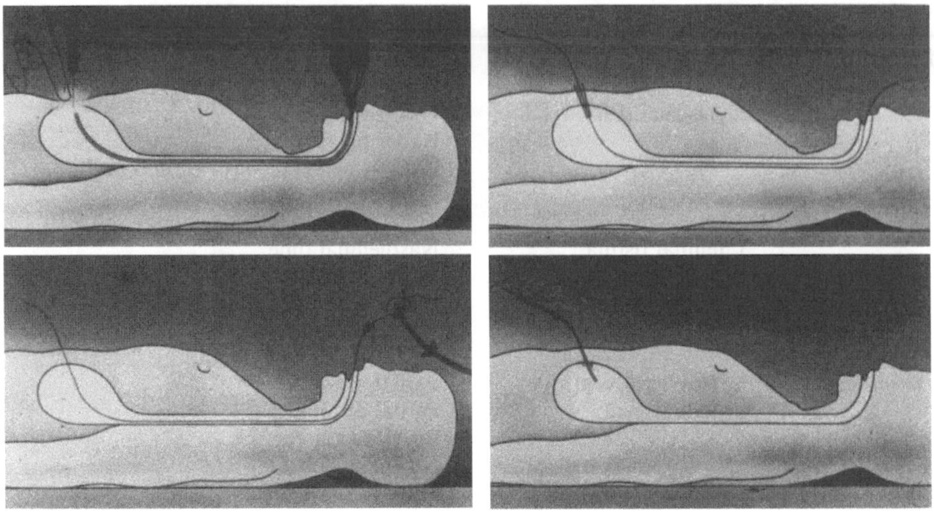

Fig. 4. Principle of percutaneous endoscopically guided gastrostomy (PEG)

1. With loss of over 10% of the initial weight
2. With extensive tumors interfering with swallowing
3. When the patient has undergone extensive surgery in the past
4. When aggressive radiotherapy is planned (large volume, including oropharynx and salivary glands, high dose, accelerated fractionation)
5. With temporary implantation of iridium-192-seeds in the ENT areas

In the case of ambulatory tumor patients placed on long-term enteral or parenteral feeding, patient care by a nutrition team in conjunction with a comprehensive nutritional service called "home-enteral nutrition" or "home-parenteral nutrition" ("Erlanger Modell") has provided good results. This solution brings about a desirable reduction of cost, to say nothing of the social and psychological advantages for the patient.

Outlook

Malnutrition is liable to impair organ functions and to augment morbidity and mortality (Table 11) [66]. Therefore it is necessary and reasonable that all malnourished tumor patients are administered the missing essential nutrients. This brings about a marked amelioration of the Karnofsky performance status and of the general quality of life [18, 52, 64]. Moreover, most retrospective studies have testified to the favorable influence of nutritional therapy on the loss of weight and on the gastrointestinal side-effects of irradiation [8, 12, 35, 38, 45, 53, 83].

Unfortunately, to date no prospective randomized study has been able to demonstrate an improvement in the local tumor control or in the survival rate (Table 12) [9, 10, 11, 24, 26, 31, 42, 67, 82]. This may be attributable to methodological problems, such as:

Table 11. Clinical effects of malnutrition. (Shils [66])

Weight loss	Protein depletion
Fat utilization	Progressive weakness
Skin breakdown	Apathy, irritability
Prolonged bedrest	Impaired wound healing
Endocrine changes	Electrolyte-fluid imbalance
Secondary nutrient depletion	Decreased hypoxic response

Depressed immune mechanisms:
- Impaired phagocytosis
- Decreased macrophage mobilization
- Depressed lymphocyte function

Delay in diagnostic and therapeutic program

Increased morbidity and mortality

Table 12. Summary of prospective randomized studies evaluating oral elemental diets and intravenous hyperalimentation in patients receiving abdominal and/or pelvic irradiation. (Modified from Pezner and Archambeau [53])

Author	Year	No. of patients		Chemo-therapy	Potential benefits of nutritional therapy			
		Study popul.	Control popul.		Avoids weight loss	Lessens GI toxicity	Better able to complete XRT	Improves survival or local tumor control
Oral elemental diets								
Bounous et al.[a]	1975	9	9	No	Yes	Yes	Yes	–
Douglas et al.[b]	1978	13	17	Yes	No	–	Yes	No
Brown et al.[c]	1980	51	17	No	No	No	No	–
Intravenous hyperalimentation								
Valerio et al.	1978	11	9	No	Yes	Yes	Yes	–
Bothe et al.	1979	17	15	No	Yes	Yes	Yes	–
Kinsella et al.	1981	17	15	No	Yes	Yes	Yes	–
Solassol et al.	1980	42	39	No	Yes	Yes	Yes	No
Donaldson et al.	1982	12	13	Yes	Yes	No	No	No
Ghavimi et al.	1982	11	13	Yes	Yes	No	No	No

[a] Flexical (Mead Johnson).
[b] Vivonex HN (Norwich-Eaton).
[c] Vivonex HN (not tolerable for 42% of patients).

1. Too few patients
2. A broad spectrum of tumor types and stages
3. Malnutrition nonexistent or not to be expected
4. Primary palliative therapy on account of the tumor site
5. Noncompliance by many patients

In the future, studies related to improvement in the local tumor control and the survival rate by means of adequate nutrition should only be carried out with patients who are treated with *curative intent*. Particular attention should be focused on the feeding tube management of ENT patients and PEG as a new possibility as well as on the permanent application of new and better tolerated oligopeptide diets to be administered by portable nutrient pumps to ambulatory tumor patients.

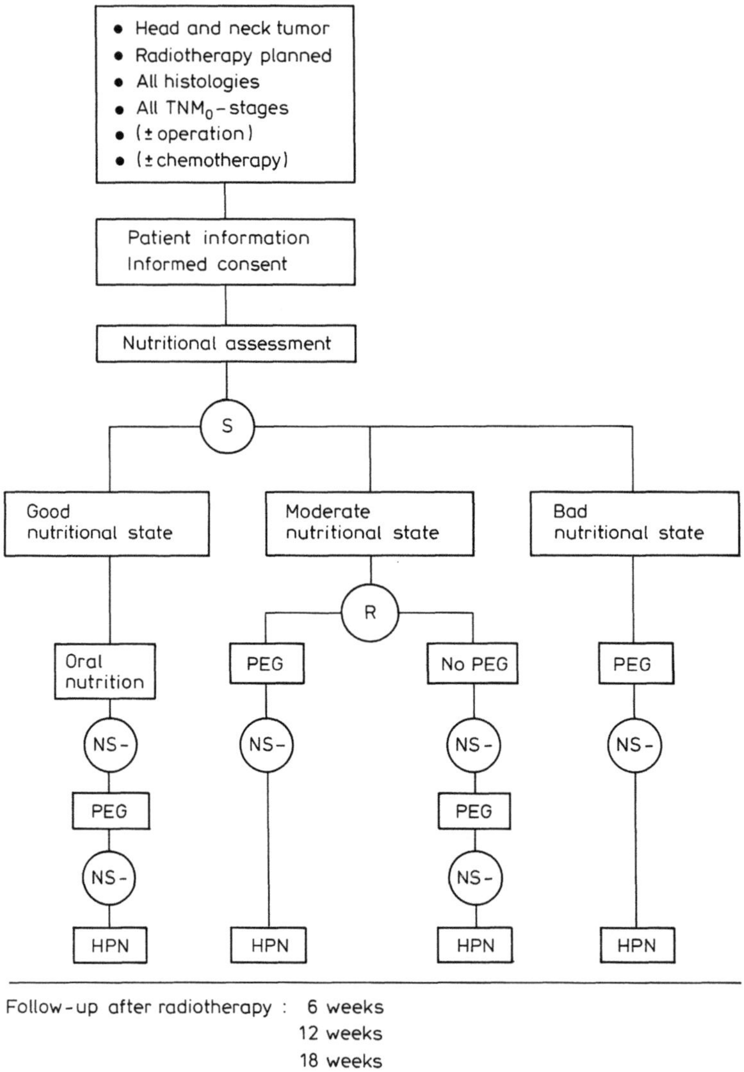

Fig. 5. Multidisciplinary, prospective, partly randomized study to investigate the significance of an adequate long-term nutritional therapy for head and neck cancer patients. *S*, stratify; *R*, randomize; *NS*, nutritional state; *PEG*, percutaneous endoscopic gastrostomy; *HPN*, home parenteral nutrition

In order to be able to investigate the significance of an adequate nutritional therapy for patients with tumors in the ear, nose, and throat regions, a multidisciplinary, prospective, partly randomized study is now in progress at our institution (Fig. 5). The patients are stratified according to their nutritional status and in the case of a moderate status, they are randomized between oral food intake and PEG-mediated feeding. We hope that this study will enable us to demonstrate that an efficacious nutritional therapy over 18 weeks and longer eliminates malnutrition and tends to diminish the incidence and severity of the acute radiation-induced reactions, thus allowing the patients to live an active and worthwhile life despite the severity of the disease.

Conclusions

With Shils [66] we draw the following conclusions:

1. Nutrition is a vital function. Malnutrition induced by cancer and its treatment is a risk factor leading to alteration of organ functions and increased morbidity and mortality and complicating further treatment of the disease.
2. Malnutrition is *not* an obligatory response of the host to cancer.
3. A rational nutritional therapeutic program for a patient requires analysis of the factors inducing depletion in that patient.
4. Early and periodic nutritional evaluation should be made a routine, integral part of therapy for every cancer patient.
5. Nutritional therapy, when indicated, should be instituted early.
6. The application and effectiveness of therapeutic programs must become part of the medical audit and general clinical procedure for inpatients and outpatients.
7. The objectives of nutritional therapy are:
   a) supportive: to maintain good status or to rehabilitate the debilitated while the patient awaits more definitive treatment,
   b) adjunctive: where nutrition therapy becomes a part of the therapeutic program,
   c) definitive: where nutrition therapy becomes the modality upon which the existence of the patient depends.
8. Nutritional status, tumor growth, and antitumor treatment are intimately related.
9. Nutritional therapy has the potential for difficulties and complications as well as benefits.
10. The provision of optimal nutritional care requires a competent multidisciplinary approach (team work) with adequate administrative and financial support.
11. The outpatient care of long-term nutritionally supported patients by a "nutritional team" operating within a care-providing system serving a wide area and involving home enteral nutrition and/or home parenteral nutrition ("Erlanger Modell") has proved highly successful. Apart from the desirable lowering of costs, the social and psychological advantages for the patient deserve special mention.

12. Within the framework of such a system, we are presently investigating, in a multidisciplinary prospective study, the value of ambulatory enteral long-term alimentation via percutaneous endoscopically guided gastrostomy (PEG) in patients with tumors of the head and neck region.

Summary

The nutritional status of a tumor patient can be negatively influenced by the local and systemic effects of the malignant tumor (tumor cachexia, anorexia, difficult oral food intake), by the effects of the various antitumoral therapy modalities (surgery, radiotherapy, chemotherapy), and by the complications associated with such modalities (anorexia, nausea, vomiting, mucositis, xerostomia, alterations of the smell and taste sensations, odynophagia, dysphagia, maldigestion, malabsorption, diarrhea, steatorrhea, conditioned aversions, radiogenic late effects), as well as by the psychological reactions of the patient to the real or feared existence of his tumor. The radiation-induced nutritional disorders depend on the tumor localization, the region irradiated, the dose and length of radiotherapy, the fractionation, the volume irradiated, and the combination with other therapeutic modalities ("combined modality therapy").

The acute radiation-induced reactions are usually of limited duration and for this reason tend to interfere with the nutritional status to a lesser extent than the permanent chronic consequences of irradiation. Weight loss and malnutrition tend to develop particularly in patients in whom segments of the gastrointestinal tract are subjected to irradiation. The incidence and severity of deficient nutrition depend not only on the region irradiated (head-neck region, thorax, abdomen, pelvis) but also, and most particularly, on the volume of the digestive tract irradiated. Chemotherapy and radiotherapy combined act very strongly on rapidly proliferating cell populations (skin, mucosa, epithelium of the gastrointestinal tract). In this context, actinomycin D and adriamycin act like real sensitizers, whereas the majority of the other drugs are likely to produce only an additive effect. The first named cytostatics give rise to the so-called recall phenomenon, i.e., the reactivation of latent radiation effects in response to the subsequent administration of the drug.

Malnutrition impairs organ function and ultimately results in increased morbidity and mortality. For this reason it has proven mandatory and reasonable that the organism of all tumor patients suffering from malnutrition is provided with the missing essential nutrients (especially amino acids for protein synthesis). This tends to clearly improve the Karnofsky performance status, with a positive effect on response rates, toxicity, and survival rates in retrospective studies. So far the prospective randomized studies have demonstrated a favorable influence of the nutritional therapy on the weight loss and on gastrointestinal side-effects in patients undergoing radiotherapy, but they have failed to evidence an improvement in the local tumor control or in the survival rate. However, this may be attributable to methodological problems. Future studies regarding amelioration of local tumor control and the survival rate by adequate nutrition should only be carried out on patients who are treated with curative intent.

References

1. Aker SN (1979) Oral feedings in the cancer patients. Cancer 43: 2103-2107
2. Andersson H, Bosaeus J, Nyström C (1978) Bile salt malabsorption in the radiation syndrome. Acta Radiol [Oncol] 17: 312
3. Archambeau JO, Maetz M, Jesseph JE, Bond VP (1965) The effects of bile diversion and pancreatic duct ligation on the gastrointestinal syndrome in dogs receiving 1500 rads whole body irradiation (abstract). Radiat Res 25: 173
4. Berk RN, Seay DG (1972) Cholerheic enteropathy as a cause of diarrhea and death in radiation enteritis and its prevention with cholestyramine. Radiology 104: 153-156
5. Blackburn GL, Bistrian BR, Maini BS, Schlamm HT, Smith MF (1977) Nutritional and metabolic assessment of the hospitalized patients. JPEN 1: 11-22
6. Blackburn GL, Benotti PN, Bistrian BR, Bothe A, Maini BS, Schlamm HT, Smith MF (1979) Nutritional assessment and treatment of hospital malnutrition. Infusionsther Klin Ernahr 6: 238-250
7. Bonanni G, Perazzi F (1963) Variations of taste sensitivity in patients subjected to high energy irradiation for tumors of the oral cavity. Nunt Radiol 131: 383-397
8. Bonomi P, Morrin B, Wilbanks J, Slayton R (1978) Phase II trial of hexamethylmelamine (HMM) in ovarian carcinoma after alkylating agent failure. Proc Am Soc Clin Oncol 19: 335
9. Bothe A, Valerio D, Bistrian BR, Blackburn GL (1979) Randomized control trial of hospital nutritional support during abdominal radiotherapy. JPEN 3: 292
10. Bounous G, LeBel E, Shuster J, Gold P, Tahan, WT, Bastin E (1975) Dietary protection during radiation therapy. Strahlentherapie 149: 476-483
11. Brown MS, Buchanan RB, Karren SJ (1980) Clinical observations on the effects of elemental diet supplementation during irradiation. Clin Radiol 31: 19-20
12. Cater SK (1977) Clinical trials and their interpretation. Presentation to Division of Oncology, Standford University Medical School
13. Chencharick JD, Mossman KL (1983) Nutritional consequences of the radiotherapy of head and neck cancer. Cancer 51: 811-815
14. Chung CT, Sagermann RH, King GA, Yu WS, Johnson JT, Cummings CW (1978) Complications of high dose preoperative irradiation for advanced laryngohypopharyngeal cancer. Radiology 128: 467-470
15. Conger AD (1973) Loss and recovery of taste acuity in patients irradiated to the oral cavity. Radiat Res 53: 338-347
16. Cooper GP (1968) Receptor origin of the olfactory bulb response to ionizing radiation. Am J Physiol 215: 803-806
17. Copeland EM, Daly JM, Dudrick SJ (1977) Nutritions as an adjunct to cancer treatment in the adult. Cancer Res 37: 2451-2456
18. Copeland EM, MacFadyen BV, Lanzotti VJ, Dudrick SJ (1975) Intravenous hyperalimentation as an adjunct to cancer chemotherapy. Am J Surg 129: 167-173
19. De Wys WD, Walters K (1975) Abnormalities of taste sensation in cancer patients. Cancer 36: 1888-1896
20. Donaldson SS (1977) Effect of nutrition as related to radiation and chemotherapy. In: Winick M (ed) Nutrition and cancer. Wiley, New York, pp 137-153
21. Donaldson SS (1977) Nutritional consequences of radiotherapy. Cancer Res 37: 2407-2413
22. Donaldson SS, Jundt S, Ricour C, Sarrazin D, Lemerle J, Schweisguth O (1975) Radiation enteritis in children. A retrospective review, clinicopathologic correlation, and dietary management. Cancer 35: 1167-1178
23. Donaldson, SS, Lenon RA (1979) Alterations of nutritional status: impact of chemotherapy and radiation therapy. Cancer 43: 2036-2052
24. Donaldson SS, Weslay MN, Ghavimi F, Shils ME, Suskind RM, De Wys WD (1982) A prospective randomized clinical trial of total parenteral nutrition in children with cancer. Med Pediatr Oncol 10: 129-139

25. Donaldson SS (1982) Effects of therapy on nutritional status of the pediatric cancer patient. Cancer Res 42: 729-736
26. Douglas HO, Milliron S, Nava H et al. (1978) Elemental diet as an adjuvant for patients with locally advanced gastrointestinal cancer receiving radiation therapy: a prospectively randomized study. JPEN 2: 682-686
27. Dwyer JT (1979) Dietetic assessment of ambulatory cancer patients. With special attention to problems of patients suffering from head-neck cancers undergoing radiation therapy. Cancer 43: 2077-2086
28. Eggert JH, Dumbach J, Steinhäuser EW (1985) Zur Ätiologie und Therapie der Osteoradionekrose des Unterkiefers. Dtsch Zahnarztl Z 40: 2-11
29. Eneroth CM, Henrikson CO, Jakobsson P (1972) Effect of fractionated radiotherapy on salivary gland function. Cancer 30: 1147-1153
30. Fletcher GH (1980) Textbook of radiotherapy. Lea and Febiger, Philadelphia
31. Ghavimi F, Shils ME, Scott BF, Brown M, Tamaroff M (1982) Comparison of morbidity in children requiring abdominal radiation and chemotherapy with and without total parenteral nutrition. J Pediatr 101: 530-537
32. Goldgraber MB, Rubin CE, Palmer WL, Dobson RL, Massey BW (1954) The early gastric response to irradiation. A serial biopsy study. Gastroenterology 27: 1-20
33. Henkin RJ, Graziadei PPG, Bradley DF (1969) Clinical Staff Conference. The molecular basis of taste and its disorders. Ann Intern Med 71: 791-821
34. Hofmann AF, Poley JR (1972) Role of bile acid malabsorption in pathogenesis of diarrhea and steatorrhea in patients with ileal resection. I. Response to cholestyramine or replacement of dietary long chain triglyceride by medium chain triglyceride. Gastroenterology 62: 918
35. Holoye PY, Goepfert H, Samuels ML (1978) Combination chemotherapy of head and neck carcinoma. Proc Am Soc Clin Oncol 19: 358
36. Jervis HR, Donati RM, Stromberg LR, Sprinz H (1969) Histochemical investigation of the mucosa of the exteriorized small intestine of the rat exposed to x-radiation. Strahlentherapie 137: 326-343
37. Johnson CH (1980) Nutritional care of cancer patients receiving radiotherapy. In: Fletcher GH (ed) Textbook of radiotherapy. Lea and Febiger, Philadelphia, pp 92-102
38. Jones SE, Coltman CA, Fisher R (1978) Comparison of 3 combination drug programs for advanced Hodgkin's disease (HD): a preliminary report of the Southwest Oncology Group (SWOG) MOPP 5 Study. Proc Am Soc Clin Oncol 19: 333
39. Karmiol M, Walsh R (1975) Dental caries after radiotherapy of the oral regions. J Am Dent Assoc 91: 838-845
40. Kashima HK, Kirkham WR, Andrews JR (1965) Postirradiation sialadenitis: a study of the clinical features, histopathologic changes and serum enzyme variations following irradiation of human salivary glands. AJR 94: 271-291
41. Kinsella TJ, Bloomer WD (1980) Tolerance of the intestine to radiation therapy. Surg Gynecol Obstet 151: 273-284
42. Kinsella TJ, Malcolm AW, Bothe A, Valerio D, Blackburn GL (1981) Prospective study of nutritional support during pelvic irradiation. Int J Radiat Oncol Biol Phys 7: 543-548
43. Kleinberg I, Jenkins GN (1964) pH of dental plaques in the areas of the mouth before and after meals and their relationships to the pH and rate of flow of resting saliva. Arch Oral Biol 9: 493
44. Kokal WA (1985) The impact of antitumor therapy on nutrition. Cancer 55: 273-278
45. Krikorian JG, Daniels JR, Brown BW, Hu MS (1978) Variables for predicting serious toxicity (vinblastine dose, performance status and prior therapeutic experience): chemotherapy for metastatic testicular cancer with cisdichlorodiamine platinum (II), vinblastine and bleomycin. Cancer Treat Rep 62: 1455-1463
46. Larson DL, Lindberg RD, Lane E et al. (1983) Major complications of radiotherapy in cancer of the oral cavity and oropharynx: a 10-year retrospective study. Am J Surg 146: 531-536

47. Lawrence W (1979) Effects of cancer on nutrition: impaired organ system effects. Cancer 43: 2020-2029
48. Mossman KL, Henkin RJ (1978) Radiation-induced changes in taste acuity in cancer patients. Int J Radiat Oncol Biol Phys 4: 663-670
49. Mossman KL, Chencharick JD, Scheer AC, Walker WP, Ornitz RD, Rogers CC, Henkin RJ (1979) Radiation-induced changes in gustatory function. Comparison of effects of neutron and photon irradiation. Int J Radiat Oncol Biol Phys 5: 521-528
50. Mossman KL, Shatzman A, Chencharik JD (1982) Long-term effects of radiotherapy on taste and salivary function in man. Int J Radiat Oncol Biol Phys 8: 991-997
51. Nichini FM, Tansy MF, Kendall FM (1973) Serum magnesium fall in radiation-induced gastrointestinal symptomatology. Radiology 108: 413-415
52. Pareira MD, Conrad EJ, Hicks W, Elman R (1955) Clinical response and changes in nitrogen balance, body weight, plasma proteins and hemoglobin following tube feeding in cancer cachexia. Cancer 8: 803-808
53. Pezner R, Archambeau JO (1985) Critical evaluation of the role of nutritional support for radiation therapy patients. Cancer 55: 263-267
54. Phillips TL, Fu KK (1978) The interaction of drug and radiation effects on normal tissues. Int J Radiat Oncol Biol Phys 4: 59-64
55. Phillips TL, Fu KK (1976) Quantification of combined radiation therapy and chemotherapy effects on critical normal tissues. Cancer 37: 1186-1200
56. Phillips TL, Wharam MD, Margolis LW (1975) Modification of radiation injury to normal tissues by chemotherapeutic agents. Cancer 35: 1678-1684
57. Poyton HG (1968) The effects of radiation on teeth. Oral Surg 26: 639-646
58. Reeves RJ, Cavanaugh PJ, Sharpe KW, Thorne WA, Winkler C, Sanders AP (1965) Fat absorption studies and small bowel X-ray studies in patients undergoing ^{60}Co teletherapy and/or radium application. AJR 94: 848-851
59. Reeves RJ, Sanders AP, Isley JK, Sharpe KW, Baylin GJ (1959) Fat absorption from the human gastrointestinal tract in patients undergoing radiation therapy. Radiology 73: 398-401
60. Roswit B (1974) Complications of radiation therapy: the alimentary tract. Semin Roentgenol 9: 51-63
61. Roswit B, Malsky SJ, Reid C (1972) Severe radiation injuries of the stomach, small intestine, colon and rectum. AJR 114: 460-475
62. Rubin P, Casarett GW (1972) A direction for clinical radiation pathology: the tolerance dose. In: Vaeth J (ed) Frontiers of radiation therapy and oncology, vol 6. University Park Press, Baltimore, pp 1-16
63. Schein PS, MacDonald JS, Waters C, Haidak D (1975) Nutritional complications of cancer and its treatment. Semin Oncol 2: 337-347
64. Schwartz GF, Green HL, Bendon ML, Graham WP, Blakemore WS (1971) Combined parenteral hyperalimentation and chemotherapy in the treatment of disseminated solid tumors. Am J Surg 121: 169-173
65. Sell A, Jensen TS (1966) Acute gastric ulcers induced by radiation. Acta Radiol [Oncol] 4: 289-297
66. Shils ME (1979) Principles of nutritional therapy. Cancer 43: 2093-2102
67. Solassol C, Joyeux H, Dubois JB (1980) Total parenteral nutrition (TPN) with complete nutritive mixtures: an artificial gut in cancer patients. Nutr Cancer 1: 13-18
68. Stryker JA, Hepner GW, Mortel R (1977) The effect of pelvic irradiation on ileal function. Radiology 124: 213-216
69. Stryker JA, Mortel R, Hepner GW (1978) The effect of pelvic irradiation on lactose absorption. Int J Radiat Oncol Biol Phys 4: 859-863
70. Tarpila S (1971) Morphological and functional response of human small intestine to ionizing radiation. Scand J Gastroenterol [Suppl 12] 6: 9-52
71. Thiel HJ (1981) Strahlennebenwirkungen. Prophylaxe und Therapie. Musik und Medizin 18: 7-26

72. Thiel HJ, Raab W (1982) Die Zahnprophylaxe und -behandlung von Bestrahlungspatienten. MMW 124: 319-322
73. Thiel HJ (1985) Ist die Ernährungsbehandlung von Tumorpatienten vor, während und nach Radiotherapie eine medizinisch notwendige Maßnahme? Aktuel Onkol 23: 223-234
74. Thiel HJ (1986) Sondenernährung von Patienten mit HNO-Tumoren unter Strahlentherapie. Beitr Infusionsther Klin Ernahr 14: 117-136
75. Thornton C (1979) Nutritional management with radiotherapy. In: Wollard (ed) Nutritional management of the cancer patient. Raven, New York, pp 43-56
76. Trier JS, Browning TH (1966) Morphologic response of the mucosa of human small intestine to x-ray exposure. J Clin Invest 45: 194-204
77. Troidl H (1980) Adäquate enterale Ernährung des Langzeitliegers. Die Schwester/Der Pfleger 19: 16
78. Tsujii H (1985) Quantitative dose-response analysis of salivary function following radiotherapy using sequential RI-sialography. Int J Radiat Oncol Biol Phys 11: 1603-1612
79. Van der Brenk HA (1969) Radiation damage to salivary glands. Br J Radiol 42: 799
80. Vatistas S, Hornsey S (1966) Radiation-induced protein loss into the gastrointestinal tract. Br J Radiol 39: 547-550
81. Wescott WB, Mira JG, Starcke EN, Shanon IL, Thornby JI (1978) Alterations in whole saliva flow rate induced by fractionated radiotherapy. AJR 130: 145-149
82. Wiernik G (1966) Radiation damage and repair in the human jejunal mucosa. J Pathol 91: 389-393
83. Yatvin MB, Hinke DH (1968) Influence of host protein nutrition on the response of various tumors to ionizing radiation. Proc Soc Exp Biol Med 128: 200-206
84. Zelen M (1973) Keynote address on biostatistics and data retrieval. First international workshop for therapy of lung cancer. Cancer Chemother Rep (part 3) 4: 31-42

*Vitamins and Cancer**

H. B. Stähelin

Medizinisch-geriatrische Klinik Markgräflerhof, Kantonsspital, 4031 Basel, Switzerland

The profound impact of vitamins on growth and differentiation led even shortly after their discovery to speculation that they might play a role in carcinogenesis. In the last decade this question has again received more attention. In this short overview the focus is on four aspects of the vitamin-cancer relationship schematically shown in Table 1.

The topic may be divided into cancer prevention and cure of already established neoplasms. The mechanisms are either a general function of certain vitamins (e.g., antioxidant properties or cell differentiation) or particular effects like the inhibition of *N*-nitrosamine formation by vitamin C in the stomach or the "rescue" effect of folinic acid. Vitamins influence many functions of the living organism which are important in the induction or promotion of neoplasms; a list of vitamins and their mechanism of action proposed to be important in carcinogenesis is given in Table 2.

Prevention

Data from our own study indicate that the antioxidant properties may be important in cancer prevention [1, 2]. In fact, the molar product of the plasma concentration of the antioxidant vitamins C, E, and *β*-carotene is inversely associated with

Table 1. Vitamins and cancer

Mechanism	Prevention	Cure
General	e.g. antioxidants (vit. C, E, *β*-carotene)	e.g. cell differentiation (vit. A, vit. D)
Particular	e.g. *N*-nitrosamine (vit. C)	e.g. "rescue" (citrovorumfactor)

* This work was supported in part by the Swiss National Research Foundation, grant no. 3.805.0.84 and by the regional Krebsliga, Basel.

Table 2. Vitamins and their proposed mechanism of action in carcinogenesis

Vitamin		Proposed mechanism of action in carcinogenesis
Retinol	A	Cell differentiation
β-Carotene[a]	Provitamin A	Growth of organism
		Membrane properties
		Free radical scavenger
		Immune function
Thiamine	B_1	
Riboflavin	B_2	
Biotin		
Niacin		
Pyridoxine	B_6	
Cyanocobalamin		
Folic acid		- Citrovorum factor "Rescue" effect
Panthothenic acid		
Ascorbic acid	C	- *N*-nitrosocompounds Antioxidant properties Collagen synthesis Immune function
Calciferol	D	- Cell differentiation Ca-metabolism
α-Tocopherol	E	- Antioxidant Synergistic action with vitamin A, β-carotene, and Selenium
Menadione	K	

[a] The effect of other carotene compounds is less well explored.

cancer death in the Prospective Basle Study (Fig. 1). The inverse association of β-carotene and lung cancer [3] is now well recognized (Fig. 2). β-Carotene is known to be a highly active singlet oxygen scavenger, thus protecting cellular structures from oxidative damage [4].

As well as β-carotene, plasma vitamin A levels are highly predictive for stomach cancer (Fig. 3). In western societies with an affluent diet the two isoprenes behave independently. In several studies [1] dietary vitamin A intake is inversely correlated with cancer incidence. It is tempting to speculate that vitamin E protects the lipids in the membranes from peroxidation. However, in order to be an effective antioxidant, α-tocopherol requires vitamin C in the plasma. Vitamin C, on the other hand, was found to be related to gastric cancer incidence (Fig. 3) and is a convincing example of a particular vitamin action preventing cancer formation [2]. The inhibition of N-nitrosamine formation by vitamin C as suggested by Tannenbaum [5] is consistent with our results. Incidently, recently it was shown that *N*-nitrosamine formation is involved in the immune system, thus explaining the effect of vitamin C on immune function [6].

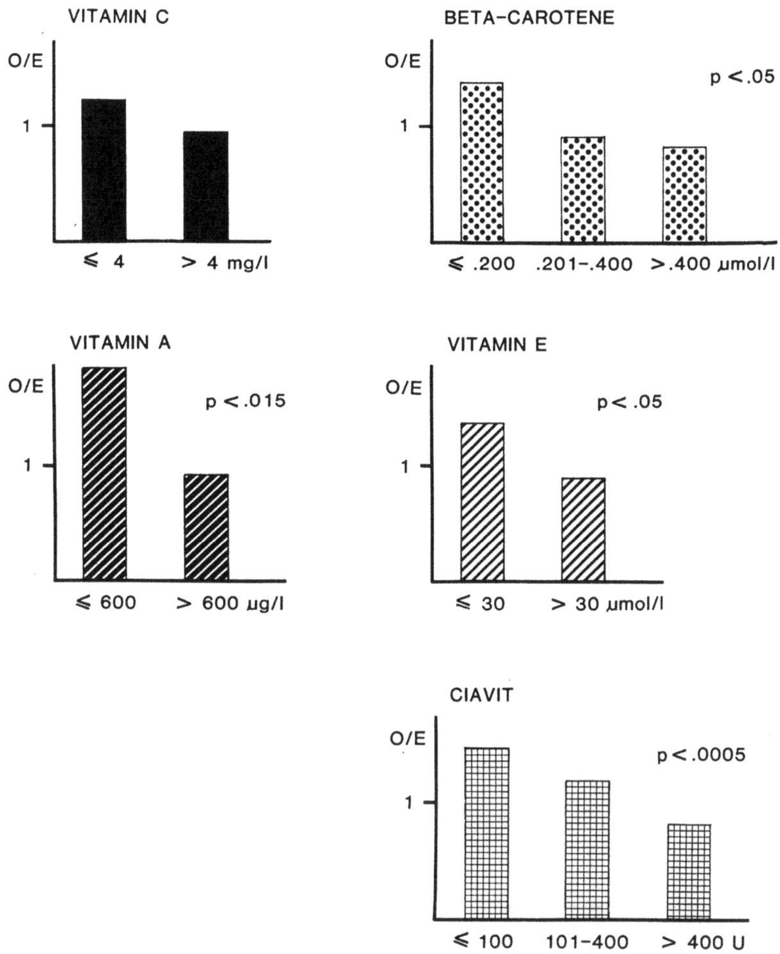

Fig. 1. The observed over expected *(O/E)* ratio of death from all 102 cancers in the Prospective Basle Study is given after adjustment of the different plasma vitamin concentrations for smoking and age. *CIAVIT* denotes the cumulative index of antioxidant vitamins and is computed as a molar product of the plasma concentrations of vitamin C, vitamin E, and β-carotene

Cure of Advanced Cancer

Whether or not vitamins in physiological, pharmacological, or even megadoses indeed affect advanced cancer remains controversial. In one particular case vitamin therapy became an important adjuvant. The "rescue" effect of folinic acid or citrovorum factor was hailed by Burchenal as a giant step forward [7] and dominates the literature. Originally introduced with methotrexate, it is now used in different combinations and lately with 5-fluorouracil [8, 9].

The effects of other vitamins have been less explored. Great hopes were raised by Pauling's hypothesis that megadoses of *vitamin C* might be beneficial [10].

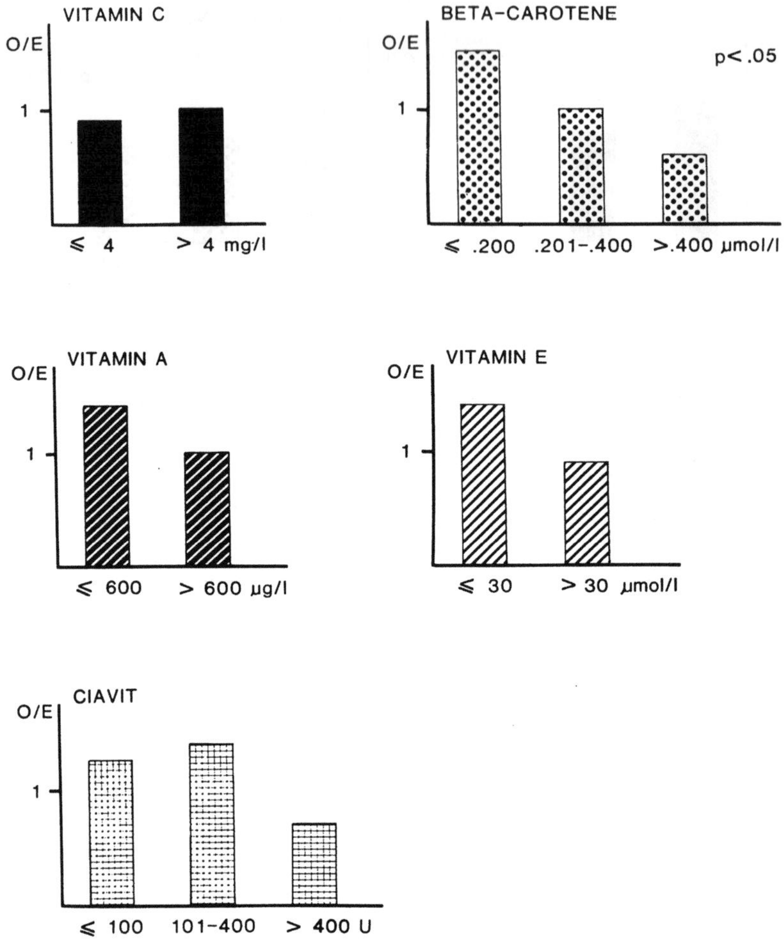

Fig. 2. Lung cancer death cases ($n = 37$) in relation to the different plasma vitamin concentrations. For further explanation see Fig. 1

However, the initial positive results reported by Cameron and Pauling [11] were not validated in subsequent trials [12, 13]. According to Jaffey [14] and Pauling [15], megadoses of vitamin C are probably valuable in the treatment of patients with cancer, but such claims are controversial.

Bussey and co-workers [16] observed that 3 g ascorbic acid daily significantly reduces familial polyposis and suggested it may play a role in chemoprevention. At present, this observation is more of theoretical than practical interest.

High doses of *vitamin A* are reported to be beneficial in mycosis fungoides [17] and are thought to enhance immune function in subjects with lung cancer. A synergistic effect of vitamin A together with chemotherapy or radiation therapy has been proposed [18, 19]. Oral retinol at a dosage of 200000 IU/m^2 appears to have limited activity in patients with advanced cancer [20]. Vitamin A is probably more effective in benign neoplasms, as suggested by the reported complete or partial re-

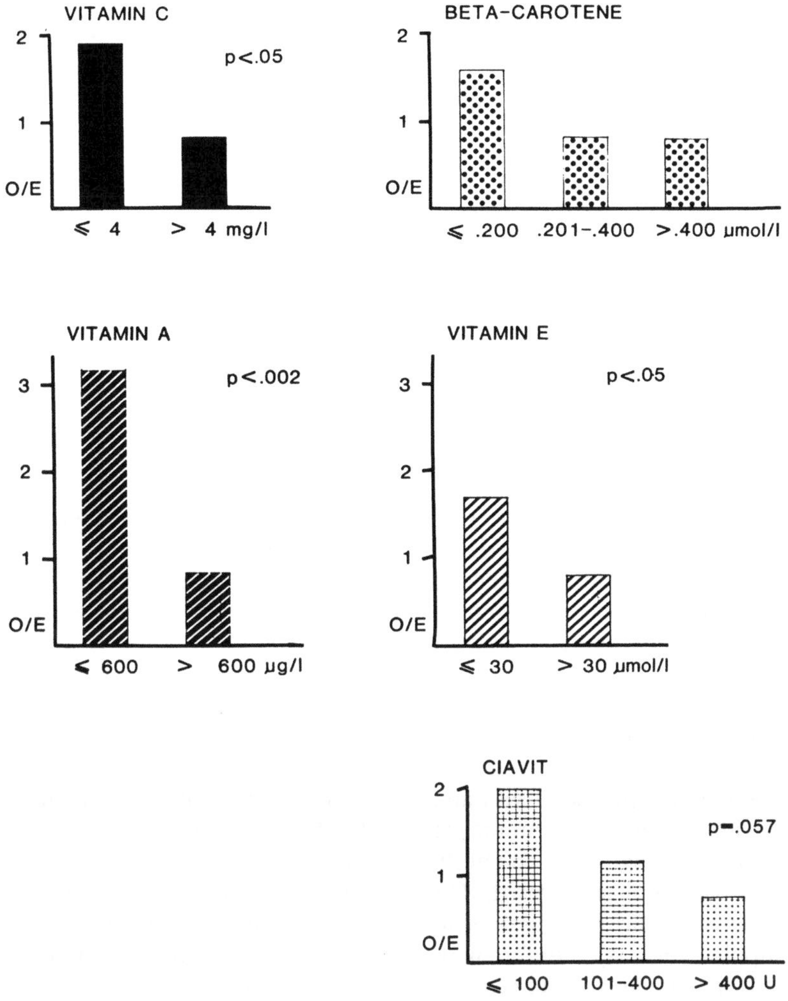

Fig. 3. Gastrointestinal cancer cases in relation to the different plasma vitamin concentrations (17 stomach, 9 large bowel + rectum). For further explanation see Fig. 1

sponse in females with benign breast disease [21]. Since it is difficult to increase vitamin A level by oral supplementation [22], retinoids offer a more promising route which does not depend on liver regulation and retinol binding proteins [22]. Further studies are still needed to establish the clinical benefit of this therapy [23, 24, 25].

More recent research has been directed toward the effect of *vitamin D* on lymphoma [26] and leukemia cells in vitro. Again, metabolic effects preclude an effective elevated dosage of vitamin D in vivo and a search for suitable vitamin D analogues seems rewarding [27].

Vitamin E offers a theoretically interesting pharmacology, although intervention studies have been disappointing both in patients with mammary dysplasia [28,

Table 3. Causes of anorexia. (After Hardy et al. [35])

Gustatory:	Decreased threshold for bitter flavor, increased for sweet flavor
Gastrointestinal:	Strength of contraction diminished Decreased hypothalamic stimulation GI secretion, insulin response decreased
Metabolic:	Lactic acid FFA increased Imbalance of amino acids
Neurotransmission:	Serotonin and tryptophan concentration Increased in brain stem
Depression	
Learned aversion reactions	
Nausea, vomiting	
Malabsorption	
Obstruction	

29] and in established cancer [30]. However, the mechanism of vitamin E might depend on the presence of vitamin C or other reducing agents. This mechanism is probably of great importance in the prevention of cancer but of minor influence in advanced cancer, where immunological and metabolic events are more important in controlling the neoplastic growth.

Supportive Care

The therapeutic use of vitamins raises the question of whether the administration of vitamins enhances tumor growth [31]. In the numerous studies with citrovorum factor after high dose chemotherapy there is no evidence of an unfavorable influence on neoplastic growth. One report concerning folic acid supplementation in 6-mercaptopurine remission maintenance therapy in leukemia suggests that folate supplements may interfere with therapy [32]. On the other hand, nutrients as therapy for patients with cancer are important as adjunctive therapy [33]. In patients with cancer numerous mechanisms lead to anorexia (Table 3) and diminish the quality of life. One interesting mechanism is related to the fact that the tumor derives its energy mainly from glucose and thus increases the thiamine demand. In fact a neurological paraneoplastic syndrome responsive to thiamine was reported [34], and thiamine supplementation should be considered in cancer patients.

Supplementation with vitamins, minerals, and certain trace elements is recommended by Hoffmann [31] for the cancer patient who is supported by prolonged parenteral nutrition.

In conclusion: The preventive effect of certain vitamins has been reasonably well established by clinical, epidemiological, and experimental work. Whether physiological or elevated dosages of vitamins C and A can have a curative effect is still controversial. The most effective use of vitamins in cancer therapy is the "rescue" operation with folinic acid after chemotherapy. Patients with cancer will profit from an adequate diet rich in vitamins, minerals, and trace elements.

References

1. Gey KF, Brubacher GB, Stähelin HB (1987) Plasma levels of antioxidant vitamins in relation to ischemic heart disease and/or cancer. Am J Clin Nutr 45: 1368-1377
2. Stähelin HB, Gey KF, Brubacher GB (1987) Plasma vitamin C and cancer death: the Prospective Basle Study. Ann NY Acad Sci 498: 124-131
3. Stähelin HB, Rösel F, Buess E, Brubacher G (1984) Cancer, vitamins and plasma lipids. Prospective Basle Study. JNCI 73: 1463-1468
4. Gey KF (1986) On the antioxidant hypothesis with regard to atherosclerosis. Bibl Nutr Dieta 37: 53-91
5. Tannenbaum SR (1983) *N*-nitroso compounds. A perspective on human exposure. Lancet 1: 629-632
6. Tannenbaum SR (1987) Inhibition of nitrosamine formation by ascorbic acid. Ann NY Acad Sci 498: 354-363
7. Burchenal JH (1974) Editorial: A giant step forward - if. N Engl J Med 291: 1029-1031
8. Cunningham J, Bukowski RM, Budd GT, Weich JK, Purvis J (1984) 5-Fluorouracil and folinic acid: a phase I-II trial in gastrointestinal malignancy. Invest New Drugs 2: 391-395
9. Bertrand M, Doroshow JH, Multhauf P et al. (1986) High-dose continuous infusion folinic acid and bolus 5-fluorouracil in patients with advanced colorectal cancer: a phase II study. J Clin Oncol 4: 1058-1061
10. Cameron E, Pauling L (1974) The orthomolecular treatment of cancer. I. The role of ascorbic acid in host resistance. Chem Biol Interact 9: 273-283
11. Cameron E, Pauling L (1976) Supplemental ascorbate in the supportive treatment of cancer: prolongation of survival times in terminal human cancer. Proc Natl Acad Sci USA 73: 3685-3689
12. Creagan ET, Moertel CG, O'Fallan JR et al. (1979) Failure of high dose vitamin C (ascorbic acid) therapy to benefit patients with advanced cancer. A controlled trial. N Engl J Med 301: 687-690
13. Moertel CG, Fleming TR, Creagan ET, Rubin J, O'Connell MJ, Ames MM (1985) High-dose vitamin C versus placebo in the treatment of patients with advanced cancer who have had no prior chemotherapy. A randomized double-blind comparison. N Engl J Med 312: 137-141
14. Jaffey M (1982) Vitamin C and cancer: examination of the Vale of Leven trial results using broad inductive reasoning. Med Hypotheses 8: 49-84
15. Pauling L (1986) A proposition: megadoses of vitamin C are valuable in the treatment of cancer. Nutr Rev 44: 28-32
16. Bussey HJ, DeCosse JJ, Deschner EE, Eyers AA, Lesser ML, Morson BC, Ritchie SM, Thomson JP, Wadsworth J (1982) A randomized trial of ascorbic acid in polyposis coli. Cancer 50: 1434-1439
17. Schimpf A, Jansen KH (1972) Hochdosierte Vitamin A-Therapie bei Psoriasis und Mycosis fungoides. Fortschr Med 90: 635-639
18. Komiyama S, Hiroto I, Ryu S, Nakashima T, Kuwano M, Endo H (1978) Synergistic combination therapy of 5-fluorouracil, vitamin A and cobalt-60 radiation upon head and neck tumors. Oncology 35: 253-257
19. Kucera H (1980) Vitamin A als Zusatztherapie bei der Bestrahlung des fortgeschrittenen Gebärmutterhalskarzinoms. Wien Klin Wochenschr [Suppl] 92 (118): 1-20
20. Goodman GE (1986) Phase II trial of retinol in patients with advanced cancer. Cancer Treat Rep 70: 1023-1024
21. Band PR, Deschamps M, Falardeau M, Ladouceur J, Cote J (1984) Treatment of benign breast disease with vitamin A. Prev Med 13: 549-554
22. Goodman DS (1984) Vitamin A and retinoids in health and disease. N Engl J Med 310: 1023-1031

23. Weber W, Hartmann D, Obrecht JP (1982) Die Bedeutung von Vitamin A und Vitamin-A-Derivaten (Retinoide) in der onkologischen Therapie. MMW 124: 29-31
24. Hill DL, Grubbs CJ (1982) Retinoids as chemopreventive and anticancer agents intact animals (review). Anticancer Res 2: 111-124
25. Sporn MB, Roberts AB (1983) Role of retinoids in differentiation and carcinogenesis. Cancer Res 43: 3034-3040
26. Cunningham D, Gilchrist NL, Cowan RA, Forrest GJ, McArdle CS, Soukop M (1985) Alfacalcidol as a modulator of growth of low grade non-Hodgkin's lymphomas. Br Med J 291: 1153-1155
27. Koeffler HP, Hirji K, Itri L (1985) 1,25-Dihydroxyvitamin D3: in vivo and in vitro effects on human preleukemic and leukemic cells. Cancer Treat Rep 69: 1399-1407
28. London RS, Sundaram GS, Murphy L, Manimekalai S, Reynolds M, Goldstein PJ (1985) The effect of vitamin E on mammary dysplasia: a double-blind study. Obstet Gynecol 65: 104-106
29. Ernster VL, Goodson WH, Hunt TK, Petrakis NL, Sickless EA, Miike R (1985) Vitamin E and benign breast "disease": a double-blind, randomized clinical trial. Surgery 97: 490-494
30. Committee on Diet, Nutrition and Cancer (1982) Diet, nutrition and cancer. National Academic Press, Washington DC
31. Hoffman FA (1985) Micronutrient requirements of cancer patients. Cancer 55: 295-300
32. Lennard L, Lilleyman JS, Maddocks JL (1986) The effect of folate supplements on 6-mercaptopurine remission maintenance therapy in childhood leukaemia. Br J Cancer 53: 115-119
33. Bertino JR (1979) Nutrients, vitamins and minerals as therapy. Cancer 43: 2137-2142
34. Nausieda PA, Tanner CM, Weiner WJ (1981) Opsoclonic cerebellopathy: a paraneoplastic syndrome responsive to thiamine. Arch Neurol 38: 780-781
35. Hardy C, Wallace C, Khansur T, Vance RB et al. (1986) Nutrition, cancer and aging: an annotated review II. Cancer cachexia and aging. J Am Geriatr Soc 34: 219-228

Unproven Dietary Methods of Treatment of Oncology Patients

M. Hunter

The Royal Marsden Hospital, Fulham Road London SW3 6JJ, Great Britain

"Unproven dietary methods of treatment" refers to any unorthodox or unconventional modification of a normal diet which is claimed to treat or cure cancer. These diets may be used in conjunction with, or istead of conventional anti-cancer therapies. Most derive from either the United States or the Far East, and they are becoming increasingly popular amongst cancer patients in the United Kingdom. They have, however, been received with great scepticism by both the medical and the dietetic professions. I was fortunate to be granted a Winston Churchill travel fellowship in 1985 to visit the United States and Japan to investigate the philosophies and efficacy of the most popular regimes as practised in the original centres.

The most popular regimes in the United Kingdom at present are:

- The Bristol Diet - originated by Dr. Alec Forbes at the Bristol Cancer Help Centre.
- Macrobiotics, as formulated by Michio Kushi at the Kushi Institute, Boston, Mass.
- The Gerson Therapy, originated by Max Gerson in Germany and now practised by Charlotte Gerson, his daughter, at the Gerson Therapy Centre, Tijuana, Mexico.

The reasons for the popularity of such regimes are mass media publicity, good sales technique and dramatic claims of cures. Health food stores are a major source of literature on dietary regimes. The promoters of such regimes invest much more time, money and effort in public relations and media presentations than do ordinary health scientists, and the media love sensation and will always report so-called new cures for cancer. Claims of cures are always dramatic. The literature available on such regimes varies widely in the reliability of the nutritional information published.

All regimes share a common philosophy - that is that poor diet causes cancer, so a good diet can cure it and that diet and changes in diet can be used to correct physical and emotional illness. Most regimes also share the same common principles:

- Strict vegan or vegetarian diets
- Large amounts of raw foods

Recent Results in Cancer Research, Vol. 108

- Sugar free
- Low in salt
- Use of vegetable/fruit/liver juices
- High doses of vitamins/minerals/enzymes

It is fair to say that most unproven dietary regimes apply themselves to all illnesses and not just cancer. Successes have been reported for arthritis, asthma, heart disease, migraine, diabetes and a host of other illnesses. It is fair to say that there is no doubt that these regimes can be of benefit to some people suffering from these illnesses. It is, however, on the use of these regimes in the treatment of cancer patients that I wish to concentrate. Again, there is no doubt that these regimes can be of benefit to a small percentage of cancer patients. The reason for this is unclear but it is likely to be associated with the psychological support offered by the diet and by the other holistic therapies which are usually closely linked with the dietary advice, such as counselling, relaxation, visualisation etc. Also, by following such a dietary regime, the patient feels that he is doing something positive for himself and thereby having some personal control over at least one aspect of his treatment. It is perhaps a poor reflection on conventional treatments that we do not involve patients enough in their own treatment, nor support them enough throughout their treatment.

In short, there is no doubt that some patients feel better on these regimes. If the regime is doing the patient no harm, then I see no reason why they should not continue with it. However, in looking at these treatments in cancer patients, we need to ask ourselves one fundamental question relevant to any proposed treatment, dietary or otherwise. That it - does the potential for benefit exceed the potential for harm? I would like to focus on some of the harmful effects that can result from these unproven dietary regimes. The outcome of most of these dietary regimes is:

- Weight loss
- Weakness
- Depression
- Guilt
- Anger

Why? Let us examine the treatments in more detail:

- No meat, fish or fowl
- No dairy products
- No animal protein

The result of this is a diet high in fruits and vegetables and cereals, high in bulk and low in calories - the basic of all good slimming regimes. This is the exact opposite to the needs of most cancer patients, who we know have a higher energy requirement due to a higher resting metabolic rate.

Patients experiencing loss of appetite or eating difficulties resulting from their disease or treatment find it impossible to eat a high fibre, mostly raw food diet. For most patients it is impossible to maintain an adequate intake of energy on such regimes. Often patients undertake these regimes as a last resort, when they are already weak and malnourished. These diets further exacerbate their problems. Dramatic weight loss is most common on such regimes. Such diets do not provide adequate intakes of protein, iron, calcium or vitamin B_{12}. As many patients may follow these regimes for 1-2 years or more, these factors are important.

High doses of vitamins C and E are recommended on most regimes. Although vitamin C is water soluble and excess is excreted, high doses of vitamin C (20 g plus daily) have resulted in kidney damage and kidney stones. Such high doses of vitamin C are of no known value in cancer treatment. There is also no known value in the megadoses of vitamin E often prescribed. Some regimes suggest large doses on vitamin A in the form of B carotene capsules or carrot juice. Again, there is no value in this and vitamin A toxicity following such high intakes is not uncommon.

Pancreatic enzymes, as prescribed on the Gerson Therapy, have no value except when necessary as a replacement for pancreatic dysfunction. Coffee enemas are very popular and according to Gerson are said "to dilate the bile ducts to facilitate secretion of toxic cancer breakdown products by the liver and dialysis of toxic products from blood across the colonic wall."

The evidence to support these treatments is minimal and unsound and the burden of proof is on those who propose the treatment, especially if it involves such strange concepts. As well as the high bulk, low energy content of these diets, they are mostly:

- Unpalatable. In most cases the diets involve a drastic change in cooking and eating habits, with most patients having to eat food they have never eaten before. The low salt, low fat content of the diet often makes them very bland and unpalatable to western palates.
- Difficult to prepare. Quite a long time is also required to learn how to prepare and cook various cereal grains, sprouting grains, pulses etc.
- Costly to follow, involve expensive. They often organically grown foods and vitamin or mineral supplements.

In addition, some of the diets offer conflicting advice.

This leaves patients:

- Confused
- Depressed, if they do not enjoy the diet or find it too difficult to prepare or too costly to follow.
- Guilty, if they have to abandon the diet for any reason and give up their "hope of a cure".
- Angry, if they see no result for their dietary sacrifices and physical effort.

The question I posed was "Does the potential for benefit outweigh the potential for harm?" The answer to this in respect of cancer patients is no. The harm that can and does result from these regimes far exceeds possible benefits. For this reason, these regimes cannot be openly recommended for cancer patients. In practice, patients I see who are following such regimes have their nutritional intake carefully assessed regularly. If they have an adequate intake, then they continue the regime if they wish, and continue being assessed. If the patient has an inadequate intake, which is usually the case, then I advise and encourage them to widen their range of foods eaten so as to improve their nutritional status. The patient may decide, however, to remain strictly on the regime. That is their choice.

If patients enquire whether they should start such regimes, I encourage them to read all they can about the regime but recommend that they follow good general healthy eating guidelines. The disadvantages of dietary modifications are discussed fully with the patients. If they choose to follow a regime, I advise that they try it for 1 month and then return for reassessment and further discussion. This way there is no pressure on the patient and no guilt at abandoning the diet if it proves impractical to follow.

In conclusion, at best, unproven dietary treatments make the patient feel better. At worst, they offer false hope to patients who are at their most vulnerable. Who can blame patients for wanting to try such regimes. The responsibility for making the decision to follow an unproven dietary treatment rests with the patient. The responsibility for providing sufficient, balanced information on which they make that decision rests with dietitians.

Psychosocial Care in Cancer Patients

Liaison Psychiatry on an Oncology Ward

F. Meerwein

Mühlebachstraße 82, 8008 Zürich, Switzerland

In this chapter I shall describe the liaison psychiatric service as now organized on the oncology ward of Zurich University Hospital. It is operated by a physician, who is also a psychotherapeutically trained psychologist, two clinical psychologists, and the author (Training Analyst of the Swiss Psychoanalytical Association). The clinical psychologists and the supervisor function on an hourly basis, the physician, delegated by the psychiatric outpatient clinic, on an all-day basis. Neither the Cantonal Government nor the Swiss or the Zurich Cancer Society was prepared to finance the activity of the two psychologists. For this purpose it was necessary for the Foundation of Psycho-oncology to be established, which collects private donations and in this way guarantees the effectiveness of our liaison-psychiatric activity.

Liaison-psychiatric activity can be defined as an attempt to unite and to bind together whatever, in the cancer patient's understanding of himself or in his life and in his familial and clinical milieu, has been separated owing to the outbreak of the illness. Such separations or severings can arise, for example, between the patient's physical and his emotional life, between his past and his present, between the patient and his family, and between the patient and his doctor concerning their ideas about the cause and method of treatment of the illness, and can lead to conflicts which are detrimental to the treatment and to the chances of recovery. However, emotional tension can also give rise to such severings; this can be tension between patients, doctors, and nurses, between doctors and members of patients' families, between winners and losers in the struggle to cure the patient, or between survivors and the dying. Finally, severance can result between the conscious and the unconscious experience of patients, between love and hate, between hope and despair. Wherever such severings make their appearance, they influence the functioning of the oncology ward as a diagnostic and therapeutic system and often have a negative effect on the quality of life of the patients.

The liaison psychiatrist or psychologist does not regard himself as a rival of the oncologist and his nursing team and would not like to be so regarded. As far as his professional competence is concerned, he is the equal of the oncologist. However, his competence operates at a level of understanding that is quite distinct from that of somatic medicine. He is concerned not only with the patient's cancer as a dis-

Recent Results in Cancer Research, Vol. 108

ease but also with the cancer as a metaphor expressing a total threat to the patient's individual life and with its effect on the patient, his family, and the clinical team treating him. It is the task of the liaison psychiatrist or psychologist to reestablish the connection between these different levels of understanding, no matter where and how this connection has been interrupted or has collapsed. The liaison psychiatrist is, so to speak, a "communication specialist." Owing to his presence on the oncology ward, at presentations of cases, reports on patients' social milieus, and at team conferences, he makes himself available as such a contact man, with advisory and interpretive functions. At the request or instigation of the oncologist, he can also concern himself with individual patients in separate psychotherapeutic sessions. On the oncology ward of the Zurich University Hospital, art therapy can also be administered in individual, especially appropriate cases. How this functions has been described in several more detailed publications. Thus although the activity of the liaison psychiatrist is conceived to be complementary to and not in competition with that of the oncologist, tensions and conflicts are inevitable even between these members of the clinical team. These conflicts make necessary a continuous supervision of the activity of the liaison psychiatrist by a trained supervisor. I would like at this point briefly to set down a number of these possible conflicts.

1. Conflicts can arise when the oncologist fears that the liaison psychiatrist claims a higher human competence for himself than that possessed by the oncologist. Such apprehensions, however, are as a rule wholly unfounded. As already described, the competence of the liaison psychiatrist is *different* from that of the oncologist but not of higher worth. What it has in view is complementary and not competitive activity. This is often not sufficiently taken into consideration.
2. Tensions between oncologists and liaison psychiatrists can come about when the oncologist succumbs to the erroneous notion that the psychiatrist wishes to "psychiatrize" the patient, i.e., psychically to pathologize and clinically label him. There is no basis whatsoever for such a misgiving, which stems from an unconscious hyperidentification by the oncologist with the problems of his patients and a simultaneous defence against them. The liaison psychiatrist regards the cancer patient as, in the first instance, a psychically healthy human being whose psychological equilibrium has possibly been disturbed by the onset of the illness. This disturbance, however, is in most cases not to be equated with a psychic illness.
3. Numerous psycho-oncological examinations have repeatedly revealed that cancer patients display a marked tendency to what is known as harmonization, i.e., a denial of conflicts, and a "high social desirability score" [13]. This means that they have a strong tendency to adapt quietly to given situations and to appear complaisant. This can result in their internal suffering remaining concealed and, owing to its denial, in their making excessive energetic and emotional demands on themselves. In my experience this overexertion is often easier for the liaison psychiatrist to recognize than for the oncologist, so that differences of opinion between the oncologist and the liaison psychiatrist can arise regarding the nature and the scope of the assistance to be offered.
4. Cancer patients, like many markedly regressive patients, often have the tendency to divide up their "objects," that is, the persons immediately surrounding

them, including doctors and the therapeutic team, into "all good" or "all bad" objects and to cling emotionally to the "all good" persons, but to reject the "all bad" [11]. In this way considerable problems of jealousy can often make their appearance in the clinical environment. Thus the oncologist can become "all bad," the liaison psychiatrist, on the other hand, "all good." The reverse situation, however, is also conceivable. It is the task of the liaison psychiatrist to recognize the mechanisms and the genesis of such severing processes in good time and to prevent them by taking appropriate steps, preferably in case and team conferences.

5. Once such severing processes have become established they may induce paranoid developments on the part of the oncologist. The oncologist may begin to fear that patient and liaison psychiatrist have been conspiring against him during his absence, and he may sense a desire to penetrate this conspiracy, from which he feels excluded, and to disrupt it. Here again it is the task of the liaison psychiatrist, by suitably clarifying the situation for all concerned, to prevent such unfavorable developments, which in the end are detrimental to the patient. What the liaison psychiatrist does with the patient is in fact like any other kind of psychotherapeutic activity in that it entails a certain degree of discretion over third persons. If this discretion is missing, the liaison psychiatrist's activity is in most cases detrimental to the patient.
6. Cancer may frequently assume a symbolic meaning in the life of patients, i.e., the tumor can signify persecution, destruction, or punishment, among other things, and symbolically represent the irruption and the action of such vitally significant factors. This kind of symbolization occurs for the most part unconsciously, but in exceptional cases consciously. The action of unconscious factors in the progress of the illness, however, often arouses astonishment and defensive reactions in those who take the positivistic approach of the natural sciences. The consequence is that the liaison psychiatrist, in conversation with the oncologist, had better avoid any reference to the unconscious motivations of the patient, unless he wants to risk being laughed at and derided as a "spinner of yarns." Unfortunately, present-day medical men still remain almost entirely inaccessible to the unconscious dimension. Having to make allowance for this fact imposes considerable demands on the liaison psychiatrist.
7. Somatic medicine is, essentially, a manipulatory, action-oriented discipline. Psychology, on the contrary, relies on the effect of the spoken word. Its mode of operation is often puzzling and incomprehensible to the somatic medical man. This lack of understanding can have the consequence that the spoken word, as he sees it, is either vested with magical omnipotence and thus feared, or wholly depreciated, which may lead to conflicts with the liaison psychiatrist and psychologist. Liaison psychiatrists who apply training procedures such as autogenous training, behavioral therapy, or meditation exercises do not so often become involved in conflicts with somatic physicians, and psychopharmacological medicaments can also be prescribed, in a conflict-free zone between oncologist and liaison psychiatrist.

The liaison psychiatrist or psychologist ought to be a member of the oncological team. He should be present as frequently as possible on the ward and be available there to all members of the team. If possible, he should take part in all team conferences. Members of the therapeutic team feel a need to call in a liaison psychiatrist or psychologist for the patient especially if their own emotional reactions render difficult their dealings with the patient, if the patient or the members of his family do not comport themselves in accordance with the roles expected of them, if the adaptive denial or the terminal personality split [11] is falsely assessed, or if the patient inwardly withdraws and the therapeutic team becomes baffled by this [9, 12]. On the oncology ward of the Zurich University Hospital, around 400 new patients are registered each year and around 400 patients are seen on a consultative basis by the physicians of the ward on other wards. In 1985 45 patients were specially dealt with by the liaison psychiatrist and/or psychologists during 580 h.

To sum up: Liaison psychiatry on an oncology ward, in the form of team consultation and complementary treatment of the patients, can decisively contribute to the improvement of the quality of life of those on the oncology ward. Continually arising conflicts, which are immanent in the nature of the given situation, between the therapeutic team and the liaison psychiatrist (or psychologist), can in most cases be resolved if there is a constant readiness to communicate. The fact that in Zurich neither the Government nor the various cancer societies are prepared financially to assist this activity and that the establishment of a private foundation became necessary for this purpose is regrettable, indeed incomprehensible, and deserves treatment in a separate study.

References and Further Reading

1. Alby N (1985) Die Zusammenarbeit von Psychologen und Onkologen. In: Bräutigam W, Meerwein F (eds) Das therapeutische Gespräch mit Krebskranken. Huber, Bern
2. Bräutigam W, Meerwein F (eds) (1985) Das therapeutische Gespräch mit Krebskranken. Huber, Bern
3. Burkhardt-Murbach R (1987) Kunsttherapie als psychotherapeutischer Zugang bei Krebspatienten. Zum Wesen ihrer Sprache-Indikationsprobleme. Schweiz Rundschau Med (Praxis)
4. Dreifuss E (1981) Die Bedeutung der Kunstpsychotherapie in der Behandlung Krebskranker. Schweiz Rundschau Med (Praxis) 70: 1095
5. Dreifuss E (1982) Der Krebspatient und seine Familie. Erfahrungen aus der Klinik. Schweiz Rundschau Med (Praxis) 71: 1927
6. Dreifuss E (1986) Praxis der klinischen Kunsttherapie. Huber, Bern
7. Dreifuss-Kattan E, Honsalek-Blaschegg I, Meerwein F (1985) Angewandte Psychoanalyse in der medizinischen Klinik. In: Leuzinger-Bohleber (ed) Psychoanalytische Kurztherapien. Westdeutscher Verlag, Opladen
8. Honsalek I (1983) Das Behandlungsteam des Karzinom- und des Leukämie-Patienten. Schweiz Rundschau Med (Praxis) 72: 44
9. Meerwein F (1985) Einführung in die Psycho-Onkologie, 3rd edn. Huber, Bern
10. Meerwein F (1986) Das ärztliche Gespräch. Grundlagen und Anwendungen, 3rd edn. Huber, Bern
11. Meerwein F (1987) Bemerkungen zur Metapsychologie chronischer Krebskrankheiten. Bull Schweiz Ges Psychoana 23: 2
12. Nehmkis AM et al. (1981/82) Consultation issues on a cancer ward: The Hidden Agenda. Int J Psychiatry Med 11 (4): 353
13. Schmale A, Morrow G, Ader R (1977) Cancer, leukemia and related diseases. In: International encyclopedia of neurology, psychiatry, psychoanalysis and psychology. Van Nostrand Reinhod, New York

Psychological Issues in Patients with Hematological Malignancies

L. M. Lesko and J. C. Holland

Memorial Sloan-Kettering Cancer Center, 1275 York Avenue, New York, NY 10021, USA

The past two decades have witnessed major advances in the treament and supportive care (newer antibiotics, Broviac catheters, total parenteral nutrition) of hematological malignancies, resulting in longer survival and potential cure by conventional and innovative (bone marrow transplantation) treatment regimens. With this improved survival, greater attention has been given to the normal and abnormal emotional reactions patients have to their diagnosis, its treatment, and survivorship. Likewise, quality of life issues are extremely important for patient and family when treatment can only be palliative.

This paper will address the psychological issues encountered by patients with hematological malignancies through a review of (a) the psychological responses and syndromes associated with diagnosis and treatment, (b) pharmacological, psychotherapeutic, and behavioral interventions, and (c) special issues concerning treatment (transplantation, germ-free isolation, survivorship, and finally, supportive care during terminal illness).

Psychological Issues Assocsiated with Diagnosis and Treatment

Normal Concerns

Hematological cancer has remained a disease especially equated with hopelessness, pain, fear, and eventual death. For most patients, the universal human problems they deal with are what we have called the 6 D's [20] involving issues of *death*; *dependency* on family, spouse, and physician, balanced against the need for independence; *disfigurement* and changes in body appearance and self-image, sometimes resulting in loss or changes in sexual functioning: *disability* that interferes with achievement of age-appropriate tasks in work, school, or leisure roles; *disruption* in interpersonal relationships; and lastly *discomfort* and pain in later stages of illness. Recently, treatment has employed multimodal treatment regimens, i.e., drugs used in high doses, via various routes, or innovative procedures such as bone marrow transplantation, all adding to a larger number of cancer survivors. Consequently as we begin to study survivorship, we can add a seventh D –

Recent Results in Cancer Research, Vol. 108

disengagement (from the cancer diagnosis/treatment) towards reentry into a near-normal life-style.

When patients receive a diagnosis of cancer, anticipate unfamiliar treatment, learn that treatment has failed or that a relapse has occurred, or mark various anniversaries of these events, they show a characteristic emotional response: a period of shock and disbelief, followed by a period of emotional unrest with anxiety or depression, irritability, and disruption of appetite and sleep. The ability to concentrate and carry out usual daily patterns of life can be impaired; intrusive thoughts about the disease and fears about the future are present. These responses to crisis or transitional points in the course of cancer resemble the response to stress which has been described in relation to other traumatic or catastrophic losses. These normal psychological symptoms usually resolve in 2 weeks with support from family/friends and a physician who outlines a realistic plan aimed at patient education and offers hope.

The patient's ability to manage these stresses depends on factors determined by medical, psychological, and social issues. These include: (a) the disease itself (i. e., symptoms, clinical course, type of treatment required, number of relapses), (b) prior level of adjustment, especially to medical illness, (c) the threat that cancer poses in attaining age-appropriate developmental tasks and goals (i. e., adolescence, career, family), (d) cultural and religious attitudes, (e) the presence of emotionally supportive persons in the patient's environment, (f) the patient's potential for physical and psychological rehabilitation, and finally (g) the patient's personality and coping style [17, 18]. Intervention beyond that provided by empathic physicians, nurses, health care professionals, and clergy is generally not required unless symptoms of emotional distress interfere with patient function, patient compliance with cancer treatment is jeopardized or prolonged, or intolerable pain and discomfort interfere with the patient's ability to manage his/her treatment. When the cancer patient's emotional distress exceeds what would seem expectable or normal, the psychiatric symptoms must be evaluated and a therapeutic plan instituted.

A Developmental Model for Understanding the Impact of Cancer upon Patient and Family

The normal psychological concerns that patients with hematological malignancies confront are felt differently at various stages of the life cycle. We have tried to conceptualize different developmental tasks for patients of each age group and to outline the disruption in these tasks that cancer threatens [17, 18]. All patients should be informed of their diagnosis and treatment irrespective of their developmental stage. Selective information depending on age and circumstance aids in coping and in psychological control over the unknown. Realistic goals blended with hope aid both patient and family.

The *young child* has as his/her tasks the development of ties to family. Illness disrupts these patterns by slowing the ability to carry out motor and speech and cognitive activities. At times, a milestone of development may be lost and there may be regression to an earlier stage of development. The child becomes fearful of treatment, needles, and the things that are done to him/her in the hospital and clinic. On the emotional side, anxiety might occur from being separated from parents by hospitalization. Sometimes there is a withdrawal and lack of emotional involvement in surroundings. The *older child* at prepubertal stages is often going through increasing relatedness to peers and begins to become very interested as a latency child in athletic and intellectual prowess. For these children the disruption of illness is apt to involve problems of looking different, by virtue of hair loss and radiation side-effects. Being different also leads to lack of ability to perform both physically and intellectually. It is not surprising that school phobias appear in this age group. Fears of both injuries to the body and of death become much more common as children reach the stages where their understanding of death is more realistic. The *adolescent* is going through the changes of puberty and sexuality. Here, extra family relationships take on even greater importance and the normal adolescent wants to look as nearly like his peers as possible. The adolescent is beginning to seek autonomy and differentiation from his family, and is beginning to experiment with the sexual feelings. Cancer causes major disruption to adolescence. Feelings of dependence upon family by virtue of illness causes major conflicts in the ability to develop autonomy. This group suffers most from looking and being different in appearance, particularly by virtue of hair loss, Broviac catheters, and inability to perform usual athletic activities. They are at risk for poor school attendance. For the adolescent, illness can often be experienced as a kind of punishment for thoughts, feelings, or actual activities that are considered transgressions beyond parental approval. The *young adult* has tasks that relate to developing intimacy and heterosexual adjustment. The development of a marital relationship, a parental relationship with offspring, and identification of a career area are all significant tasks for this period of the life cycle. Cancer causes major disruption by diminishing attractiveness and by causing insecurity in the sexual role and the ability to maintain heterosexual relationships. The problems that arise from sterility, impotence, and inability to carry the sexual marital role may be significant, as are concerns about insurance and job security. *Middle-aged individuals* are going through certain important life tasks that indicate approaching older age. They experience children growing up and leaving home. Careers are at a peak and career goals have either been attained or the patient is adjusting to the fact that he has not been able to meet expected job-related goals. Illness is a particularly painful disruption because of declining physical and emotional stamina that impinge on sexual dysfunction and disrupted family and work roles. The *older person* is beginning to experience adjustment to losses (physical and emotional) and limitations on activities. There is an emphasis on the nurturing role by becoming a grandparent, concerns for the nuclear family, a diminishing of the physical aspects of sexual activity, and an increase in problems related to retirement and decreased income. Illness simply accentuates all of these tasks by putting additional strain on income and on the already decreased ability to carry out work and family roles.

Families, like patients, go through several stages of a life cycle. A developmental model of the family can provide an understanding of the stresses upon its members and a framework upon which to plan psychosocial interventions. Psychological stress on the family with a cancer is particularly complex since the disease occurs at all ages.

Diagnostic and Management Considerations

The most frequent disorders in patients with hematological malignancies are anxiety, depression, delirium, pain, and anorexia. Each is discussed below with guidelines in pharmacological management.

Anxiety

Anxiety in the cancer setting is either acute anxiety related to disease/treatment or chronic anxiety related to disorders which antedate the cancer diagnosis and are exacerbated by illness. *Acute* anxiety occurs at several points in the illness: (a) while awaiting the diagnosis of cancer; (b) while awaiting procedures (bone marrow aspiration, wound debridement, lumbar puncture), (c) prior to major treatment (surgery, chemotherapy radiation); (d) while awaiting test results; (e) upon learning of relapse; (f) upon change of treatment; and (g) on the anniversary of illness-related events. Pain, hypoxia, metabolic abnormalities, drug withdrawal (alcohol, narcotics, benodiazepines, barbiturates), and medications (e.g., steroids and neuroleptic drugs) also produce symptoms of anxiety. The *chronic* anxiety states which cause problems during cancer are generalized anxiety disorders, simple phobias (e.g., claustrophobia during radiological diagnostic scanning, fear of needles), and panic states with stressful events. All may require use of anxiolytic drugs along with reassurance, support, and behavioral techniques of relaxation or distraction.

Acute and chronic anxiety states in cancer are usually treated with benzodiazepines. Commonly used anxiolytics are listed in Table 1. Smaller doses than are

Table 1. Commonly prescribed benzodiazepines in patients with hematological malignancies

Drug (trade name)	Approximate dose equivalent	Initial dosage p.o. (mg)	Elimination half-life, drug and metabolites (h)	Active metabolites
Short acting				
Alprazolam (Xanax)	0.5	0.25–0.5 mg t.i.d.	10– 15	yes
Oxazepam (Serax)	10	10–15 mg t.i.d.	5– 15	no
Lorazepam[a] (Ativan)	1	0.5–2.0 mg t.i.d.	10– 20	no
Moderately long acting				
Chlordiazepoxide (Librium)	10	10–25 mg t.i.d.	10– 40	yes
Long acting				
Diazepam[a] (Valium)	5	5–10 mg b.i.d.	20–100	yes
Clorazepate (Tranxene)	7.5	7.5–15 mg b.i.d.	30–200	yes

[a] Available for i.v. use.

used in a psychiatric population are recommended for cancer patients. Patients with hepatic dysfunction will tolerate anxiolytics with shorter half-lives and those without active metabolites. Antipsychotic medications in low doses (e.g., thioridazine 10 mg t.i.d.) are used in severe anxiety when the therapeutic dose of a benzodiazepine is not effecitve. Occasionally, antihistamines are used for patients in whom physicians have grave concerns about suppression of central respiratory mechanisms by the benzodiazepines. Concerns about compromising respiratory function should not preclude a trial of an anxiolytic since the patient's shortness of breath may be markedly improved when anxiety is improved.

Since all benzodiazepines are metabolized by the liver, patients who have impaired hepatic function should be treated with the short-acting compounds that are primarily metabolized by conjugation and excreted by the kidney (oxazepam and lorazepam). In control of anxiety before chemotherapy or painful procedures, the short-acting benzodiazepine, lorazepam, is useful because it produces anterograde amnesia after intravenous administration. As in noncancer psychiatric patients, β-blockers (e.g., propranolol) and tricyclic antidepressants (e.g., imipramine) are used for both generalized panic and phobic symptoms, although drug doses may be lower.

Profound anxiety during terminal illness is seen in patients who are hypoxic or whose pain is poorly controlled. They respond very successfully to intravenous morphine sulfate. Recommended starting doses of morphine sulfate are highly variable and the maximum varies widely [39].

Depression

Depression in cancer patients results from (a) the stress related to the cancer diagnosis and treatment; (b) medications (steroids, interferon, or other chemotherapeutic agents); (c) a biologically determined depression (endogenous depression) which is not related to a precipitating event; and (d) recurrence of a bipolar affective disorder. The first two are the most common.

While the diagnosis of depression in physically healthy patients depends heavily on the somatic symptoms of fatigue, anorexia, and weight loss, these indicators are of little value in the assessment of a cancer patient, since they are common to both cancer and depression. Diagnosis must rest upon psychological (not somatic) symptoms: presence of dysphoric mood, loss of self-esteem, and feelings of helplessness or hopelessness, worthlessness, suicide, or guilt. Psychotic depressions are rare in the cancer patient, except when associated with steroids or previous psychiatric illness. Canter patients who are at higher risk for depression are those with a poor physical state, advanced stages of illness, inadequately controlled pain, or preexisting depressive syndromes.

In addition to supportive psychotherapy, the pharmacological agents that are used in the oncology setting for depression are (a) the tricyclic antidepressants, (b) lithium carbonate, (c) monoamine oxidase inhibitors (MAOIs), and (d) sympathomimetic stimulants. The tricyclic antidepressants are most commonly used. For reasons that are unclear, patients with neoplasms respond to doses far below those which are effective in physically healthy depressed patients. The starting dose is low, beginning with 10–25 mg at bedtime, increased by 25 mg every 2–3 days until a therapeutic effect is seen. Usually this is achieved by 125 mg/day. Patients are maintained on the tricyclic antidepressant for 4–6 months after their symptoms have improved, after which the dose is tapered gradually and discontinued.

The choice of the tricyclic antidepressant depends upon the nature of the depressive symptoms, side-effects of the medication, concurrent medical problems, and the route of administration. As with other medically ill patients, the depressed patient who is agitated or has insomnia will benefit from a tricyclic antidepressant with sedating effects (amitriptyline, doxepin). Patients with psychomotor retardation will benefit from compounds with the least sedating effects, such as nortriptyline or desipramine. The patient who has stomatitis secondary to radiotherapy or chemotherapy, urinary retention, or slow intestinal motility secondary to narcotic pain medication should be given a tricyclic antidepressant with little anticholinergic effect, such as nortriptyline or desipramine. Patients who are unable to take medication in pill form, because of restricted oral intake or severe esophagitis, may be able to take an elixir (nortriptyline, doxepin) or an intramuscular form (amitriptyline, imipramine, doxepin) available in Europe. Patients who have been receiving lithium carbonate for depression or mania prior to their cancer diagnosis may be maintained on it. Close monitoring is especially important during pre- and postoperative periods when fluid intake is low, during chemotherapy when hydration is mandatory, and when patients are receiving a nephrotoxic chemotherapy drug. The use of lithium to stimulate granulocyte production in neutropenic patients or to prevent leukopenia during chemotherapy has been attempted; however, these stimulation effects appear to be minimal and transient. Corticosteroids, prednisone, and dexamethasone, commonly used in leukemia and lymphoma therapy, can cause a range of psychiatric symptoms, including affective changes with manic and depressive symptoms. There are several reports in the literature regarding the potential usefulness of lithium carbonate for prevention of steroid-induced mood changes. Neuroleptics should be used when psychotic symptoms appear. We have not found lithium helpful in preventing steroid-related affective symptoms.

If a cancer patient has responded to an MAOI prior to medical illness, its continued use is appropriate. However, most psychiatrists in the oncology setting are reluctant to prescribe an MAOI in patients who often already have dietary restrictions or subsequent nutritional deficiencies. The psychostimulants dextroamphetamine and methylphenidate are sometimes used with terminally ill cancer patients who are depressed. Used in this situation, amphetamines often improve appetite, promote an increased sense of well-being, and counter the sedative effects of opiates. The starting dose is 2.5 mg dextroamphetamine given twice daily (in the morning and early afternoon). Electroconvulsive therapy (ECT) can be used for hematological cancer patients in remission in whom treatment with antidepressants involves unacceptable side-effects or in patients with psychotic or dangerously suicidal features.

Delirium

Delirium is common in cancer, due both to the direct effects of cancer on the CNS and to the indirect effects of changes related to disease and treatment. The prevalence of delirium in the general cancer patient population has been noted to range from about 5% to 25% in various studies. Variations in populations sampled, age, preexisting dementia, and levels of physical disability are confounding factors; all prohibit interpretation of data to arrive at a uniform prevalence.

As in other medical settings, early symptoms of delirium are often unrecognized or misdiagnosed by medical or nursing staff. Yet early recognition of delirium is important since the underlying etiology may be a treatable complication of cancer. When faced with an abrupt behavioral change in a cancer patient, the physician must begin to search for one or more (Table 2). These may be the "direct" result of the tumor itself or of metastatic spread to the CNS via hematogenous or lymphatic routes. Of equal importance are the "indirect" effects of infection, vascular complications, metabolic changes, organ failure, treatment effects, nutritional state, and remote effects. Some are potentially reversible and the patient will be able to return to the prior level of mental function following successful treatment.

Table 2. Prevalence of delirium in hospitalized cancer patients

Author	Number of patients	Stage/type of disease	% OMS	Comments
All hospitalized patients				
Davies et al. [8]	46	Advanced cancer	27	Patients screened for OMS and depression
Folstein et al. [14]	83	Consecutive admissions	26	
Derogatis et al. [9]	215		8	Included delirium, dementia with depression, organic affective syndrome, atypical organic brain syndrome, organic personality disorder
Posner (1979)		CNS complication	15	
Hospitalized patients (referred for psychiatric consultation)				
Massie et al. [29]	334	All stages	25	
Levine et al. [24]	100	All stages	40	All OMS, "chronic" and "acute", DSM-II
Shevits et al. [44]	1000	Cancer and noncancer (gen. hosp.)	16	All OMS, "chronic" and "acute", DSM-II
Massie et al [28]	546	All stages	20	
Hinton [16]	50	Terminal illness	10	
Massie et al. [29]	13	Terminal illness	85	

OMS, organic mental syndrome.

Failure of vital organs, especially the liver, kidneys, and lungs, or the metabolic changes that result from thyroid or adrenal failure are common. Electrolyte imbalance, especially sodium, potassium, and calcium, may constitute a metabolic cause of altered mental status. Hepatic encephalopathy will prevent a patient from metabolizing drugs, thereby precipitating CNS complications.

Adequate use of narcotic analgesics to manage cancer pain may sometimes result in oversedation and hallucinatory experiences. Medications with anticholinergic effects as well as other agents such as amphotericin B, acyclovir, and interferon are associated with encephalopathy. All steroid compounds may cause psychiatric disturbances, ranging from affective changes (emotional lability, euphoria, depressed mood), anxiety, and fear, to paranoid interpretation of events, suspiciousness of others, illusions, delusions, and hallucinations. Symptoms can develop 4–5 days after beginning high-dose steroids or when the dose is rapidly tapered, but psychiatric symptoms can also develop while patients are on a maintenance dose. No relationship has been shown between the development of steroid psychosis and prior psychiatric history.

Among the more than 60 chemotherapeutic agents now available for treatment of cancer, central nervous system symptoms are not a prominent feature. Those which cause delirium are methotrexate, 5-fluorouracil, vincristine and vinblastine, bleomycin, BCNU, cisplatin, asparaginase, and procarbazine. The newest chemotherapy agents include biological response modifiers: α- and γ-interferon, interleukins, tumor necrosis factor (TNF), and B cell growth factor (BCGF). To date, interferon has been successfully used in clinical studies in patients with hairy cell leukemia, chronic myelocytic leukemia, and some lymphomas. Intramuscular administration of interferon in dose ranges of 2–50 million units per day produces influenza-like symptoms of lethargy, anorexia, and nausea, or depression, somnolence, confusion, and paresthesia. These symptoms appear to be dose dependent and to disappear upon discontinuation of the drug. Symptoms of fatigue, malaise, and depression are sometimes severe enough to compromise patient compliance. The psychological side-effects of the other agents have been less carefully studied and documented.

Amphotericin B is used regularly in cancer patients who are immunologically compromised for the treatment of fungal infections. It can cause anaphylaxis, fever, rigors, anorexia, and impaired renal function. Various neurological side-effects, including delirium, have been reported with intrathecal administration. Patients treated with the methyl ester of amphotericin B may be particularly susceptible to CNS effects [11]. The same study reported on 14 patients who developed progressive severe neurological dysfunction including dementia, akinesia, mutism, hyperreflexia, tremor, and white matter degeneration. Symptoms were dose dependent; they were most severe with doses greater than 9.0 g. Often it is difficult to distinguish CNS effects of antifungal medication from those of fever, CNS infection, or metabolic abnormalities.

Acyclovir is a relatively new antiviral drug which has proved efficacious for the prophylaxis and treatment of herpes simplex and varicella zoster virus. It is used widely in patients who are immunologically compromised (bone marrow transplantation and leukemia). Wade and Meyers [49] reported reversible neurotoxicity in 6 of 143 bone marrow transplant recipients studied. Symptoms which develop in a median of 8 days after the initiation of treatment included lethargy ($n=5$), agitation ($n=5$), tremor ($n=5$), disorientation ($n=1$), and transient hemiparesthesias ($n=1$). The authors notet that these patients may have been predisposed to neurological side-effects by previous intrathecal methotrexate therapy, total body irradiation, preexisting CNS leukemia, herpes virus infections, or the concurrent use of interferon. However, improvement in all patients upon discontinuation of acyclovir suggested that the transient CNS toxicity was secondary to the antiviral agent rather than to other causative agents.

Whole brain radiation, combined with intrathecal methotrexate, enhances the development of encephalopathy. Rowland et al. [41] retrospectively studied children with acute lymphocytic leukemia who were treated with intrathecal methotrexate and cranial radiation as prophylaxis against CNS recurrence. They found that children who received both radiation and intrathecal methotrexate had a mean 10-point lower IQ than children who received only intrathecal methotrexate. Abnormalities in growth hormone and soft neurological signs were also evident. Radiation causes a transient syndrome in children known as the radiation somnolence syndrome. This occurs several weeks after radiation and is caused by demyelinization. The doses of radiation required to treat brain tumors at times produce cognitive impairment and occasionally progressive dementia.

As in other medically ill patients, antipsychotic drugs are the mainstay in the management of delirium. The same principles apply for their use, administration, and dosage in cancer except that patients who are debilitated require a lower starting dose. Haloperidol is the most commonly prescribed antipsychotic drug in a U.S. cancer setting because of its low incidence of cardiovascular and anticholinergic effects, and the availability of elixir, pill, and parenteral forms. It is often administered intravenously when patients are thrombocytopenic, unable to take medications orally secondary to stomatitis, or agitated (and rapid sedation is needed).

Pain

Psychological symptoms of anxiety or depression may be either a consequence of or a contributor to pain; treating both usually has the effect of reducing pain [38]. The data from these authors confirm clinical observations that the psychiatric symptoms (anxiety, depression) of patients who are in pain must initially be considered as a consequence of uncontrolled pain. Acute anxiety, depression, despair (when the patient believes the pain means disease progression), irritability, agitation, uncooperativeness, anger, and altered sleep patterns are common emotional and behavioral symptoms of pain. Psychiatrists could first assist in the management of the patient's pain and then reassess the patient's mental state *after* pain is adequately controlled to determine whether the patient's symptoms are psychiatric in nature. In summary, the cancer patient with pain has an enhanced risk of developing psychiatric disorders commonly seen in cancer. Clearly, depression, anxiety, or mixed symptoms of depression and anxiety are the most common of these problems.

Pharmacological therapy remains the mainstay of treatment of acute and chronic pain. The analgesic medications most commonly used are divided into these major categories [35]: (a) aspirin, acetominophen, and nonsteroidal anti-inflammatory drugs which peripherally produce analgesia via inhibition of the enzyme prostaglandin synthetase; (b) narcotic agonists and antagonists which act centrally and peripherally by binding to opiate receptors and activating endogenous pain suppression; and (c) adjuvant drugs (antidepressants, antipsychotics) which act centrally to control pain by poorly understood mechanisms [13]. Excellent guidelines for pharmacological management of pain are available [13]. The principles include:

1. Treat the psychological as well as the physical symptoms of the pain.
2. Use a specific drug for specific pain (aspirin or a nonsteroidal anti-inflammatory drug is used for mild to moderate pain, and an oral or parenteral narcotic for moderate to severe pain).
3. Learn the pharmacology of the specific pain medication - equivalent analgesic dose per route of administration, peak time and duration of analgesia, pharmacokinetics, and toxic side-effects (sedation, respiratory depression, nausea, vomiting, constipation).
4. Administer analgesics regularly.
5. Be flexible in changing medications but allow each analgesic an adequate trial.
6. Watch for development of analgesic tolerance, physical dependence, and withdrawal.
7. Do not use placebos to assess cancer pain.
8. Consider use of combinations of drugs to enhance analgesia, i.e., narcotic analgesic with nonnarcotic analgesic, dextroamphetamine, hydroxyzine, or amitriptyline [41].
9. Adequately manage pain in terminal illness by morphine infusions when possible [39].

Anorexia

Anorexia is one of the most common symptoms of cancer and is one of the most difficult to treat since it and related weight loss may be caused by disease, treatment, and/or psychological disorders. Medical causes of appetite loss are related to tumor burden, fever, bowel obstruction, metabolic abnormalities (hepatic and renal dysfunction), and treatment (radiation and chemotherapy). Radiation produces acute side-effects of stomatitis, esophagitis, and an altered sense of taste, all making it difficult to eat. Many of the chemotherapeutic agents, besides causing nausea and vomiting, can produce ulcerations of the gastrointestinal tract and alter the taste of food and the pleasure of eating. Antibiotics, antifungal agents, and pain medication can produce gastrointestinal distress and anorexia.

Psychiatric syndromes and behavioral dynamics are often overlooked as a cause of appetite loss. Sometimes anorexia occurs in the context of depression or anxiety and in the rare instance can emerge as a symptom of a previous psychiatric illness, such as anorexia nervosa or bulimia. Anorexia may also result from anticipatory anxiety or worry about poor intake. Fear, anxiety, worry, and anorexia may become behaviorly coupled to one another. In these situations, techniques such as relaxation and self-hypnosis can lower anticipatory anxiety related to eating. Learned food aversions may also play an important role in cancer-related anorexia. "Learned food aversions are acquired aversions to specific foods or tastes which develop as a result of the association of those foods with unpleasant internal responses (nausea and vomiting)" [2]. This behavioral phenomenon is similar to classical conditioning paradigms.

Management of anorexia involves educational, behavioral, and pharmacological approaches. Consultation with a nutritionist provides very valuable ideas for patients, i.e., small frequent meals with high caloric content, appetizing recipes, visually appealing presentations, and avoidance of strongly flavored foods. The "ambiance" of the meal time can be very important in encouraging eating; having a family member share a meal, serving a favorite wine or beer, and special table settings add social aspects that all individuals associate with a pleasant meal. Such simple behavioral techniques are overlooked by the disinterested patient or distraught family member. Operant conditioning, with rewards such as family visits or watching TV or movies being contingent upon weight gain or caloric intake, is usually unsuccessful in physically ill patients with cancer.

Psychological and Behavioral Interventions

Over the last few years, as attention to psychological aspects of cancer has grown, so has the interest in developing psychological interventions to treat that distress. Some advocate treating all cancer patients on the assumption that all patients need or want psychological intervention. Worden and Weisman [51], however, have stated that many cancer patients adapt well to their illness and treatment and do not need psychological intervention. However, early identification of patients at high risk for psychological morbidity is essential. In addition to identifying which patients and families are vulnerable, attempts are being made to develop various psychotherapeutic and psychosocial treatment modalities specific to cancer: individual groups, family support programs, and self-help or patient-to-patient volunteer programs.

Individual psychotherapy with cancer patients is largely supportive, utilizing educational techniques, answering questions about laboratory results, treatment options, and the predicted side-effects of treatment, correcting facts and giving reassurance, and assisting the patient and family in negotiating the medical system. Explanation of psychological dynamics often leads to exploration of "more effective coping mechanisms." The therapist (a) should offer support in short visits (20 min for the seriously ill), focusing on current issues of illness or hospitalization, (b) should be knowledgeable of various psychotherapeutic techniques, i.e., the principles of crisis intervention and supportive psychotherapy, as well as understanding issues of family dynamics, and (c) must be knowledgeable of the medical aspects of the patient's disease.

Group psychotherapy for the cancer patient may be advantageous, allowing him/her to receive support from others (patients or nonpatients) who have experienced and have conquered similar problems of illness and treatment. The patient in a group setting can easily learn that there are a range of "normal reactions" to illness and a range of "healthy adaptive coping styles" which others have employed to make adjustment to illness easier. Group participation decreases a sense of isolation and alienation. The general principles of group therapy for the nonmedically ill person apply for group therapy with cancer patients.

Self-help and Patient-to-Patient Volunteer Programs

Self-help and patient-to-patient volunteer programs are an alternative form of support for patients and families. Historically, life crises, such as bereavement, divorce, or drug addiction, often provided the impetus for individuals to seek emotional support from others experiencing the same trauma. In cancer, self-help and patient-to-patient volunteer programs started after World War II, when the American Cancer Society began a "visitors" program offering practical help for patients at home. Most self-help support networks for cancer patients work closely with the medical profession. At our hospital volunteers in the patient-to-patient volunteer program visit every newly admitted cancer patient. The veteran patient volunteer facilitates coping in the newly diagnosed patient by (a) being a source of "credible" information based on his or her own past cancer experience, (b) encouraging patient participation in their own treatment; (c) demonstrating constructive ways of managing and living despite illness; (e) serving as a "surrogate patient" who spouses and family members can question and express feelings to [30].

Sexual Counseling

It is well known that treatment for hematological malignancies may result in infertility and sexual dysfunction. Increasingly, there is recognition of the need for psychosexual rehabilitation for patients, irrespective of age. A psychological consultant trained as a sex rehabilitation specialist brings special expertise to teams caring for such patients. Auchincloss [1] suggests it is the job of the oncological professional to initiate the subject of sexuality with all patients. Patients are often embarrassed or even may assume that after cancer, one's sex life should no longer exist. Married patients may have had precancer sexual problems which are compounded by cancer treatment. Single patients face dating and potential marriage (partner) issues. Evaluation includes obtaining a sexual history, including the partner, noting preexisting sexual problems, and addressing the patient's current treatment-specific questions and fears. The therapist must be informed about the physical sequelae of radiation or chemotherapy in order to supply information and practical suggestions. Patients with persistent concerns about body image, sexual desire, and sexual function should be referred to professionals who are trained in sexual rehabilitation. In the United States, sperm banking for patients undergoing cancer treatment is routine practice.

Behavioral Interventions

Behavioral techniques include passive relaxation with visual imagery, progressive muscle relaxation, electromyographic (EMG) biofeedback, systematic desensitization, and cognitive distraction. These methods are useful as adjuvant treatments combined with pharmacological agents for pain and discomfort during chemotherapy infusions, bone marrow biopsies, or venipunctures. Research efforts at our hospital are directed toward study of passive relaxation and cognitive distraction during chemotherapy infusions and for anticipatory nausea and vomiting (ANV) which occur before hospital visits. ANV before chemotherapy or radiation follows a classical behavioral conditioning pradigm and is a far more common symptom than has been previously recognized [32]. ANV can occur hours or even days before chemotherapy administration and often occurs in patients who (a) receive repeated cycles of a chemotherapy regimen or highly emetogenic drugs, (b) experience severe posttreatment nausea and vomiting, and (c) have high levels of anxiety or alterations of taste and smell associated with the chemotherapy infusion. In some patients ANV has persisted for 12 years after treatment [5].

Special Issues

Patients with hematological malignancies may undergo unique treatment regimens, such as bone marrow transplantation and germ-free isolation, compared to other cancer patients. Psychological concerns with such treatment and management guidelines will be discussed. General therapeutic principles will also be presented for those patients whose treatment is palliative, being aimed at comfort during terminal illness, or who have completed successful curative treatment and begin reentry into family, job, or school.

Bone Marrow Transplantation

Bone marrow transplantation (BMT) is an increasingly frequent alternative treatment utilized for acute and chronic leukemia and more recently for lymphoma. In the 1970s, BMT was an experimental regimen reserved for end-stage disease; however, clinical experience has found improved results (a) with transplantations done in remission, while patients are medically stable, and (b) early in the course of disease (i.e., in the chronic phase of chronic myelocytic leukemia, during first remission for acute nonlymphocytic leukemia, and during second remission for acute lymphocytic leukemia). Today, BMT can be divided into two types: (a) BMT from a twin (syngeneic) or a histocompatible donor (allogeneic) and (b) refusion of the patient's own purged bone marrow (autologous). The latter procedure is now being used for advanced lymphoma patients and leukemia patients who have no compatible donors. Newer and improved methods for marrow purging will herald and secure this treatment option as a standard modality for patients without an appropriate matched donor.

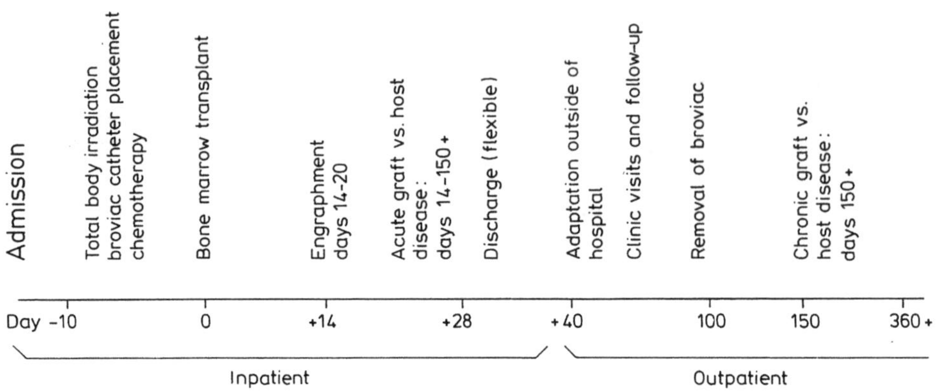

Fig. 1. Bone marrow transplant schema

Both allogeneic and autologous transplants necessitate 2-3 months' hospitalization in a reverse isolation room or laminar airflow (sterile) unit. Complications may arise from immediate and delayed effects of the transplant: graft rejection, infection, graft-versus-host disease (in those receiving marrow from a donor), and neurological and psychological complications. Convalescence, both physical and psychological, requires at least 6-12 months and can be stressful for patients and family, especially when it entails return to school or work.

The BMT procedure can be devided into several stages which encompass both the medical treatment and its psychological sequelae [4, 21]. The medical stages of BMT are shown in Fig. 1, and the psychological states associated with each of these stages are described below.

Often the decision to accept the transplantation procedure is made against a background of chronic illness and, at times, organ failure. Patients may have experienced months or years of feeling ill, and fears of death/uncertainty are coupled with hope of possible cure. The decision to have a transplant may be made many miles from the transplantation center and is often made quickly due to urgent medical complications, the physical status of the patient, and bed availability. The patient's and family's decision to accept the recommendation for transplant is always preceded by the stress of medical tests and tissue typing of family members.

The *medical consultation* usually takes place on an outpatient basis at the patient's own hospital and/or at the transplant center. Along with the medical evaluations, some form of psychological assessment is often undertaken to evaluate the patient's social supports and ability to cope with the procedure. This is a time when the prospective patients should be encouraged to visit the transplant unit and meet the staff who will care for them. Families find housing, especially if they are a great distance from home, and learn what may be brought from home to make the patient's hospital stay more pleasant. Since there is concern that relapse may occur before the treatment can be instituted, anticipation and waiting can be difficult.

Hospitalization for the transplant requires more tests and is accompanied by mixed feelings of anxiety and hope. Patients enter the sterile germ-free or reverse isolation room relatively soon to avoid infection. They then undergo a 10-day pretransplant conditioning regimen comprising high dose immunosuppressive drugs and hyperfractionated total body irradiation. A Broviac/Hickman catheter is placed, making possible the drawing of blood samples and administration of blood products, medications, antibiotics, and total parental nutrition without the need for frequent peripheral sticks. These days are marked by physical discomfort: nausea, vomiting, and fatique secondary to radiation and chemotherapy. This is "the point of no return," for unlike kidney transplantation, there is no dialysis to fall back on.

The *transplantation* is brief and anticlimatic compared to the lengthy "pretransplant treatment" and the "convalescent period." It is usually uncomplicated and is paradoxically undramatic, involving only an infusion of one or several packets of concentrated bone marrow.

In the *immediate recovery period,* concerns regarding marrow engraftment or rejection, continuation of immunosuppressive drugs, the risk of infection and high fever, and the specter of graft-versus-host disease are paramount. Currently, researchers are virtually eliminating patients' risk of developing graft-versus-host disease by employing newer techniques of T cell depleted grafts. The requisite convalescent period in the hospital is usually 1-2 months post-transplant, during which time the patients must undergo several weeks of supportive care: hyperalimentation, antibiotics, and blood products. It is a trying time for families who are usually asked to visit daily to provide emotional and physical support. Family disruption may be quite obvious at this time when the stresses of the seemingly endless hospitalization do not relent.

Preparation for discharge usually takes 1-2 weeks. Patients have renewed hope of picking up their lives where they left off and show a heightened interest in the world outside the hospital. However, as they begin to learn the self-care which will be necessary at home, the excitement over the anticipated discharge is mixed with fear of leaving the security of their room and the transplant unit. At this time patients commonly have difficulty with their appetite, particularly if they are being weaned from hyperalimentation.

Convalescence and adaptation outside the hospital is protracted and lasts almost 6-12 months. Transplantation does not guarantee immediate or total restoration of preillness health, and thus the transplant patient requires considerable support from staff throughout discharge and convalescence. Weekly visits to the transplant clinic occur for at least the first 2 months. As time following transplantation increases, patients turn their concerns from "living as a patient" to "living as a survivor." They have profound fatigue and may show signs of actual inability to "reenter" normal activities related to home and work. Young adults who have undergone BMT may in particular need help managing their small, active children. Children resume normal life more rapidly than adults. Rehabilitation is as much a psychological process as a physiological process; the two must proceed hand-in-hand.

Total Body Irradiation. TBI is used in combination with chemotherapy in the transplant protocol. TBI is given in the range of 1000-1300 rads, usually divided into 12 treatments over 3-4 days. This irradiation may lead to acute transient nausea and vomiting or delayed sequelae of infertility and delayed growth and maturation in small children.

Broviac/Hickman Catheterization and Total Parenteral Nutrition (TPN). TPN was introduced by Dudrick et al. in 1968 [10]. The continuous infusion via an intravenous catheter of a hypertonic solution of protein hydrolysates, glucose, vitamins, minerals, and lipids requires an indwelling catheter placed in the large vessels and right atrium. The catheter is also used as a route for blood products, immunosuppressive drugs, and other medications. TPN is currently being used routinely in all BMT patients for nutrition in the hospital and is usually stopped 2 weeks before discharge but catheters may stay in place for up to 3-6 months after transplantation. Broviac/Hickman line catheterization can cause anxiety, depression, fear, and negative body image. The positive side, however, is that this special type of venous access decreases anxiety related to the multiple painful venipunctures which would otherwise be necessary for amphotericin and antibiotics. Minor adjustment problems of transplant patients related to TPN reflect four major areas of concern: (a) the temporary loss of the basic function of eating and controlling nutrition; (b) dependence on nurses for the TPN care, which results in separation anxiety on discharge; (c) the high level of technical care of the catheter which must be learned for maintenance at home; (d) the psychological dependence on the line itself for food and fluids. Expressions such as, "Is it a chain, a lifeline, an umbilical cord?" show the dependence, frustration, and problems for patients in adjusting to its presence and removal.

Graft-Versus-Host Disease. Engraftment of donor bone marrow in the patient is a sign of hematological success, but it sometimes paradoxically brings with it the life-threatening problem of graft-versus-host disease (GVHD). Approximately 50% of recipients develop acute mild to moderate GVHD; it is fatal in 20% of patients. Chronic GVHD may develop after 150 days, with chronic skin pigmentation and debilitating contractures. Both the acute and the chronic form result in psychological ramifications of added uncertainty of chronic illness, physical deformity, long-term medication, and altered life-style. Future progress in T cell depleted grafts will make this sequela nonexistent.

Emotional Disturbances Related to Transplantation. Chronic anxiety and depression are by far the most common psychiatric sequelae of the transplantation procedure. Frequent outpatient visits, repeated blood tests, prophylactic medication for GVHD and infections, transfusions, and bone marrow biopsies, coupled with fatigue, decreased stamina, and concerns about relapse, disability, and job status foster chronic anxiety and depressive symptoms. Psychological convalescence is particularly difficult for those patients who have delayed or disrupted important developmental life tasks. Patients must make the philosophical transition from living one day at a time to anticipating the future. "Aiming at short-term goals" and "not looking beyond tomorrow," which were adaptive against immediate stresses of relapse, now result in difficulties in dealing with longer-term goals.

Sexual dysfunction, associated with premature menopause, vaginal dryness, painful intercourse, and sterility, is seen in women following transplantation.

These symptoms are secondary to radiation and subsequent endocrine imbalances and most women are placed on estrogen replacement. Decreased sexual desire may also be related to depression and the patient's altered self-image.

Coping mechanisms and psychological techniques (conscious and unconscious) to master such BMT stresses, i.e. intellectualization, repression, displacement, regression, and rationalization, are means by which the individual copes with the transplant environment. Three features are central to successful adaptation: (a) the need to gather information about the transplant process and subsequently intellectualization/rationalization, (b) the ability to temporarily delegate much of his or her own control and authority ot others, and (c) the capacity to establish a close, trusting relationship with the staff.

Germ-Free Environments

Certain oncological conditions, including BMT and aggressive administration of cancer chemotherapy, may require treating a patient in a germ-free environment. Although therapeutically useful to decrease the risk and severity of infection in such patients, these environments (whether reverse isolation or sterile laminar airflow) impose prolonged physical and psychological isolation from family and staff. Information from a variety of sources provides insight into the psychological issues, which are similar to those experienced by patients treated in protected isolation environments. This information includes literature on the intensive care unit (ICU) syndrome, social isolation in novel or extreme environments, sensory deprivation, parental separation from children, long-term isolation of children, and the importance of oral and maternal stimulation for early behavioral development. Of particular interest is the ICU syndrome, characterized by disorientation and defects in memory, attention, and concentration. This syndrome was originally observed in cardiac surveillance facilities, recovery rooms, and intensive care units. Organic brain dysfunction caused by the underlying medical illness, sleep deprivation, and the use of artificial assistance (ventilation, vasopressor medication, feeding tubes, suctions) are the main contributors to this state. Continual bombardment of unfamiliar auditory and visual stimuli and the unfamiliar environment of mechanized units, foreign to the patient's usual life-style, are stressful. On the other hand, Holland et al. [19] believe that ICU environments have positive effects, providing the patient with a feeling of being attentively cared for.

Many of the descriptions of the psychological consequences of isolation come from the pediatric literature. Many researchers feel that, while patients may at times exhibit symptoms of regression, as well as affective sensory and behavioral changes, these symptoms tend to be transient and isolation environments do not fundamentally interfere with normal development. Most research on psychological reactions of adults to protected environments was begun with the expectation that severe psychological disturbances might result from prolonged isolation, a natural extension from the earlier work on sensory deprivation and the ICU syndrome. Authors studying adult patients cared for in germ-free isolation have in fact concluded that while most patients are anxious and apprehensive before entering isolation, almost all adapt well to the psychological stress despite the serious nature of their illness, their unusual environment, and the range of premorbid personalities. Psychological equilibrium is influenced *only* by the severity of the patient's physical illness or by the presence of an organic delirium, not by isolation itself. Perceptual and cognitive disturbances such as those described in sensory deprivation experiments are not found.

The patient's primary psychological difficulty lies in adjusting to the diagnosis of a life-threatening illness, and germ-free environments tend to attenuate or aggregate this difficulty. Every patient brings to the treatment their own character and coping mechanisms; these influence tolerance of a restricted environment. Depression, anxiety, irregular sleep, regression, withdrawal from one's surroundings, and occasional disorientation are noted. Several management principles are mentioned below and are summarized in Table 3 [22].

1. *Patient education.* Knowledge about one's illness, its severity, and its treatment enhances emotional stability and cooperation in such a restricted environment. An honest and open relationship with nurse and physician allows the patient to gather more information about his/her illness and at the same time affords the health care giver an opportunity to obtain more information about the patient's character, psychological functioning, modes of coping with past illness, and capacity for dealing with stress.
2. *Preparation.* It is recommended that all patients with a family tour the isolation unit or room prior to hospitalization. Meeting the unit's personnel, especially the nursing staff, can be comforting for children and will also provide an opportunity for family members to ask questions about items they can bring from home for the patients. Many units develop an orientation pamphlet which includes procedural as well as psychological preparation for reverse isolation.

Table 3. Patient management guidelines

1. *Patient education*
Knowledge about one's own illness and treatment
2. *Preparation*
Visiting the isolation unit
Meeting staff (nurses, social workers)
Patient information booklets
3. *Environmental manipulation*
Orientation
Access to windows, clocks, calendars, TVs, radios, natural light
Personal belongings from home
Stable daily schedule
Single rooms, with monitoring equipment outside of room
Patients participating in own care
4. *Psychological support*
Nurturing but structured support from all staff
Liberal visiting hours
5. *Medication*
Anxiolytics used to control anxiety, neuroleptics rarely indicated except for delirium

3. *Environmental manipulation.* Patients are encouraged to bring personal belongings (books, hobbies, paintings, posters, pictures, stereos, radios, stuffed animals, albums, and clothes) to brighten up the isolation area, providing a sense of familiarity. Access to natural light, windows, clocks, radios, calendars, and TVs are helpful in orienting patients and maintaining a stable daily and diurnal rhythm. Monitoring equipment is best kept outside the patient's room when possible and exposure to monotonous noises should be kept to a minimum. Regression, due to psychological stress and illness, should be discouraged by encouraging patients to participate in their own care and to remain as self-sufficient as possible (e.g., managing their own hygiene and schedules, operating radios and televisions).
4. *Psychological support.* Support from the staff is a more valuable tool than psychotropic drugs in improving a patient's and family's capacity to cope with illness, physical concerns, and the stress of isolation. Liberal visiting privileges for family and friends will help to maintain the necessary contacts with the outside world. All staff should meet regularly to assess how patients and families are coping and to devise interventions when appropriate. Preparation for leaving the isolation unit should take place a few days before the actual move to a "step down" unit or discharge. Patients are encouraged to talk about feelings of leaving the hospital and "reentry" to home. Once leaving, patients may develop anxiety about being out of their special environment. This may take the form of worries about family and/or somatic concerns about new aches, pains, and symptoms. Patients in these environments have been accustomed to being monitored and supervised very closely. After discharge minor aches and pains can produce acute anxiety and some patients may for a period need constant reassurance that they are progressing as expected.
5. *Medication.* Anxiolytics can be used to modulate excessive anxiety, relieve insomnia, and serve as an adjunct in control of pain. Major tranquilizers (neuroleptics) are rarely indicated and could mask recognition of an acute confusional state secondary to metabolic abnormalities. Antidepressants can be utilized when patients experience major depressive symptomatology in the post hospital convalescent period.

Terminal Illness

The "terminally ill" patient with a hematological malignancy has not responded to known curative measures, and treatment is aimed at providing maximal comfort. In such patients, the science and art of medicine and psychiatry must be integrated. The "art" is guided by the health care giver's own personality/philosophy and the history that the family and patient bring with them (i.e., their psychosocial and cultural values) [17, 18]. Conflicts regarding decisions about terminal or supportive care may lead to requests for psychiatric consultation and intervention.

We often forget that the patient who is dying has not changed; only their physical status has changed and their emotional and psychological needs only intensify. Physicians', patients', and family attitudes define the period of "terminal" from a few hours to weeks to months. As more effective life support and resuscitative measures have become available in critical care medicine, "terminal illness" has become much harder to define. When the label "terminal" is assigned to a patient, the behavior and attitudes of staff, family, and friends often assume a different character. These attitudes may tend to isolate or draw the patient from those he or she most needs at an important time. As the definition of "terminal illness" has changed, so has that of "supportive" care. Today, this treatment often includes blood products, antibiotics, hydration, pain medication, palliative radiation, total parenteral nutrition, or home infusions of low dose chemotherapeutic agents.

To Tell or Not To Tell

Should patients know of their critical state? What should they be told? How? When?

In the United States there is a trend toward greater candor in disclosure about cancer and its treatment with both patient and family. Novack et al. in 1979 [36] reported that 97% of physicians favored telling cancer patients their diagnosis, in contrast to 90% of physicians who did not tell their patients in 1961 [36]. Today, most patients prefer to know about their illness. Recent articles in the lay press have again emphasized the patient's right to be told the truth. Most patients, even children, want to be told the seriousness of their illness, but also want to hear the ways in which family and professionals will help. Those patients and families who need to deny the truth will continue to do so. By discussing the availability of supportive measures such as pain control and palliative treatment and by offering flexibility in care outside the hospital, the physician communicates his pledge to provide continued care for the dying patient.

Concept of Terminal Illness

A patient's *perception* of terminal illness depend on several medical or physical factors (pain, relapse) in the course of illness. The patient's or family's first "sense" of terminal disease may result from an increase in the severity of medical problems, development of pain, delirium, organ failure, a rapid illness course irrespective of adequate medical management, or the level of care given by the health care team. A patient's and a family's *acceptance* of terminal illness depends on many psychological, cultural, and religious factors.

The psychological stages of denial, anger, depression, bargaining, acceptance, and resolution as defined by Kubler-Ross [20] never occur in any uniform progression. More uniformly, patients show daily changes in optimism and pessimism, related to the medical events of their disease and treatment. Information gathering and intellectual problem solving are coping mechanisms to provide control over unknown prognosis, side-effects, and general feelings of hopelessness. Patients who psychologically do well during terminal illness have the ability to integrate problem-solving methods with the right amount of denial and hope.

Since both views and attitudes toward death change with age, the stage of the life cycle during which terminal illness occurs has a profound impact on how death will be perceived and accepted [20]. The young adult, like the adolescent, understands the finality of death, which is apt to be viewed as the adversary that must be fought and conquered. Often, bitterness and hostility will be strong emotions in terminal stages. Mature adults have established social and family roles and are often at the peak of their intellectual work and output. At this stage, death comes at the time of feeling that one has "just made it" in terms of work, family, and children. The older adult, sensing diminishing responsibilities and thinking toward the "rewards of older age and retirement" feels that death must be faced, but "not yet." Since old age is normally a time for increased introspection and "taking stock," death is approached more realistically. The elderly adult usually has a realistic view of life expectancy and may be more concerned about the manner of dying than about death itself. Thoughts of becoming a burden, particularly to one's children, are of great concern. Again, for the elderly patient, the frequent losses of significant others - especially spouse, friends, and siblings - may contribute to a pervasive sadness, and sometimes the meaning of living is substantially reduced. Supportive sessions in which patient and therapist put past memories in order allows the reworking of past events.

It is also important to remember that while the patient has a perception of terminal illness, so does the physician and nurse. Differing attitudes toward death can become an issue because of the varying ages between patient and physician and their age-related *perceptions* of death. The physician may be somewhere between 23 and 30 (the young medical student) or 60 and 70 (the physician who practices into postretirement years). The young physician who is taking care of a child or another young adult shares the attitude, found in young patients, of anger and outrage at catastrophic illness. The young patient's terminal illness threatens the young doctor's sense of his or her own invulnerability and omnipotence. Guilt may develop for one's inability to offer curative measures. On the other hand, the same young physician may be less interested and able to mount a vigorous effort to treat older patient who is critically ill. The young professional (physician and nurse) often sees death as an appropriate life stage for the older or geriatric patient. When this is combined with culturally sanctioned negative views of the elderly, an indifferent manner may make an older patient feel less compassionately treated. The middle-aged and older professional who takes care of the young patient may appear not to be sharing the "fighting spirit" of never "giving up." The older professional will often have views toward terminal illness that are similar to his/her older patient. Shared views and a common cultural or historical past make for a natural and comforting relationship toward resolving terminal-care issues.

Traditionally, care of the terminally ill patient has been delegated to and accepted as the responsibility by various religious orders. Twenty years ago, the issue of dying patients was made publically visible by Cicely Saunders, who founded St. Christopher's Hospice. This was the beginning of the hospice movement, which has since spread to Europe and the United States. Currently, there is a trend in the United States to allow terminally ill children to die at home; this requires a sophisticated and compassionate team approach to care for the pediatric patient's medical condition and the psychological needs of family and friends. Unfortunately, the decision as to whether a terminally ill patient is cared for at home or in a hospice is often made hastily without involving the patient, with only a few family members present; it can be governed by financial restraints or job requirements of the supporting family and/or by the lack of family. Ideally, mental health professionals should be consulted at this stage to best fit the needs of the patient, family, doctor, and community resources.

Irrespective of whether a terminally ill patient is cared for at home or in the hospice setting, psychiatric consultation can be beneficial in the care of such patients. The most common reasons for a psychiatric consultation in the terminally ill are the presence of delirium, suicidal ideation, staff conflicts, family conflicts about "letting go" or "fighting on" involving heroic measures, and supportive care. Issues that should be addressed by such consultants are:

1. What is the extent of the patient's and family's understanding of terminal illness, their coping mechanisms, and their cultural or religious background?
2. Is there a preexisting psychiatric syndrome (patient and/or family), a problem with pain control, drug abuse, or delirium that makes management of such a patient complex for the physician?
3. Is there open communication between patient, family, and professional staff so that a sense of trust in care and decision making can be sustained throughout the illness?
4. Does the family have the physical and psychological stamina, financial support, and educational ability to juggle work schedules, changes in responsibilities, and physical care, besides assuming their normal day to day chores?
5. Has the pattern of family function been one that suggests ability to maintain cohesion and retain adequate social support during this period?
6. Are there internal or external family resources available to bolster the family's self-image during illness and bereavement?

Survivorship

Today, survival and cure from hematological malignancies are often achieved at significant cost. With innovative treatment such as BMT and intensive multidrug protocols, long-term physical sequelae (such as infertility, organ failure, and peripheral and central nervous system dysfunction) compound the possible emotional sequelae associated with diagnosis and treatment. Survival carries with it the stressors of possible delayed medical sequelae, fears of relapse, a lingering affinity with death, a precarious sense of longevity, and numerous demands of reentry into normal life (family, school, job). These can be divided into two broad areas - medical and psychosocial sequelae - and are outlined in Table 4.

Table 4. Sequelae of survivorship

Medical
1. Occurrence of second malignancies or relapse
2. Peripheral and central nervous system dysfunction
3. Organ failure (cardiovascular, renal, reproductive, hepatic)
4. Failure of maturation and growth
5. Decreased stamina

Psychological/social
1. Concern with termination of treatment
2. Fear of relapse
3. Preoccupation with somatic symptomatology and sense of physical damage (body image, infertility)
4. Reentry into developmental life tasks
5. Transition from patient to healthy status
6. Sense of being on one's own
7. Hidden concerns: sense of financial insecurity, job discrimination, social withdrawal, life or health insurance difficulties
8. Tenuous sense of longevity (Damocles syndrome)
9. Lingering affinity with death (Lazarus syndrome)
10. Survivors' syndrome (guilt)

Medical Concerns

Relapse and Second Malignancies. Patients with leukemia relapse in the bone marrow and three common sanctuary sites: central nervous system (CNS), testis, and ovary. Even though there have been improvements in therapy to prevent CNS relapse, testicular relapse ranges between 5% and 16% [3] during initial remission and up to 30%-40% after treatment is discontinued. Second malignant neoplasms (SMNs) as a result of radiation or chemotherapy are rare in leukemia; however, the most common are lymphoma and another type of leukemia [33]. More often, SMNs (sarcomas, thyroid carcinomas, ALL) can occur in Hodgkin's disease 3-21 years after treatment with alkylating therapy and/or radiation [27, 32, 42, 48]. Several groups have reported SMNs in adults, and it appears that Hodgkin's patients are at 2%-5% risk for lung and breast cancer and 10% risk for secondary acute leukemia.

Maturation and Organ Failure. In spite of aggressive chemotherapy and chronic illness, children with hematological malignancies grow and mature normally. However, some authors have reported growth hormone deficiencies in leukemia patients who received cranial irradiation for CNS prophylaxis. Others have noted only temporary impairment of growth with symmetrical loss in height [46]. However, young Hodgkin's disease lymphoma and BMT patients who received radiation to specific sites especially during rapid growth periods have maturation loss. In the past, unilateral irradiation to the spine or growth centers of the long bones had caused scoliosis and short stature.

Survivors also can experience delayed toxicity to peripheral nervous, cardiovascular, endocrine, pulmonary, hepatic, and renal systems. Patients may have residual and permanent vincristine peripheral neuropathy, anthracycline-related cardiomyopathy, hepatic fibrosis secondary to methotrexate, and antibiotic-related renal failure. Occasionally, when chemotherapy is given in combination with radiation, organ damage is enhanced. Radiotherapy for Hodgkin's disease can result in pneumonitis, pericarditis, pleurisy, and thyroid dysfunction.

The delayed effects of cytoreductive treatment on fertility and sexual function have been under closer study for psychological repercussions. Young adult men who undergo chemotherapy and pelvic irradiation for Hodgkin's disease or rigorous chemotherapy for BMT often become aspermic and remain sterile.

Intravenous chemotherapy regimens may be less gonadal toxic compared to oral drugs taken daily or weekly. Even though three-fourths of men may have poor sperm quality prior to treatment, sperm-banking is important and is believed to reduce some of the long-term psychological sequelae. Fertility in men with acute leukemia is less well studied. Evenson et al. [12] have noted that men treated at the Memorial Sloan-Kettering Cancer Center on the L-10 protocol remain fertile. The success of this treatment may rely, according to the authors, on its use of intrathecal methotrexate rather than on cranial irradiation providing salvage to the hypothalamic pituitary gonadal system.

Treatment-related ovarian failure and subsequent amenorrhea, diminished libido, painful intercourse, and sexual dysfunction have occurred in a number of young women survivors of Hodgkin's disease. Radiation of less than 2000 rads and/or relocation of the ovaries during treatment of lymphoma may prevent reproductive damage. Siris et al. [45] found that most young women aggressively treated for leukemia in childhood have a relatively good prognosis for normal CNS controlled ovarian function. However, preliminary research at the Memorial Sloan-Kettering Cancer Center [23] reveals that women surviving aggressive leukemia treatment may be at more psychological risk of developing decreased sexual drive, satisfaction, and body image than their male counterparts. In summary, it appears that for fertile couples in whom one survives cancer, neither chemotherapy nor radiation has an oncogenic or mutagenic effect on progeny. However, many young adult survivors are unaware of or are unprepared for possible treatment-related sexual dysfunction, adding further stress and problems in adjustment. This is particularly true of adolescents who have survived a pediatric cancer illness.

Peripheral and Central Nervous System Dysfunction. Young [52] has noted that neurological toxicity from chemotherapy regimens has increased. Chemotherapy is often given as part of a "multimodality" (drug, radiation, immunotherapy) or "multiagent" approach. High doses with "rescue" techniques and innovative routes of administration (intrathecal) can also add to possible toxicity. Also, children and young adults survive longer, with more opportunity for CNS side-effects to develop. The well known immediate CNS side-effects of chemotherapeutic agents are nausea, vomiting, anorexia, generalized fatigue and weakness, confusion, and irritability. These symptoms are disruptive to work, home, and school routines, and can cause depressive symptoms. Late sequelae include mild cognitive dysfunction (learning disorders) in children treated for acute leukemia; these vary considerably relating to whether intrathecal methotrexate, systemic chemotherapy, and/or cranial irradiation were given. Studies of children undergoing all three forms of prophylaxis suggest subtle neurological impairment evidenced by seizures, lack of coordination, minor gait and motor abnormalities, and language and behavioral difficulties [31]. Some studies report normal psychological and neurological development in spite of cerebral atrophy on CT scan [37], while other studies note a number of structural abnormalities and cognitive deficits in 25%-30% of survivors [15, 34].

Psychological Concerns

The psychological sequelae of cancer survivorship are listed in Table 4. There have been a few psychological studies in patients with mematological malignancies and the necessity for longitudinal follow-up of young adults cured of leukemia has been demonstrated by Sherins and Devita [43], Chapman et al. [6, 7], and Sutcliffe [47] on Hodgkin's disease survivors and by Li and colleagues [25, 26] on childhood cancer survivors. They highlighted important areas of: threats of physical damage, risk of a second neoplasm, duration of remission, length of survival, and physiological sequelae. Remission brings near normal appearance and stamina. Consequently, there can be a precarious balance of fear of future disease and the specter of unsure health. Depressive mood, increased anxiety, anticipatory grief, insults to self-worth and control, somatic preoccupations, fears of relapse and death, and social stigma are all seen. Cure imposes the difficult task of discarding the patient role, separating from the hospital-family, and reentry into job and family while attending regular clinic visits. Patients with hematological malignancies often have greater psychological distress ast the end of their lengthy treatment than at the beginning of their illness. This is related to the uncertainty of when maintenance prophylaxis will end ("how many cycles of treatment were necessary, how much treatment was enough"), loss of frequent visits by staff and of close monitoring of their physical condition, and a sense of increased vulnerability to relapse in the context of professionals encouraging them to go back to "being normal." Patients often need to figure out what "is normal."

Follow-up visits and minor physical symptoms also increase anxiety and at times precipitate anniversary reactions. This inability to ignore usual aches and pains adds to a survivor's preoccupation with loss of control over their health. This is particularly evident in patients with hematological malignancies because the initial cancer symptoms are vague and systemic, and relapse often is not heralded by a prodromal syndrome other than an abnormal bone marrow. Finally, these kinds of malignancy are invisible after the completion of treatment and often be invisibility can aid in the patient's denial that he/she is chronically ill and precariously in remission. Patients frequently reevaluate old life-styles and values. Certain job-related issues no longer take on the same meaning. Survivors routinely merge preillness normalcy with postillness expectations.

References

1. Auchincloss S (1984) Gynecological cancer: psychological and sexual sequelae and management. In: Massie MJ, Lesko LM (eds) Current concepts in psycho-oncology. Gold, New York
2. Bernstein I (1986) Etiology of anorexia in cancer. Cancer 58: 1881-1886
3. Bowman WP, Aur RJA, Hustu HO, Rivera G (1984) Isolated testicular relapse in acute lymphocytic leukemia of childhood: categories and influence on survival. J Clin Oncol 2 (8): 924-929
4. Brown HN, Kelly MJ (1976) Stages of bone marrow transplantation: a psychiatric perspective. Psychosom Med 38: 439-446
5. Cella D, Pratt A, Holland JC (1986) Persistent anticipatory nausea, vomiting and anxiety in cured Hodgkin's disease patients after completion of chemotherapy. Am J Psychiatry 143: 641-643
6. Chapman RM, Sutcliffe SB, Malpas JS (1979a) Cytotoxic-induced ovarian failure in women with Hodgkin's disease: I. Hormone function. JAMA 242: 1877-1881
7. Chapman RM, Sutcliffe SB, Malpas JS (1979b) Cytotoxic-induced ovarian failure in women with Hodgkin's disease. II. Effects on sexual function. JAMA 242: 1882-1889
8. Davies RK, Quinlan DM, McKegney FP, Kimball CP (1973) Organic factors and psychological adjustment in advanced cancer patients. Psychosom Med 35: 464-471
9. Derogatis LR, Morrow GR, Fetting J, Penman D, Piasetsky S, Schmale A, Henricks M, Cornicke Jr CL (1983) The prevalence of psychiatric disorders among cancer patients. JAMA 249: 751-757
10. Dudrick SJ, Wilmore DW, Vars HM, Rhodes JE (1968) Long term parenteral nutrition with growth development and positive nitrogen balance. Surgery 64: 134-142
11. Ellis WG, Sobel RA, Nielsen SL (1982) Leukoencephalopathy in patients treated with amphotericin B methyl ester. J Infect Dis 136 (2): 125-137
12. Evenson D, et al. (1984) Male reproductive capacity may recover following drug treatment with the L-10 protocol for acute lymphocytic leukemia. Cancer 53: 30-36
13. Foley K (1986) Non-narcotic and narcotic analgesics: applications. In: Foley K (ed) Management of cancer pain: MSKCC. Gold, New York
14. Folstein MF, Fetting JH, Lobo A, Niaz U, Capozzoli K (1984) Cognitive assessment of cancer patients. Cancer 53 (suppl): 2250-2255
15. Goff JR, Anderson HR, Cooper PF (1980) Disractability and memory deficits in long-term survivors of acute lymphocytic leukemia. J Dev Behav Pediatr 1: 158-163
16. Hinton J (1972) The psychiatry of terminal illness in adults and children. Proc R Soc Med 65: 1035-1040
17. Holland JC (1982) Psychological aspects of cancer. In: Holland JF, Frei E (eds) Cancer medicine. Lea and Febiger, Philadelphia
18. Holland JC (1982) Psychological issues in the care of the terminally ill. In: Flach F (ed) Directions in psychiatry. Hatherleigh, New York
19. Holland J, Sgroi SM, Marwit SJ, Solkoff N (1973) The ICU syndrome: fact or fancy. Int J Psychiatry Med 4: 241-249
20. Holland JC, Rowland J, Lebovits A, Rusalem R (1979) Reactions to cancer treatment: assessment of emotional response to adjunct radiotherapy. Psychiatr Clin North Am 2: 347-358
21. Kubler-Ross E (1969) On death and dying. Macmillan, New York
22. Lesko LM, Hawkins DR (1983) Psychological aspects of transplantation medicine. In: Akhtar S (ed) New psychiatric syndrome: DSM-III and beyond. Jason Aroson, New York, pp 265-309
23. Lesko LM, Kern J, Hawkins DR (1984) Psychological aspects of patients in germ free isolation: a review of child, adult, patient management literature. Med Ped Oncol 12: 43-49
24. Lesko L, Mumma G, Mashberg D, Holland J (1987) Psychological adjustment and sexual functioning of acute leukemia survivors (Abstract). Leukemia 1: 278

25. Levine PM, Silberfarb PM, Lipowski ZJ (1978) Mental disorders in cancer patients: a study of 100 psychiatric referrals. Cancer 42: 1385-1391
26. Li FP, Jaffe N (1974) Progency of childhood cancer survivors. Lancet 2: 707-712
27. Li FP, Stone R (1976) Survivors of cancer in childhood. Ann Intern Med 84: 551-553
28. List A, Doll DC, Greco A (1985) Lung cancer in Hodgkin's disease: association with previous radiotherapy. J Clin Oncol 3: 215-221
29. Massie MJ, Holland JC (1987) Psychiatric diagnoses among patients with cancer. In: Silberfarb PM (ed) Psychiatric medicine. (in press)
30. Massie MJ, Holland J, Glass E (1983) Delirium in terminally ill cancer patients. Am J Psychiatry 140: 1048-1050
31. Mastrovito R, Moynihan R (1987) Self help and mutual support programs in cancer. In: Holland JC, Rowland JH (eds) Handbook of psychiatric oncology. Oxford University Press, New York
32. Meadows AT, Evans AE (1976) Effects of chemotherapy on the central nervous system. Cancer 37: 1079
33. Meadows AT, Baum E, Fossati-Bellani F et al. (1985) Second malignant neoplasms in children: an update from the late effects study group. J Clin Oncol 3: 532-538
34. Mosijczwk AD, Ruymann FB (1981) Second malignancy in acute lymphocytic leukemia. Am J Dis Child 135: 313-316
35. Moss HA, Nannis ED, Poplack DG (1981) The effects of prophylactic treatment of the central nervous system on the intellectual functioning of children with acute lymphocytic leukemia. Am J Med 71: 47
36. Moulin D, Foley K (1984) Management of pain in patients with cancer. Psychiatr Ann 14 (11): 815-822
37. Novack DH, Plumer R, Smith RL, Ochitill H, Marrow GR, Bennet JM (1979) Changes in physicians' attitudes toward telling the cancer patient. JAMA 241 (9): 897-900
38. Obetz SW, Smithson WA, Groover RV et al. (1979) Neuropsychologic follow-up of children with acute lymphocytic leukemia. Am J Pediatr Hematol Oncol 1: 207-213
39. Peteet J, Tay V, Cohen G et al. (1986) Pain characteristics and treatment in an outpatient cancer population. Cancer 57: 1259-1265
40. Portnoy RK, Moulin DF, Roger A, InTurrisi CE, Foley KM (1986) Intravenous infusion of opioids in cancer pain: clinical review and guidelines for use. Cancer Treat Rep 70 (5): 575-581
41. Pratt A, Lazar R, Penman D, Holland J (1984) Psychological parameters of chemotherapy-induced conditioned nausea and vomiting: a review. Cancer Nurs 1: 483-490
42. Rowland JH, Glidewell OJ, Sibley RF, Holland JC, Tull R, Berman A, Brecher ML, Harris M, Glicksman AS, Forman E, Jones B, Cohen ME, Duffner PK, Freeman AI (1984) Effects of different forms of central nervous system prophylaxis and neuropsychologic function in childhood leukemia. J Clin Oncol 2: 1327-1335
43. Schomberg PJ, Evans RG, Banks PM et al. (1984) Second malignant lesions after therapy for Hodgkin's disease. Mayo Clin Proc 59: 493-497
44. Sherins RJ, Devita VT (1973) Effect of drug treatment for lymphoma on male reproductive capacity: studies of men in remission after therapy. Ann Intern Med 79: 216-220
45. Shevits SA, Silberfarb PM, Lipowski ZJ (1976) Psychiatric consultations in a general hospital: a report of 1000 referrals. Dis Nerv Syst 37: 295-300
46. Siris ES, Leventhal BG, Vaitukaitis JL (1976) Effects of childhood leukemia and chemotherapy on puberty and reproductive function in girls. New Engl J Med 294: 1143-1146
47. Sunderman CR, Pearson HA (1969) Growth effects of long-term antileukemic therapy. J Pediatr 75: 1058-1062
48. Sutcliffe SB (1979) Cytotoxic chemotherapy and gonadal function in patients with Hodgkin's disease: facts and thoughts. JAMA 242: 1898-1899
49. Tester WJ, Kinsella TJ, Waller B et al. (1984) Second malignant neoplasms complicating Hodgkin's disease: The National Cancer Institute experience. J Clin Oncol 2: 762-769
50. Wade JC, Meyers JD (1983) Neurological symptoms associated with parenteral acyclovir treatment after marrow transplantation. Ann Intern Med 98: 921-925

51. Walsh TD (1986) Controlled study of imipramine and morphine in chronic pain due to advanced cancer (abstract). Proc Am Soc Clin Oncol vol 5, Abstract 237
52. Worden JW, Weisman AD (1980) Do cancer patients really want counseling? Gen Hosp Psychiatry 2: 100-103
53. Young D (1982) Neurological complications of cancer chemotherapy. In: Silverstein A (ed) Neurological complications of therapy: selected topics. Futura, New York, pp 57-113

Psychotherapy in Support of Patients Undergoing Antineoplastic Chemotherapy

R. Schwarz and M. Kaufmann

Psychosoziale Nachsorgeeinrichtung und Fortbildungsseminar,
Chirurgische Universitätsklinik Heidelberg, Ernst-Moro-Haus,
Im Neuenheimer Feld 155, 6900 Heidelberg, FRG

Anticancer chemotherapy is used not only as palliative treatment in advanced disease but also as curative treatment either by itself or in combination with surgery or radiation. On the other hand cytotoxic drugs can produce some of the most adverse side-effects of any cancer treatment [1]. Apart from the pharmacological side-effects, such as nausea and vomiting, patients experience increased negative emotions (anxiety, depression, restlessness, etc.) which again cause nausea and vomiting, forming a vicious circle. Some patients develop these symptoms even in anticipation of the therapy as a conditioned response which is usually refractory to antiemetic medications [2].

In a collaborative study with the Heidelberg Department of Gynecology we questioned 44 women who had finished adjuvant chemotherapy, following surgery for stage II carcinoma of the breast [3]. We found a typical set of psychological and physical symptoms forming a psychosomatic or somatopsychic syndrome [4]. Out of a list of 24, the seven symptoms listed in Table 1 were mentioned most frequently. It is striking that next to nausea and vomiting, psychological and psychophysiological symptoms ranked highest [5]. Table 2 shows the frequency of conditioned responses. Two-thirds of the respondents suffered from pretreatment nausea and on-third from conditioned vomiting.

In order to select theoretically meaningful clinical interventions we tried to identify predictors of the development of the distressing side-effects. Controlling

Table 1. Frequency of seven predominant side-effects during adjuvant chemotherapy ($n=44$)

Nausea	43
Vomiting	39
Restlessness	38
Feeling nervous	35
Loss of energy	31
Anxiety	31
Sudden outbursts of crying	31

Recent Results in Cancer Research, Vol. 108

Table 2. Frequency of conditioned responses ($n=44$)

	Pretreatment nausea	Pretreatment vomiting
Never	34%	68%
Sometimes	34%	25%
Always	32%	7%

for age and chemotherapy regimen, high levels of anxiety, repression, inhibited coping style, and poor social support contributed markedly to the overall stress connected with chemotherapy.

The application of chemotherapy shortly after a mastectomy is very unfavorable from the point of view of adjustment to the altered psychological and physical situation of the patients. When undergoing chemotherapy the attention and emotional engagement of patients are distracted from the social surroundings, being strongly tied to the immediate reality. Patients are incapable of recognizing and describing any conflicts or emotions and are not at all motivated to enter into a psychotherapeutic dialogue, apparently being unable to find appropriate words to express their feelings. The clinical appearance resembles the alexithymia syndrome as described by Nemiah and Sifneos [6, 7, 8].

In order to reduce the strain on patients, psychotherapy has to fulfill the following tasks:

1. To interrupt the vicious circle of anxiety, tension, and nausea or vomiting as conditioned responses
2. To help the patient to cope adequately
3. To offer a supporting relationship

Two methods of therapy used in the Psychosocial Aftercare Unit for Cancer Patients of Heidelberg University are presented below. The first is encouraging patients to paint pictures related to their illnesses; the second is systematic desensitization and relaxation training.

Painting seems to be a possibility for some patients to communicate stressful and sometimes preconscious thoughts, perceptions, and emotions in a symbolic manner. By interpreting the pictures together with the therapist, verbalization is facilitated, reasonable decisions taken, and adequate action prepared. Figures 1-3 give an impression of the pictures painted.

Another therapeutic approach is focused on the symptoms leading to conditioned nausea and vomiting, such as anxiety, tension, and passivity, and on the conditioning process itself. The kind of psychotherapeutic intervention appropriate to the clinical syndrome and the psychological impairment is, we believe, an active relaxation training combined with systematic desensitization [9].

In an exploratory study we compared two groups of patients of the Gynecology Department undergoing chemotherapy after surgery for stage II carcinoma of the breast who had developed nausea and/or vomiting. The groups were equated for age, chemotherapy regimen, antiemetic medication, and severity of side-effects according to a baseline measurement. The *experimental group* was treated with ac-

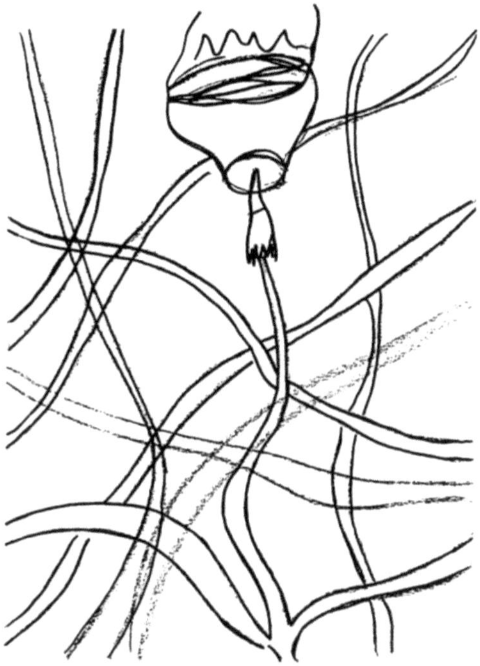

Fig. 1. "On the drip" from the perspective of a young woman; her irritation at an early stage of Hodgkin's disease is clearly evident

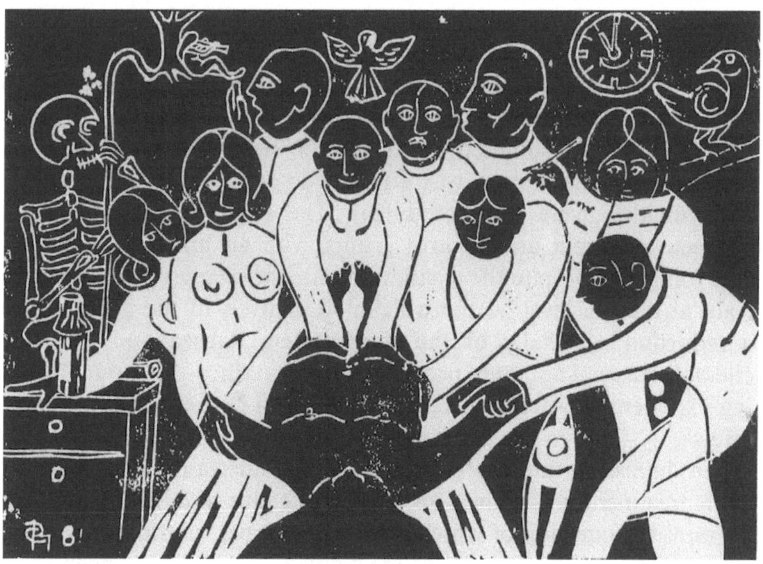

Fig. 2. "The ward round" as experienced by a 38-year-old man, whose fear of dying is symbolically represented in many details of the picture

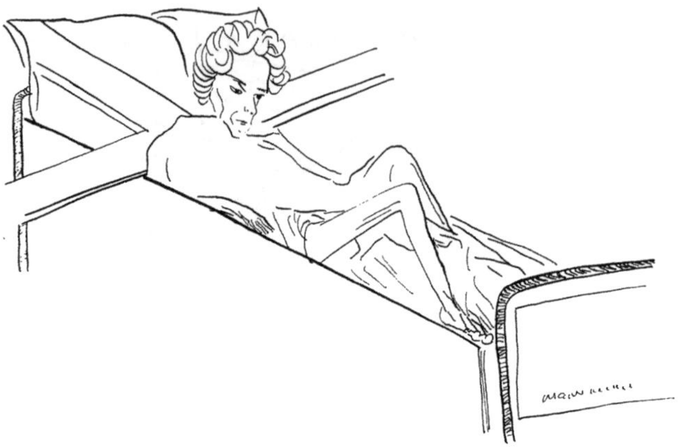

Fig. 3. A seriously ill fellow patient as depicted by the patient who drew Fig. 2. The fear of death is again evident

tive progressive muscle relaxation training according to Jacobson [10], followed by systematic desensitization. Thereby these patients were gradually exposed to more anxiety-provoking chemotherapy-related stimuli in their imagination [2]. This training was carried out immediately before the injections were given. Additionally patients were asked to practice daily at home. The *second group* received individual supportive counselling to control for nonspecific factors like the therapist's attention and expectancy effects.

Sixty percent of the patients referred to the study agreed to participate: ten women took part, five in each group. One of them dropped out during the study. In the course of six chemotherapy cycles, lasting about 3 months in total, patients daily rated the frequency and severity of nausea and vomiting on a 6-point scale. These ratings did not differ from the observations made by the attending nurse shortly before and during the infusions.

The results, as summed up in Table 3, suggest that relaxation combined with systematic desensitization was effective in reducing the distress as far as nausea and vomiting were concerned [11]. The third column shows the differences between treatment and control group, with an up to 96% reduction in nausea and vomiting! Despite the small numbers, the changes exceeding 40% were significant at the 5% level. A more detailed analysis of the group differences reveals a reduction especially of the pretreatment nausea and the symptoms during chemotherapy. The latter presumably will reduce the strength of the conditioning experience by weakening the connection between the infusions and the side-effects.

In discussing the results we have to consider a methodological problem. Even if the treatment procedure seems to be effective in reducing the distress of chemotherapy, the question of which factors may have contributed to the positive results remains to be answered. Three mechanisms have usually been mentioned:

1. The sedative and anxiety- and tension-alleviating effect of the relaxation; this could be viewed as a psychophysiological effect

Table 3. Effects of desensitization on chemotherapy-related nausea and vomiting[a]

		Counselling (n=5)	Treatment (n=4)	Improvement
Before chemotherapy				
Nausea	- Frequency	4.4	1.5	2.9 (65%)
	- Severity	4.8	1.2	3.6 (75%)
During chemotherapy				
Nausea	- Frequency	2.4	0.5	1.9 (79%)
	- Severity	4.8	0.2	4.6 (96%)
Vomiting	- Frequency	0.4	0.5	-
	- Severity	0.8	0.7	0.1 (13%)
After chemotherapy				
Nausea	- Frequency	3.3	1.9	1.4 (42%)
	- Severity	3.9	3.4	0.5 (13%)
Vomiting	- Frequency	1.6	1.0	0.6 (38%)
	- Severity	4.1	3.5	0.6 (15%)

[a] The figures represent mean values (range 0–5) related to the particular period.

2. Counterconditioning effects by means of the desensitization
3. Giving the patients a feeling of self-control and the ability to counteract the symptoms themselves as a cognitive effect

We want to add of fourth source of influence:

4. The personal involvement of the therapist – as an object-relational or interpersonal effect.

Since we distrusted the capacity of the control group design to equate for the relationship between the therapist and the patient, the therapist documented the length of the contact, the emotional status, the patient's interest in the contact, and the content of the conversation. Despite the therapist's endeavor to spend about the same length of time with all patients, the contact with the members of the relaxation group was found to be significantly longer. After the training these patients engaged the therapist in an intensive dialogue, whereas the conversation with the counseling group remained rather laborious and superficial. The patients in the treatment group had established close interpersonal relationships that enabled them to talk about their feelings and thoughts toward cancer and chemotherapy as well as about personal problems. At the same time their ability to express their fantasies and emotions increased. Therefore the alexithymic appearance could perhaps be viewed as part of a coping style to prevent fearful and dreading thoughts, that is, as a reaction to illness and treatment [12] rather than as a personality trait, as some authors suggest [13].

These observations are relevant to the question of how to establish a beneficial patient-therapist relationship with cancer patients, especially with those undergoing painful medical procedures. In order to overcome the patients' alexithymic state of mind, it appeared useful to arrange the sessions in a way that allowed them to gradually gain confidence under cover of the rather technical behavioral procedure, and relying on this confidence, to loosen their inner defence. Thus behavioral interventions can facilitate a supporting relationship that we believe is badly needed by these patients and is helpful in enabling them to achieve a better quality of life.

References

1. Holland JC, Mastrovito R (1980) Psychologic adaption to breast cancer. Cancer 46: 1045-1052
2. Morrow GR, Morrell C (1982) Behavioral treatment for the anticipatory nausea and vomiting induced by cancer chemotherapy. N Engl J Med 307: 1476-1480
3. Kaufmann M, Kubli F (1983) Adjuvante Chemotherapie und Modalitäten beim Mammakarzinom an der Universitätsfrauenklinik Heidelberg. In: Diehl V, Jonat W, Maas H, Nagel GA (eds) Adjuvante Therapie des Mammakarzinoms. Kehrer, Freiburg
4. Michel U, Schwarz R, Kaufmann M (1986) Compliance bei adjuvanter Chemotherapie. Rehabilitation 25: 17-23
5. Knobf T (1986) Physical and psychological distress associated with adjuvant chemotherapy. J Clin Oncol 4: 678-684
6. Nemiah JC, Sifneos PE (1970) Psychosomatic illness: a problem of communication. Psychother Psychosom 18: 154-160
7. Sifneos PE (1973) The prevalence of alexithymic characteristics in psychosomatic patients. Psychother Psychosom 22: 255-263
8. Sifneos PE (1975) Problems of psychotherapy of patients with alexithymic characteristics and physical disease. Psychother Psychosom 26: 65-70
9. Burish TG, Carey MP (1984) Conditioned response to cancer chemotherapy. In: Fox BH, Newberry B (eds) Impact of psychoendocrine systems in cancer and immunity. Hogrefe, New York
10. Jacobson E (1938) Progressive relaxation. University of Chicago Press, Chicago
11. Egly S, Müller A (1984) Systematische Desensibilisierung bei Brustkrebspatientinnen unter adjuvanter Chemotherapie. Heidelberg: unpublished
12. Schwarz R, Geyer S (1984) Social and psychological differences between cancer and noncancer patients: cause or consequence of the disease? Psychother Psychosom 41: 195-199
13. Bahnson CB, Bahnson MB (1960) Role of the ego defenses: denial and repression in the etiology of malignant neoplasm. Ann NY Acad Sci 125: 827-845

*Psychotherapy in Patients Cured of Gynecological Cancers**

G. Bos-Branolte, E. M. Zielstra, Y. M. Rijshouwer, and H. J. Duivenvoorden

Department of Gynecology, University Hospitals Rijnsburgerweg 10, 2333 AA Leiden, The Netherlands

Psychological morbidity in cured cancer patients is seriously underestimated [1-8]. Little research has been done on the long-term psychologic consequences of gynecological cancer, whereas a relatively large number of studies have been done on breast cancer. The latter work has shown that the psychological morbidity in cured patients is high (22%-33%) and that the psychological distress often does not become manifest until 6-9 months after medical treatment [9].

Until now no research has been done to determine whether professional psychotherapy can reduce the psychological distress or improve the quality of survival. The survivors' need for help in coping with the emotional effects of the disease and its treatment has only recently begun to be realized and more attention is now being given to the enhancement of the quality of life.

Several investigators underscore the point that aftercare should not be based solely on referral by surgeons [7, 10], whereas others [1, 5, 11] emphasize that help should not be delayed until the patient asks for it.

So far, professional psychotherapy for patients with cancer has been virtually restricted to newly diagnosed cases [12, 13], to patients receiving medical treatment [14], to patients with recurrence [15, 16], and to patients in a terminal stage of the disease [17]. It has not been offered to cured patients.

The part of the study reported here was designed to yield information about late psychological effects of gynecological cancer and cancer treatment, and about the severity of the psychological distress. Attention is given to a number of medical and psychological variables. In addition, the need for psychotherapy is assessed and the power of psychological variables to differentiate between acceptors and nonacceptors is estimated. Finally, the effects of psychotherapy are evaluated by comparing the psychotherapy patients with a reference group (patients not accepting psychotherapy).

* This study was supported by the Netherlands Cancer Foundation.

Material and Methods

Patients

Patients were selected from the files of the Department of Gynecology of the Leiden University Hospital in consultation with the medical staff. The following selection criteria were applied: the patient had to be (a) in complete remission for at least 6 months after medical treatment; (b) not older than 70; (c) able to speak the Dutch language; (d) informed about the cancer diagnosis; (e) without any other type of cancer; (f) free of manifest psychiatric pathology.

Of the 90 patients who participated in the study so far, complete sets of data were collected from 83. The sites of the gynecological malignancy were the ovaries (34 cases), the cervix (29), the corpus uteri (16), and the vulva (4). The forms of treatment were surgery (29 cases), combined surgery and chemotherapy (25), combined surgery and radiotherapy (22), or a combination of surgery, chemotherapy, and radiotherapy (7). At the time of entry to the study, the patients' ages ranged from 14 to 70 years, with a mean of 49 years; the duration of remission ranged from 6 to 86 months, with a mean of 36 months.

Design of the Study

In the period between 1985 and 1986 patients were invited by letter to participate in the study. Appointments were entirely separate from the medical follow-up visits. The initial assessment (M_1) consisted of filling in a questionnaire and this was followed by a diagnostic interview. Psychotherapy was then offered to all patients. Psychotherapy was given during the first 3 months after M_1 (Fig. 1). Follow-up measurements 6 (M_2) and 9 months (M_3) later included the same questionnaire and a follow-up interview (Fig. 1). Because we were especially interested in the long-term effects of psychotherapy, we compared M_3 with M_1. Consequently, M_2 fell beyond the scope of this part of the study.

Basic Oncology Scale (BOS)

The BOS is a self-rating scale constructed specifically for gynecological cancer patients [18]. The six variables included in the present study are anxiety, depression, body image, self-esteem, partner/proximity relation, and general feeling of well-being. The questionnaire took about 30 min to complete and was filled in individually in our consulting room in the hospital in the presence of a member of the research team.

Diagnostic Interview

According to the protocol of the study, semistructured in-depth interviews were conducted by the psychotherapist (GBB) with all the patients ($n=90$). These interviews dealt with the same six variables, were individually tailored, and included

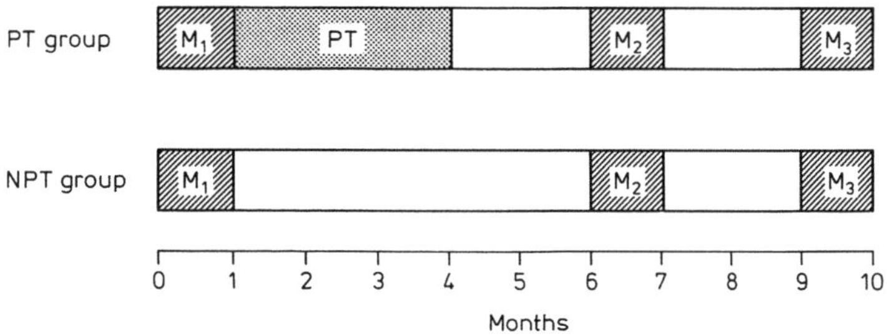

Fig. 1. Time schedule of the two groups. *PT,* psychotherapy; *NPT,* nonpsychotherapy; *Mi,* measurements

the more sensitive issues such as partner relationship, sexual functioning and general feeling of well-being. The diagnostic interviews took 30–45 min each and were recorded on tape. Patients who accepted the offer of psychotherapy at the end of the interview had already become acquainted with their future therapist during the interview.

Follow-Up Interview

The follow-up interviews took place after the filling in of the questionnaire of M_2 and M_3. They were conducted by one of the psychologists to obtain information about possible changes in the patient during the preceding months. On this occasion the patients once more had the opportunity to accept psychotherapy. The patients who had had psychotherapy evaluated their experiences. To assess the long-term effects of psychotherapy, only data from M_3 and M_1 were compared.

Psychotherapy

Group Psychotherapy

Group psychotherapy (GPT) consisted of eight 90-min sessions spaced over the course of 10 weeks. The semistructured treatment plan was based on the model of effects of gynecological cancers [9], which covers physical, psychological, and sociocultural effects pertaining to female organs and functions, female identity, and female image. In the therapy emphasis was put on the same six themes of the BOS questionnaire and in the diagnostic interview, i.e., anxiety, depression, body image, self-esteem, partner/proximity relation, and well-being. The main objective of the sessions was to generate favorable changes in the quality of life. The treatment plan included progressive muscle relaxation (each patient is given a tape to practice this method at home), role-playing, and learning-by-imitation. Use was made of two video films (each lasting about 30 min) in which cancer survivors shared their experiences. The films, which were recorded some years before the outset of this research project, served as a model for what might be expected from psychotherapeutic treatment, since the majority of the patients had harly any idea of its scope. The first session starts with the film in which the earlier group of women are talking about their emotions regarding the diagnosis and medical treatment and how they tried to cope with it. The second film, which deals with the sexual and intimate relationship with the partner, was shown during the fifth session.

Individual Psychotherapy

The number of sessions for individual psychotherapy (IPT) was not fixed in advance. As a rule, each session lasted 45 min and the series started on a weekly basis, the frequency being reduced gradually. The themes were the same as those for the GPT; however the structure was individually tailored and more insight oriented. Another important difference was that for IPT, separate sessions for the partner (or together with the partner) and for young patients for their parents, could be organized. In this study the IPT comprised 4–22 sessions with each patient, plus in most cases 1–4 sessions with her partner (or parents).

Methods Used for Data Analysis

Regarding the severity of psychological distress, the scores for the six variables (anxiety, depression, body image, self-esteem, partner/proximity relation, and well-being) were dichotomized according to the following decision rule: scores ≥ 0.50 SD below the mean - based on the initial assessment (M_1) - were labeled as negative ("severe problems"), as against moderate or slight/no problems.

Regarding change measurements, the scores for the six variables on M_1 were trichotomized as follows: scores ≥ 0.50 SD above the mean were labeled as positive ("slight/no problems"), those ≥ 0.50 SD below the mean were labeled as negative ("severe problems") and the in-between scores were labeled as intermediate ("moderate problems"). The degree of progress after 9 months (M_3) was also trichotomized, here according to the following decision rules: an increase of ≥ 0.50 SD compared to M_1 was considered positive ("improved"), and a decrease of ≥ 0.50 SD negative ("deteriorated"). An in-between change was labeled "unchanged". Comparisons were made between the psychotherapy group and non-psychotherapy group (reference group) and within the groups (i.e., differences between treated and untreated patients, separately).

For group comparison use was made of the χ^2 test, corrected for continuity in the case of 2×2 tables [19], for categorical variables (i.e., dichotomized and trichotomized); for continuous variables the Mann-Whitney *U* test was used. For measurements pertaining to (trichotomized) change, the χ^2 test was used. Throughout, the level of significance was taken at $p \leq 0.05$ (two-tailed).

Results

Psychotherapy was accepted by 27 patients (30%), six choosing individual and 21 group psychotherapy. For group therapy (GPT), four groups were formed each of

Table 1. Percentages of severe problems at M_1 with respect to six variables in patients who accepted psychotherapy (PT, $n=26$) and those who did not (NPT, $n=57$)

	Severe problems		χ^2	p
	PT	NPT		
Anxiety	54	16	11.08	≤ 0.001
Depression	42	12	7.79	≤ 0.01
Body image	35	14	3.47	NS
Self-esteem	42	25	3.04	NS
Partner/proximity relation	39	25	1.07	NS
Well-being	42	7	12.73	≤ 0.001

five or six patients. All 27 patients completed their psychotherapy treatment, but there were no follow-up measurements in one patient because of severe illness. Of the 63 nontherapy patients, there were no follow-up measurements in six; four patients had recurrences and two died. From the 90 patients therefore a complete set of data was obtained from 83 patients, 26 receiving psychotherapy and 57 not.

From the data of the first measurement (M_1), the psychotherapy patients and nonpsychotherapy patients were compared with respect to their medical characteristics: the groups showed no significant difference as to the type of cancer ($\chi^2=6.21$; NS) or medical treatment ($\chi^2=2.25$; NS). No significant difference with respect to age was found (Mann-Whitney *U* test; NS). The only difference was that patients receiving psychotherapy were significantly shorter in remission than those who did not (Mann-Whitney *U* test; $p\leq 0.05$; means 27 and 40 months respectively).

However, comparison of these groups with respect to the six variables (Table 1) showed that those patients who accepted psychotherapy suffered significantly more from anxiety and depression and that they had a significantly more negative feeling of general well-being than those not receiving psychotherapy.

Although the groups appeared to differ for body image, self-esteem and partner/proximity relation, the differences were nonsignificant. The psychological morbidity, i.e., severe psychological problems, assessed for the 90 patients on the basis of M_1, amounted to 26%, with a mean of 33% for ovarian cancer, 19% for cervical cancer, 16% for endometrial cancer, and 42% for vulvar cancer [18].

Improved

Between-Groups Comparison

A comparison was made between patients who accepted psychotherapy and those who did not, with respect to improvement of severe problems (Table 2).

The results indicated that, of the patients who had severe problems, those who accepted therapy were considerably better off than those who did not, when seen over a period of 9 months. The difference was significant for self-esteem and well-being (both $p\leq 0.01$); for the other variables the chance of improvement appeared

Table 2. Improvement of severe problems on six variables in patients who accepted psychotherapy (PT, $n=26$) and those who did not (NPT, $n=57$)

	PT		NPT		χ^2	p
	n	%	n	%		
Anxiety	14	64	9	33	1.04	NS
Depression	11	64	7	14	2.45	NS
Body image	9	56	8	13	1.81	NS
Self-esteem	11	73	14	14	6.50	≤ 0.01
Partner/proximity relation	10	40	14	14	0.91	NS
Well-being	11	91	4	25	3.58	≤ 0.01

Table 3. Improvement of moderate problems on six variables in patients who accepted psychotherapy (PT, $n=26$) and those who did not (NPT, $n=57$)

	PT		NPT		χ^2	p
	n	%	n	%		
Anxiety	7	71	23	35	1.63	NS
Depression	7	43	15	20	0.03	NS
Body image	12	50	28	14	3.97	≤ 0.05
Self-esteem	8	63	15	13	3.86	≤ 0.05
Partner/proximity relation	10	100	18	11	17.27	≤ 0.001
Well-being	8	100	24	0	26.89	$\ll 0.001$

two to four times higher in patients who accepted therapy, although differences were nonsignificant.

A comparison was also made between the groups of patients with respect to improvement of moderate problems (Table 3). With psychotherapy the chance of improvement of anxiety and depression was twice as high as without psychotherapy and on body image and self-esteem it was nearly four to five times higher than without psychotherapy (both $p \leq 0.05$). The improvements for partner/proximity relation and well-being were even more striking ($p \leq 0.001$ and $p \ll 0.001$).

Finally, an attempt was made to compare the extent to which patients with severe or moderate problems improved with respect to the six variables in GPT and IPT (Fig. 2). It can be seen that with GPT the average improvement of all six variables was 61%; the greatest improvement was on well-being (93%), followed by self-esteem (64%).

With IPT the average improvement of all six variables was 93%. As Fig. 2 shows, IPT patients improved more than GPT patients, although the number of patients in IPT was too small to permit unequivocal conclusions concerning differences in the effectiveness of IPT and GPT. An inspection of Fig. 2 also shows that improvement of severe and moderate problems after 9 months was significantly higher in patients who accepted psychotherapy on all six variables.

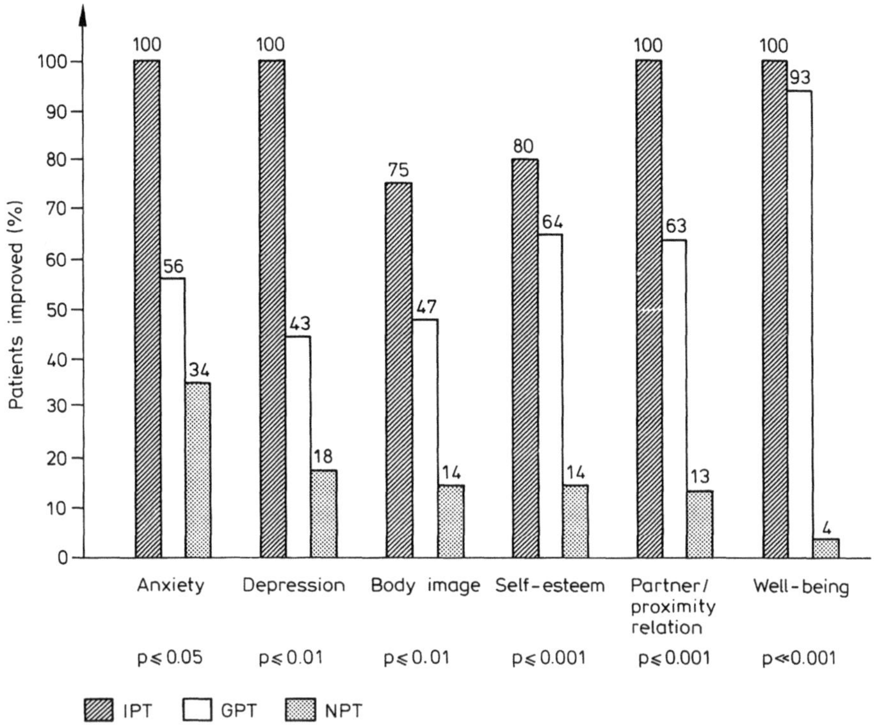

Fig. 2. Improvement of severe and moderate problems after 9 months (M_3) of patients in individual psychotherapy (*IPT; n*=5), group therapy (*GPT; n*=21), and nonpsychotherapy (*NPT; n*=57), in %

Within-Groups Comparison

Psychotherapy Patients. Results concerning improvement of severe problems in psychotherapy patients are presented in Table 2. Almost two-thirds of patients receiving psychotherapy who had severe problems improved on anxiety and depression, more than half had a better body image, and about three-fourths showed an increase in self-esteem. In the patients who had severe problems in their partner/proximity relation, 40% improved and more than 90% improved on well-being.

Results concerning improvement of moderate problems in psychotherapy patients are presented in Table 3. It can be seen that nearly half to two-thirds of patients receiving psychotherapy who had moderate problems on anxiety, depression, body image, and self-esteem improved on these variables. All patients who had moderate problems on partner/proximity relation and well-being improved (10 and 8 patients respectively).

Nonpsychotherapy patients. It can be seen from Table 2 that one-third of the nonpsychotherapy patients with severe problems improved on anxiety, 13%–14% on body image, depression, partner/proximity relation and self-esteem, and that one of the four patients with severe problems on well-being improved.

Results concerning improvement of moderate problems in nonpsychotherapy patients are presented in Table 3. It appears that one-third of them improved on anxiety, between 10% and 20% on partner/proximity relation, self-esteem, body image and depression, but that of the 24 patients with moderate well-being problems not a single patient improved.

Unchanged

Not every patient who suffered from severe or moderate problems changed for the better. A considerable number remained unchanged.

Between-Groups Comparison

It appears from Fig. 3 that most of the nonpsychotherapy patients who had severe or moderate problems could not solve these problems in the course of 9 months, whereas most of the psychotherapy patients could. The difference was significant

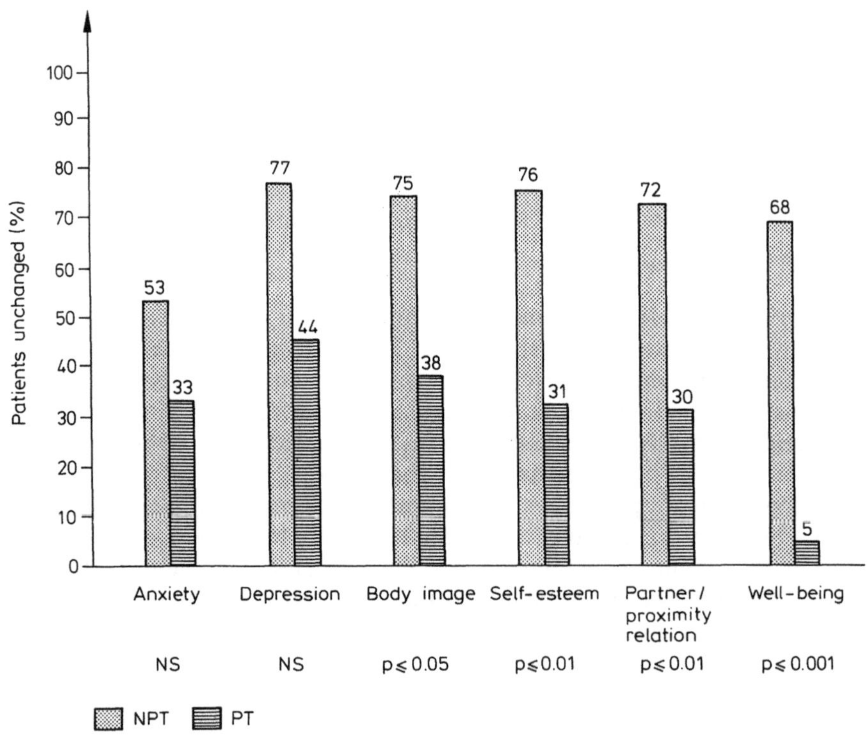

Fig. 3. Percentages of patients with severe and moderate problems who dit not change, divided into those who accepted psychotherapy (*PT*, $n=26$) and those who did not (*NPT*, $n=57$)

for body image ($p \leq 0.05$), self-esteem and partner/proximity relation (both $p \leq 0.01$), and well-being ($p \leq 0.001$). Anxiety and depression showed similar, albeit nonsignificant, trends.

Within-Groups Comparison

About one-third of the psychotherapy patients with severe and moderate problems on anxiety, self-esteem and partner/proximity relation, remained the same on these variables. For 40% there was no change on depression or body image, but on well-being only 5% remained unchanged (Fig. 3). With psychotherapy, the average of unchanged scores on all 6 variables was 31%.

Of the nonpsychotherapy patients with severe and moderate problems about half did not change on anxiety; about three-fourths did not change on depression, body image, self-esteem and partner/proximity relation, whereas more than two-thirds did not change on well-being (Fig. 3). Without treatment, the average of unchanged scores on all six variables was 68%.

Deteriorated

Finally, we investigated whether patients deteriorated after 9 months. In the psychotherapy patients deterioration occurred on one variable only: two patients with moderate problems on body image worsened. However, a deterioration occurred much more often in nonpsychotherapy patients: between 14% and 42% on all variables. These findings suggest that an average deterioration on all variables for untreated patients amounts to 18% and for treated patients 1%.

Discussion

Because it is often assumed that resistance to psychotherapy is common, it was of interest to find out how cured cancer patients felt about it. Our findings do not support the aforementioned assumption: 30% of our patients accepted the offer of psychotherapy. Another interesting finding is that their acceptance reflected their need, i.e., suffering. It became clear that patients who accepted psychotherapy suffered significantly more frequently from severe anxiety and depression and had a more negative body image than patients who refused such treatment. Self-esteem and well-being showed similar, albeit nonsignificant, trends.

The differences between psychotherapy and nonpsychotherapy patients did not relate to medical determinants and method of medical treatment, or to the age of the patients. The only significant difference between the treated and untreated patients was with respect to the length of remission, its average duration being 13 months shorter in patients who accepted psychotherapy. So, given the opportunity of getting psychotherapy, most of the cured gynecological cancer patients "knew" themselves whether they needed psychotherapy. This implies that screening for "at risk" patients can be done by way of a diagnostic interview for which cured cancer patients, i.e., patients in remission, should be invited approximately 1-2 years after the end of medical treatment.

During the diagnostic interview various patients in our study mentioned that they had made unsuccessful attempts in the past to obtain help in coping with cancer (treatment). Since about one-third of the patients wished to receive psychotherapy, it is reasonable to assume that our offer clearly fulfilled existing needs.

For an evaluation of psychotherapy by the patients, use was made of a short questionnaire as part of the follow-up measurement after 9 months. Many of those "in need of help" reported retrospectively that they would have preferred an earlier offer. Another finding was that three-fourths of the GPT patients were of the opinion that eight sessions was insufficient. The optimal time of intervention probably lies between 1 and 2 years after the cure, with slight differences between the various organ sites.

The effects of psychotherapy were evaluated approximately 6 months after the last session. The statistical analysis showed that the majority (two-thirds) of psychotherapy patients improved and less than one-third remained unchanged. With only few exceptions, deterioration did not occur. Psychotherapy patients with severe problems improved slightly more than patients with moderate problems. We found that IPT was more effective than GPT, especially with respect to anxiety and depression.

In contrast with the favourable results obtained in treated patients, the untreated patients with problems did less well. Overall, about two-thirds did not change for the better after 9 months; only a minority (14%) improved whilst the rest even worsened. The changes for worse and for better observed in the untreated patients might be explained by the impact of the diagnostic interview. It is possible that, for a number of patients, the diagnostic interview brought into the conscious their unconscious emotional problems (not to be equated with "creating" problems). Such an awareness of problems may have had a negative influence. On the other hand, about an equal number of untreated patients with problems improved. These patients did not deny their emotional problems in the personal interview, and were relieved to hear that it was "normal" to experience psychological problems as a consequence of their illness. Another, less satisfactory, explanation could be that some patients may improve spontaneously. Anyhow, psychotherapy was significantly more curative than nontreatment, and also proved to be cllearly more preventive against negative changes.

Not one of the patients who accepted psychotherapy dropped out of the study, a finding that contrasts to a substantial number of patients who reportedly leave traditional psychotherapy. Psychotherapy seemed for these patients to be sufficiently motivating for them to continue with the treatment.

All cured cancer patients seemed to appreciate the attention paid to them. This is illustrated by the high participation rate of untreated patients in the follow-up measurement, keeping in mind that these visits were mostly not combined with a medical check-up visit.

Another important finding from this study was that although one-third of the patients were in need of psychotherapy, very few of them would have been referred to us for psychosocial evaluation under "normal" circumstances (outside the context of this investigation). The need exists; recognition and referral by health care takers will not take place if no specific education in that direction is given, a finding which is also mentioned by other authors [3, 5, 6, 10, 20, 21]. Moreover, to depend on patient-initiated requests for help is to underestimate the strength of social forces which discourage self-confrontation. It can safely be concluded that psychotherapy should be offered to cured cancer patients, at the right time and in a suitable way.

Conclusions

The results of this prospective study on psychotherapy of cured gynecological cancer patients demonstrated that this treatment was effective in two-thirds of the patients. The results differed significantly from those in patients with psychological problems who were not treated by psychotherapy.

Increased cure rates and prolonged duration of remission have extended the life-years of cancer patients. The problems of living with cancer have become an important issue and brief psychotherapeutic interventions may prove valuable, also from the economic point of view. It is our conviction that high emotional distress as a consequence of cancer indicates a need for psychosocial services as well as medical treatment. Thereby, psychotherapeutic intervention may help to reduce the use of medical services for nonmedical symptoms. The costs of psychotherapy may be considered to be reasonable when one takes into account the considerable relief from distress of the patients, the increased ability to cope, and last but not least the fact that the treatment can add quality to the extended life-years.

References

1. Hersh SP (1982) Psychosocial aspects of patients with cancer. In: DeVita VT, Hellman S, Rosenberg SA (eds) Cancer: principles and practice of oncology. Lippincott, Philadelphia, pp 264-277
2. Trimbos C (1978) Mensen met kanker: de noodzakelijke ontwikkeling van een psychosociale oncologie. Van Loghum Slaterus, Deventer
3. Holland JCB (1976) Coping with cancer: a challenge to the behavioral sciences. In: Cullen JW, Fox BH, Isom RN (eds) Cancer: the behavioral dimensions. Raven Press, New York, pp 263-268
4. Akehurst AC (1972) Post-mastectomy morale. Lancet II: 181-182
5. Maguire GP, Lee EG, Bevington DJ, Küchemann CS, Crabtree RJ, Cornell CE (1978) Psychiatric problems in the first year after mastectomy. Br Med J i: 963-965
6. Morris T, Greer HS, White P (1977) Psychological and social adjustment to mastectomy: a two-year follow-up study. Cancer 40: 2381-2387
7. Luce JK (1979) Selecting patients for supportive therapy. In: Stoll BA (ed) Mind and cancer prognosis. Wiley, Chichester, pp 127-137
8. Tausch AM (1981) Gespräche gegen die Angst. Rowohlt, Reinbek
9. Bos G (1986) Gynecological cancer. In: Dennerstein L, van Hall E (eds) Psychosomatic gynecology - a total approach to women's health problems. Parthenon, Carnforth, pp 167-189
10. Borne van den HW, Pruyn JFA (1985) Lotgenotencontact bij kankerpatiënten. Van Gorcum, Assen

11. Martin LR (1982) Overview of the psychosocial aspects of cancer. In: Cohen J, Cullen JW, Martin LR (eds) Psychosocial aspects of cancer. Raven Press, New York, pp 1-8
12. Cain EN, Kohorn EI, Quinlan DM, Latimer K, Schwartz PE (1986) Psychosocial benefits of a cancer support group. Cancer 57: 183-189
13. Capone MA, Good RS, Westie KS, Jacobson AF (1980) Psychosocial rehabilitation of gynecologic oncology patients. Arch Phys Med Rehabil 61: 128-132
14. Jacobs C, Ross RD, Walker IM, Stockdale FE (1983) Behavior of cancer patients: a randomized study of the effects of education and peer support groups. Am J Clin Oncol 6: 347-350
15. Spiegel D, Bloom JR, Yalom I (1981) Group support for patients with metastatic cancer: a randomized prospective outcome study. Arch Gen Psychol 38: 527-533
16. Spiegel D (1985) Psychosocial interventions with cancer patients. J Psychosoc Oncol 3: 83-95
17. Spiegel D, Yalom ID (1978) A support group for dying patients. Int J Group Psychother 28: 233-245
18. Bos-Branolte G, Rijshouwer YM, Zielstra EM, Duivenvoorden HJ (1987) Psychologic morbidity in survivors of gynaecologic cancer. Eur J Gynaecol Oncol (in press)
19. Yates F (1934) Contingency tables involving small numbers and the χ^2-test. J Stat Soc 1: 217-235
20. Wood JV, Taylor SE, Lichtman RR (1985) Social comparison in adjustment to breast cancer. J Pers Soc Psychol 49: 1169-1183
21. Klein Poelhuis EH, Berg-Lachnit R van de, Postma-Schuit FCE, Dam FSAM van (1986) Vijf jaar ervaring met gespreksgroepen voor kankerpatiënten. Medisch Contact 41: 661-663

Music Therapy in Support of Cancer Patients

S. Porchet-Munro

Medizinische Klinik C, Kantonsspital, 9007 St. Gallen, Switzerland

The use of music in the treatment of cancer patients may seem farfetched, and the presence of a music therapist as a full-fledged member in a treatment team is a rare "luxury", to be found in very few centers around the world. However, the experiences in those centers indicate that the potential of music therapy deserves closer scrutiny.

The large spectrum of topics covered during this symposium point to the complexity of cancer and cancer care, a domain in which, even in the best of circumstances, we are invariably confronted by an infinite spectrum of difficulties and suffering which is often laborious to assess and meet. Music, the differentiating element of music therapy, in its myriad dimensions and in its connection to the life of man, can contribute in meeting some of the diverse challenges of the complexity of cancer care, and thus complement traditional care.

There would be no music and no need for it if it were possible to communicate verbally that which is easily communicated musically.

E. T. Gaston, 1958

Communication

While one recognizes that the diagnosis of cancer leads to a profound life crisis [1] and one may want to offer a patient psychological support, the patterns of communication not infrequently reflect the crisis situation and are distorted. In the life of most persons, music has some place, some connection, and in tuning into those connections verbally or directly through music we may reestablish communication and heighten our awareness of the individual's framework of thought, emotions, and reactions, which in turn can guide us in further interventions, be they of a medical or a psychosocial nature.

Case excerpt: Mr. S. was admitted to hospital for the investigation of "cold-like" symptoms which resisted the treatments prescribed by the family physician. After lengthy and extensive investigations, a poorly differentiated adenocarcinoma, probably of the lung, was diagnosed. The patient refused to believe the diagnosis and became hostile and withdrawn. He blamed the hospital for not finding the cause of what he suspected to be an infection. He

Recent Results in Cancer Research, Vol. 108

stated angrily: "all they looked for was cancer!" Pain control was problematic and he scarcely ate. He refused to see the physicians who tried to achieve better pain control.

Given that listening to music was one of his habits previous to the illness, tapes and a tape recorder were left at his disposal at the bedside. For a time he did not make use of these things. The music therapist kept visiting him, simply to maintain contact, without pushing the issue of music. After more than 2 weeks, the patient suddenly invited the therapist to listen to his music with him. Subsequently, he freely began to talk about his fears, his illness, his frustrations, and his many questions. The music had reflected much of this to him and after sharing the music listening, he could now share verbally. His account gave a succinct glimpse of his personality and his way of perceiving and thinking. From there he gained enough trust to let the physicians become more closely involved in his care again. They now had a better understanding of his perceptions and anxieties and were able to attain better pain control.

Motivation

The symptoms and/or treatments of cancer force restrictions and possibly a change of life-style on individuals. Due to advances in treatment techniques, hospital stay may be shorter and less frequent. While physical symptoms may be well controlled, the psychological adjustment to the diagnosis and prognosis can be particularly threatening when the patient returns to his own environment. Here, mustering the motivation to continue a near "normal" life in the face of a life-threatening illness, limited capabilities or troublesome symptoms often becomes difficult.

Faced with a crisis situation, thoughts rarely turn to such resources as music. Yet, with some encouragement to consider the potential of this medium, patients can find renewed motivation to continue or begin to benefit from music, which offers wide possibilities:

- Reviewing, taping, and cataloguing a record collection
- Exploring unknown music
- Instrument playing - to pick up where one left off (for someone who used to play) or to begin from scratch on an instrument that won't necessarily demand years of learning (if that is something the person used to wish for)
- Explorations in guided imagery and music
- Song or poetry writing

Such activities can be tailored to the physical status as well as the adaptation mechanism of the individual at any given time. Initially, the concreteness of the focus on equipment, records, and instruments may simply be a welcome distraction from happenings around the illness, but subsequently access to all the spheres of music, as presented in this paper, is often a very natural and helpful progression.

Expression

Cancer cannot be dissociated from suffering, suffering "in relation to any aspect of the person, whether it is in the realm of social roles, group identification, the relation with self, body, or family, or the relation with a transpersonal, transcendent source of meaning" [2]. Cassel, in this article, points poignantly to the complexity of the many spheres of suffering in relation to the goals of medicine and cites the case of a 35-year-old sculptor with metastatic disease of the breast. "This young woman had severe pain and other physical symptoms that caused her suffering. But she also suffered from threats that were social and from others that were personal and private. She suffered from the effects of the disease and its treatment on her appearance and abilities. She also suffered unremittingly from her perception of the future."

Anyone working with cancer patients could identify easily with the manifold issues surrounding such a case and will know the limitations of verbal communication and expression one is faced with. Throughout centuries, music has served as an avenue for man's expression of his plight, joys, fears, and depths of emotion. It is therefore not surprising that a person can identify his concerns and turmoil at a given time in and with music and thus find comfort or new insight. The nonverbal dimensions of this process, which transcend reason and intellect, are a unique mark of music.

Music therapy can provide or reopen channels of expression effectively. Techniques may vary from listening to music, instrumental playing, improvization, and song or music writing to music-inspired collages and can be adapted to the patient's physical status and psychological framework. Above all, interventions of this kind generally affect the patient's, the family's, and the staff's perception of issues and ease tensions and feelings of inadequacy or helplessness. For the patient, expression of "unspeakable" concerns not infrequently provides renewed creative energy that is usually lost in the process of an illness. This not only enriches the quality of life at such a time but may provide the impetus to live.

Case excerpt: N., a 28-year-old woman with metastatic disease of the breast, presented exaggerated pain symptoms while maintaining a jovial, almost aloof front of nonchalance. She refused to see a psychologist or psychiatrist with the comment: "I know my diagnosis and prognosis and am coping fine!" Her at times rather irratic behavior streched to the limit the patience of staff and friends in their efforts to support her.

The music therapist left a small harp at her bedside without much ado and instructed staff members to leave the choice of touching or not touching this instrument entirely up to the patient. In time, she began to strum it when she felt unobserved and alone and no comments were made. Then one day, she asked for the therapist and handed her a paper upon which she had written a song. The therapist handed it back to her and asked her to sing it for her. The outburst of frustration, anger, regrets, and fears bespoke her suffering far more penetratingly through her voice than her words.

This expression led to verbalization and also further song writing, events which entailed decreased pain.

Relaxation

The most remarkable attribute of music in this domain is its ability to influence the heart and the brain on a physiological and psychological level. While rhythmic pulse and musical sound waves affect pulse rate and brain functions [3, 4], the transcendent quality of music reaches the person beyond reason and analysis. If we consider the complex symptom picture of some cancer patients in tension and crisis states, it is exactly this combination of effects which break through irrationality, fear, anxiety, the intangible and inexplicable resistance to medication, etc.

Here, music must be chosen carefully, particularly with regard to rhythm. Melodic and harmonic elements which elicit associations must be of nonthreatening significance for the patient. As well, the location of the sound source and volume control are vital details to consider.

It is understood that music, in various circumstances, may induce a relaxation effect; however, the specifically tailored use of music to promote relaxation can be invaluable for certain symptom pictures or in treatment situations.

Case excerpt: Dr. G. was a 38-year-old surgeon with cancer of the pancreas. He received the most advanced treatments available in a North American teaching hospital, and the most supportive care from concerned colleagues, friends, his minister, and his wife. Despite such – what we may term optimal – circumstances, pain control remained a constant challenge and at a certain point in the course of the disease was compounded by insomnia which remained unaffected by medication. The patient's need, as a physician, to be "in control" of the illness and the treatment and his intellectualizing of circumstances and the severity of his condition complicated matters tremendously in every area of care and interaction.

After several days without sleep and with increased pain, agitation, tension, and anger, this vicious circle was finally broken into by the sound of ocean waves[1], "music" more powerful than the patient's resistance and withdrawal, yet unobtrusive enough to respect his protective shell. The sound-induced sleep was a first step toward renewed effectiveness of medication and therefore renewed pain control.

Discussion and Conclusions

It seems ironic that, to date, music therapy in cancer care is mainly accepted within palliative/hospice care settings. This tends to suggest that such therapy is acceptable for the terminally ill and dying patient only. It is interesting to note that the key feature of the palliative care services all over the world is the prime focus on genuine whole person medical care, possibly the best example of supportive cancer care and a brave attempt to understand all the known dimensions of personhood and their relations to illness and suffering in connection with the best medical care.

Music therapy in such settings as, for example, the Palliative Care Service of the Royal Victoria Hospital in Montreal, Canada, has had the chance to demonstrate its effectiveness and unique contribution not only in the realm of psychosocial support but also in the domain of pain and symptom control. There is no evidence to suggest that cancer care in earlier stages of the disease is of less staggering complexity if one considers it in terms of the whole person and not just in terms of a disease of the body. Music therapy, therefore, may contribute challenging perspectives to all stages of cancer care.

It is essential to underline once again that the element which distinguishes music therapy from other therapies is the unique scope, potential, and magnitude of

[1] Where the influence of instrumental timbres, melodies, and harmonic progressions of music as such would have provoked associations too irritating or threatening to this man, he could tolerate the sound of the ocean even in this stress situation.

music itself in relation to man. Music's intricate association with all of human experience enables it to touch the person on a physiological, psychological, and emotional and spiritual level. It cuts across barriers, it intrudes, it aggresses, it facilitates and provides a ready bridge between the tangible and the intangible [5, 6, 7]. Since symptoms in the cancer patient are invariably recognized as of biopsychosocial nature [8], the access of music to each of these spheres is particularly helpful. Thus, Munro and Mount [9] summarized the significant uses of music therapy as follows:

1. *Physical*
   - promoting muscular relaxation
   - breaking the vicious circle of chronic pain by relieving anxiety and depression of pain
   - facilitating physical participation in activities to the degree possible
2. *Psychological*
   - reinforcing identity and self-concept
   - altering the patient's mood, including easing anxiety and lessening depression
   - helping the patient recall past significant events
   - providing a nonverbal means of expressing a broad range of recognized and unconscious feelings
   - reinforcing reality
   - expressing fantasy
   - as a direct appeal to the emotions
3. *Social*
   - as a means of socially acceptable self-expression
   - as a bridge across cultural differences and isolation
   - as a bond and sense of community with family members and others, past and present, through the mental associations aroused
   - as a link to the patient's life before the illness
   - providing an opportunity to participate in a group
   - as entertainment and diversion
4. *Spiritual*
   - providing means of expressing spiritual feelings and feeling comforted and reassured
   - providing an avenue for expressing doubts, anger, fear of punishment, and questions on the ultimate meaning of life

The professionally trained music therapist bases his interventions on a thorough knowledge of all facets of music (historical, theoretical, practical), the behavioral sciences, treatment and educational models, and accepted therapeutic approaches. While music therapy is an adjunctive therapy, its potential and effectiveness are optimal if the therapist works as a full-fledged member of the treatment team and can integrate his/her interventions into the general treatment plan. Since man has no defense against the impact of music, the latter is a potent therapeutic agent which is to be used with respect, sensitivity, and humility.

Where scientific advances in cancer care have wrought significant advances, the human perspectives in this field must receive more attention if we are to speak of supportive care. For this, it will not be enough for care givers to continue to function in the traditional realms of medical action, knowledge, and control; rather we will have to respond to the challenge of the human plight and reexamine our concept of care. At that time, the potential of music therapy may be a very natural and welcome resource.

References

1. Meerwein F (1985) Die Psyche des Krebskranken. In: Glaus A, Jungi W, Senn HJ (eds) Onkologie für Krankenpflegeberufe. Thieme, Stuttgart
2. Cassel E (1982) The nature of suffering and the goals of medicine. N Engl J Med 6 (11): 639-645
3. Brama I et al. (1977) Auditory nerve and brain stem responses to sound stimuli at various frequencies. Audiology 16 (5): 402-408
4. Zinny G, Weidenfeller E (1963) Effects of music upon GSR and heart rate. Am J Psychol 76 (2): 311-314
5. Critchley M, Henson R (eds) (1977) Music and the brain: studies in the neurology of music. Heinemann, London
6. Bereznak Kenny C (1982) The mythic artery. Bidgeview, Atascadero, CA
7. Munro S (1984) Music therapy in palliative/hospice care. Magnamusic-Baton, St. Louis
8. Meerwein F et al. (1981/85) Einführung in die Psycho-Onkologie. Huber, Bern
9. Munro S, Mount B (1978) Music therapy in palliative care. Can Med Assoc J 119 (9): 1029-1034

Psychosocial Support of Cancer Patients: A Training Program for Oncology Staff

C. Hürny

Medizinische Abteilung, C. G. Lory Haus, Inselspital, Universität Bern, 3010 Bern, Switzerland

To work as a nurse or a physician in oncology is a stressful experience for a variety of reasons. Despite the fact that some malignancies are now curable even in advanced stages, a large proportion of cancers still have a bad prognosis. In this situation the professionals in the field of oncology have to acknowledge the limits of modern medicine. They may feel incompetent, helpless helpers, when confronted with an irresistibly advancing disease and ultimately death. They may not be able to cope with the multiple losses they are faced with in their daily routine. Cancer evokes anxiety and fear of death in all of us, including health care professionals. This is reflected by the fact that daily rounds with terminally ill patients are much shorter than those with patients who have curable disease [1]. In addition the staff has to apply toxic treatments. They have to make their patients sick first for an expected benefit later on. Furthermore they are confronted with a variety of complicated treatment regimens and a rapidly growing amount of knowledge in their subspecialty that is not easy to assimilate. Finally, complex issues of clinical research, where benefits for the individual patient may not be evident, have to be dealt with.

In the formal training of nursing and medical students no solid basis of psychosocial knowledge and skills is given to facilitate coping with these issues. There is a lack of education in interviewing skills, needs and coping mechanisms of patients with a chronic, potentially fatal disease, care of the terminally ill, and the impact of terminal illness on the physician-patient relationship. This lack of education is one important reason for staff "burnout", a syndrome of low performance and job dissastisfaction in health professionals increasingly described in recent years [2, 3, 4]. It is evident that burned-out staff are not able to deliver optimal patient care. To be able to give support they have to be supported. Different educational programs have been proposed for this purpose [5, 6, 7]. There is no unique solution to the problem. The methods have to be tailored to the local situation.

Design of the Program

The local situation of the Oncology Outpatient Department (OPD) in Bern is summarized in Fig. 1. In 1984 the nursing and medical staff asked for education in

Recent Results in Cancer Research, Vol. 108

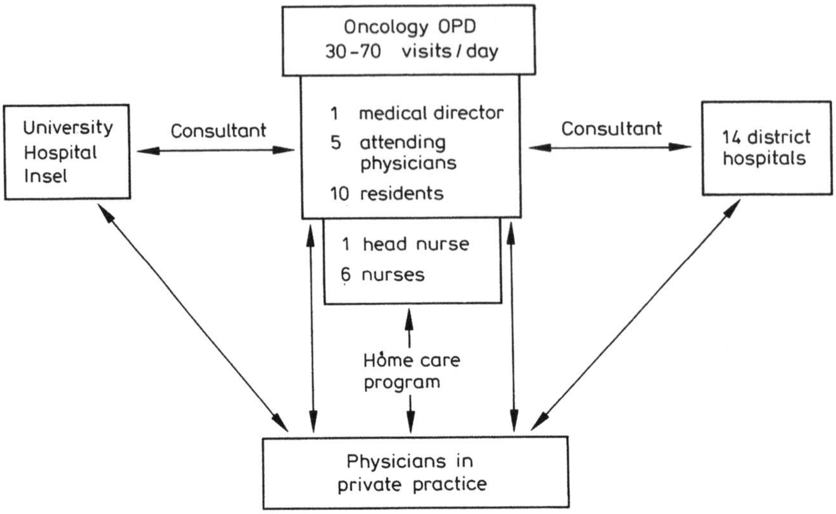

Fig. 1. Oncology Outpatient Department, University of Bern, Switzerland

Table 1. Seminar in psycho-oncology: general organization

Frequency:	Group sessions 1½ h, 1-2 times/month
Participants:	4-7 residents out of 10 } OPD 3-5 nurses out of 7 } 7-12 group members
Leader (C. H.):	Board-certified internist with special training in oncology and psychiatry/psychoanalysis
Theoretical background:	Biopsychosocial model (Engel 1980)

psychosocial aspects of oncology. As a base for optimal patient care we defined three main areas where training was needed:

- Skills in interviewing the patient
- Ability to establish a supportive relationship to the patient
- Knowledge on reactions and coping mechanisms in a potentially fatal disease

For this purpose we felt that the in-depth analysis of individual patients was more helpful than general discussions or theoretical lectures. In agreement with the medical director we decided to start a common seminar for nurses and residents. Its structure is summarized in Table 1. The biopsychosocial model of Engel serves as the theoretical background [8, 9]. In this context an interview technique is taught which allows the physician to collect and integrate biological, psychological, and social data at once [10, 11]. With time three modes of training were established:

1. The resident is asked to record an initial clinical interview with a newly referred cancer patient on videotape. The tape is then first reviewed and discussed with the leader of the seminar alone. If the resident agrees, the interview is further re-

Table 2. Seminar in psycho-oncology: sessions Feb. 1984 to Aug. 1986

	Video leader	Video residents	Balint residents/ nurses	General discussions, evaluation, follow-ups	Total
			6/4		
Patients	5	11	10		26 patients
Sessions	7	18	10	5	40 sessions within 31 months

viewed and discussed within the whole group. This method of analysis was first introduced by the Psycho-oncology Working Group (AGPO) of the Swiss Group for Clinical Cancer Research (SAKK) [12]. It allows the critical observation of a real physician-patient interaction in an everyday situation.

2. The leader of the group is asked to see a patient who creates problems for the staff. His interview is recorded on videotape and discussed in the seminar. One purpose of this mode is the demonstration of the above-mentioned interview technique.
3. According to the method of Balint [13], a staff member presents a patient to the group. In the group discussion the problems that led to the presentation are identified and if possible clarified. This mode primarily focuses on interactional problems between care giver and patient.

Evaluation of the Seminar

Between February 1984 and August 1986 a total of 40 sessions took place (Table 2). Twenty-six patients were discussed in detail. In little less than half of the sessions residents' videotapes were analyzed. Ten sessions were used to present patients according to the method of Balint; on four occasions a nurse presented a patient, while on six a resident did so. In seven sessions videotapes of patients who the leader had seen in consultation were discussed. Five sessions were used for evaluation of the program in open-ended discussions and for follow-ups.

In an attempt to evaluate the group work in the 35 sessions of in-depth analysis of individual patients, the leader (C.H.) went through the protocols he had written after each session. For every important topic discussed at length 1 point was given. Two gross categories were made: problems pertaining to the patients' reaction to cancer, defense mechanisms, and coping strategies (Table 3) and problems pertaining to the nurses' and physicians' coping with the cancer patient and his actual medical, psychological, and social situation (Table 4).

As shown in Table 3, a variety of very diverse problems of cancer patients have been observed and discussed, going far beyond the stages of coping initially proposed by Kübler-Ross [14]. It is nevertheless of interest that the question of culpability ("Why me?"), mainly adaptive denial and repression, anxiety and depression, and problems of control were most frequently observed. This largely

Table 3. Seminar in psycho-oncology: analysis of 35 group sessions (leader's protocol) – patients' reactions to cancer/defense mechanisms/coping strategies[a]

	VC (7)	VR (18)	B (10)	Total	
Anxiety (relapse/death)	3	1	1	5	9
Grief/helplessness/hopelessness/depression	1	3	1	4	
Suicide	1	1	–	2	
Search for the culpable (i.e., doctors' delay)	2	7	2	11	
Denial/repression/avoidance	2	4	1	7	
Splitting/rationalizing	–	1	1	2	
Controlling/manipulation/bargaining	1	4	5	10	
Personality style	2	5	1	8	
Impact on family	–	–	2	2	
Sexual problems	–	2	1	3	
Partner problems	–	–	2	2	
Social stigma of cancer (taboo)	1	1	1	3	
Experience with cancer in family or friends	2	2	1	5	

[a] *VC*, videotape of a consultation interview of the leader; *VR*, videotape of an initial interview of the resident; *B*, Balint session; ( ), number of sessions.

Table 4. Seminar in psycho-oncology: analysis of 35 group sessions (leader's protocol) – physicians'/nurses' problems with the cancer patient/coping strategies[a]

	VC (7)	VR (18)	B (10)	Total	
Video recording	–	7	–	7	
Interview technique	–	10	2	12	
Disclosure of information					
Diagnosis	4	12	–	16	26
Prognosis	2	7	1	10	
Treatment issues					
Toxicity (doubts)	1	2	2	5	16
Side-effects	1	1	2	4	
Patient refusal	1	1	3	5	
Unproven remedies	1	–	–	1	
Chronic pain	1	–	–	1	
Helpless helper (anger, guilt, depression)	4	2	5	11	
Death and dying	–	4	5	9	
Problems within the staff	–	1	1	2	
Psychiatric problems					
Personality disorder	2	–	5	7	13
Psychogenic symptoms	1	1	1	3	
Addiction	1	–	1	2	
Organic brain syndrome	–	1	–	1	

[a] *VC*, videotape of a consultation interview of the leader; *VR*, videotape of an initial interview of the resident; *B*, Balint session; ( ), number of sessions.

corresponds to the first four stages of Kübler-Ross. Although since this first description coping research has become much more sophisticated in the analysis of the coping process [15], I think that the Kübler-Ross stages are easy to understand and therefore appropriate to the practical training of care givers.

Table 4 summarizes the main difficulties of the staff. In seven sessions personal difficulties of the resident with being recorded on videotape were a main issue. During the first 31 months of the program 22 residents were rotating through the service. Only 11 tapes were recorded. Three patients refused to be recorded on video. It was our impression, however, that being recorded on video was much more stressful for the resident than for the patient; moreover when the patient did feel stress it was only for a short time at the beginning of the interview.

In 12 sessions technical aspects of the interview were discussed at length, in 16 sessions treatment issues, in 11 sessions the feeling of being a helpless helper or burned out, in 9 sessions issues surrounding death and dying, and in 13 sessions psychiatric problems. Only in two sessions were problems within the staff a major issue, not because problems within the staff do not exist but because the discussions were explicitly focused on patient problems. The seminar was defined as a working group, not as a therapy group. Following others with experience in this field, I think this distinction is vital for the survival of such a program [16].

Disclosure of information to the cancer patient about his diagnosis and prognosis was definitely the most important issue throughout the seminar. In 26 of 35 sessions it was a substantial point of discussion. Nowadays most physicians and the public agree that the patients have to be appropriately informed about the diagnosis, the treatment options, side-effects, and prognosis [17]. However, in the individual patient situation this is still a very difficult and subtle task for the oncologist. We have analyzed the 11 videotaped initial interviews of the residents. In discussing the diagnosis in seven interviews the word "cancer" was used by the patient or the physician, and in two interviews another word, such as "tumor," "malignant cells," or "lump." In two interviews the diagnosis was not discussed explicitly. Because of the small numbers this result is far from being representative. It shows, however, that the general agreement on the necessity of informing the patient does not necessarily mean that this is an integral part of daily practice.

No formal evaluation of the effectiveness of the program was done. In five sessions the participants were given the opportunity to discuss openly and evaluate informally the program. The frequent changes in group members and the different levels of training of nurses and physicians but also of individuals within these professional groups were mentioned as difficulties. One of the most positive effects, they felt, was the fostering of the mutual understanding of the two professional groups through the common discussions of individual patients. Another positive point was the cathartic effect of the Balint sessions, the recognition of troublesome personal emotions and the possibility to better understand patient reactions and their own reactions in caring for the patient. Furthermore they appreciated the diversity of the sessions due to the different modes of training. Although the recording of interviews on videotapes was troublesome, the self-observation and the critical appraisal of the interview technique were generally appreciated as helpful for further practice. Also important was the fact that once or twice a month 1½ hours of working time was reserved to sit back and reflect on the daily routine. Interestingly enough they did not feel that there was an accrual of knowledge, although a better understanding of the problems is evident in longstanding members of the group.

In conclusion, the program is perceived as helpful and the staff keeps attending the sessions quite regularly.

References

1. Siegrist J (1982) Asymmetrische Kommunikation bei klinischen Visiten. In: Köhle K, Raspe HH (eds) Das Gespräch während der ärztlichen Visite. Urban and Schwarzenberg, München, pp 16-22
2. Maslach L (1976) Burned out. Hum Behav 5 (9): 16-22
3. Wise TN, Berlin RM (1981) Burn-out: stresses in consultation-liaison psychiatry. Psychosomatics 22 (9): 744-751
4. Jenkins JF, Ostchega Y (1986) Evaluation of burnout in oncology nurses. Cancer Nurs 9 (3): 108-116
5. Pasnau RO (1982) Role of psychiatry in multidisciplinary cancer care, education and research. In: Holland JC (ed) Current concepts in psychosocial oncology. Memorial Sloan-Kettering Cancer Center, New York, pp 13-16
6. Richards AI, Schmale AH (1974) Psychosocial conference in medical oncology. Ann Intern Med 80: 541-545
7. Wise TN (1977) Training oncology fellows in psychological aspects of their specialty. Cancer 36 (6): 2854-2857
8. Engel GL (1977) The need for a new medical model: a challenge to biomedicine. Science 196: 129-136
9. Engel GL (1980) The clinical application of the biopsychosocial model. Am J Psychiatry 137: 535-544
10. Morgan WL, Engel GL (1969) The clinical approach to the patient. Saunders, Philadelphia
11. Adler R, Hemmeler W (1986) Theorie und Praxis der Anamnese. Der bio-psycho-soziale Zugang zur Krankheit. Fischer, Stuttgart
12. Beck D, Bernhard J, Bürgin D, Dreifuss E, Egli H, Gervasi A, Guex P, Gunn-Sechehaye A, Honsalek I, Hürny C, Meerwein F, Radanov B, Strauch I, Wildbolz A (1985) Das Erstgespräch auf der Abteilung für medizinische Onkologie. In: Bräutigam W, Meerwein F (eds) Das therapeutische Gespräch mit dem Krebskranken. Huber, Bern, pp 41-66
13. Balint M (1964) The doctor, his patient and the illness. Pitman, London
14. Kübler-Ross E (1969) On death and dying. Macmillan, New York
15. Herschbach P (1985) Psychosoziale Probleme und Bewältigungsstrategien von Brust- und Genitalkrebspatientinnen. Röttger, München
16. Lederberg M (1982) Support groups to prevent burnout. In: Holland JC (ed) Current concepts in psychosocial oncology. Memorial Sloan-Kettering Cancer Center, New York, pp 89-91
17. Goldberg RJ (1984) Disclosure of information to adult cancer patients: issues and update. J Clin Oncol 218: 948-955

Cancer in Children and Families

Supportive Care in Pediatric Oncology

H. P. Wagner

Institut für Klinisch-Experimentelle Tumorforschung, Kinderklinik, Inselspital, Universität Bern, 3010 Bern, Switzerland

Supportive care prevents and relieves a large spectrum of tumor- and therapy-induced symptoms. Since both tumors and treatment differ to a large extent in pediatric and adult oncology, it is not surprising to find that supportive care for neoplastic diseases in the young is influenced by the specificities of pediatric oncology, i.e., the preponderance of acute leukemias and sarcomas, the problems related to the necessity of treating a growing organism, and the tremendous differences between the worlds of a newborn, an infant, a toddler, children in school, and adolescents, which require different cooperative efforts between parents and those involved in treating and caring for the patient.

In pediatric oncology at least *four* separate domains can be distinguished in the large field of supportive care. These will be briefly discussed before making some more general remarks highlighting the role of supportive care in the treatment of malignant neoplasms in childhood and adolescence.

Prevention and Treatment of General Predictable Complications [1, 9]

Two categories of problems can be distinguished: Tumor- and treatment-induced.

Among the *tumor-induced* problems there are acute complications requiring immediate intervention, such as metabolic, pulmonary, cardiovascular, and neurosurgical emergencies, and more slowly arising complications, e.g., cachexia, malignant effusions, and pain.

Treatment-induced complications should be subdivided into early and late events. The former comprise phenomena such as extravasation, allergic reactions, emesis, acute renal failure, skin reactions, mucositis, diarrhea, hemorrhagic cystitis, and alopecia; the latter comprise growth retardation or arrest, hormonal, cardiovascular, pulmonary, gastrointestinal, skeletal, and muscular disturbances or defects, sterility, and, last but not least, neurological, psychomotor, intellectual, and emotional deficits, which may lead to a gradual loss of learning capabilities, stress tolerance, or psychosocial adjustment.

Since cancers grow rapidly in childhood, tumor-induced emergencies are not uncommon. In acute leukemias as well as malignant lymphomas the so-called tu-

Recent Results in Cancer Research, Vol. 108

mor lysis syndrome, characterized by high uric acid, potassium, and/or phosphate and/or low calcium may be present before therapy is initiated and will require adequate therapy. The same diseases may also present with a so-called vena cava superior syndrome characterized by venous congestion and collaterals in the head and neck area, edema, CNS symptoms, and dys- or orthopnea. After cytological or histopathological confirmation of the diagnosis, prednisone, 15 mg/m^2 p.o. q 6 h followed later by radio- and/or chemotherapy is the treatment of choice.

The main cardiovascular complications are pericarditis and venous occlusions due to tumor invasion or thrombosis.

Neuroblastoma, a tumor arising from structures of the sympathetic nervous system and affecting mainly infants and preschool children but not adults, is well known to invade the spinal canal, causing cord compression which results in motor and sensory losses, pain, biased sphincter control, and eventually transverse lesions. This complication, which may be observed in other tumors, is best controlled by dexamethasone, 50 mg/m^2 stat i.v., followed by 10 mg/m^2 q 6 h until symptoms stabilize, and later by laminectomy and radio- and/or chemotherapy.

Neuroblastomas as well as malignant lymphomas, e.g., Burkitt's lymphoma, may present initially with malignant pleural effusions and/or ascites. After biochemical or cytological confirmation of the diagnosis and drainage, no special treatment is required besides the standardized therapy for the basic disease.

Another topic evoking a lot of discussion are the indications for parenteral nutrition. Parenteral nutrition may considerably increase the patient's resistance but it may also initiate or promote untoward side-effects such as metabolic disturbances and/or infections. We have used parenteral nutrition mainly postoperatively or in children who were losing weight while on consolidation or maintenance chemotherapy, and exceptionally to avoid decubitus in terminal patients.

Cancer pain is one of the most common and occasionally one of the most difficult symptoms to control, e.g., in terminal patients with soft tissue sarcoma or bone tumor, neuro- or nephroblastoma, lymphoma, or leukemia. If aspirin, paracetamol, and related drugs are inefficient, we use metamizol-sodium, mefenamic acid, tilidine chloride and narcotics, s.c., i.m., or in form of slow-release capsules.

It is impossible, in the context of this report, to consider all the procedures for preventing treatment-induced early and late effects. Suffice it to say that with increasing survival late effects could be investigated more precisely and can now be prevented more readily, i.g., by skeletting therapy, as has occurred in patients with malignant lymphoma, nephroblastoma, or neuroblastoma. It has also been possible to reduce the late effects of surgery, radiotherapy, and chemotherapy by using sophisticated combinations of treatment modalities or by supporting the host's defense mechanism by administering i.v. immunoglobulins (0.4 g/kg every 2 weeks) and/or parenteral nutrition.

With regard to early effects, some progress has been made in preventing alopecia by using cold cap-like devices and in preventing emesis by using agents such as dexamethasone, domperidone, droperidol, and, in certain instances, scopolamine.

Prevention and Treatment of Infection [1-3, 7, 8]

Infections are the single most important factor jeopardizing the life of intensively treated children and adolescents with cancer. Iatrogenic immunosuppression, the use of prophylactic broad spectrum antibiotics, and indwelling catheters produce a rather unusual spectrum of potentially life-threatening infections, the prevention and treatment of which require special monitoring and surveillance.

A special and frequent problem is fever of unknown origin in the granulocytopenic patient. We distinguish patients with more than 0.5×10^9 granulocytes/liter in good condition, whom we treat only with cephalosporins p.o.; patients with more than 0.5×10^9 granulocytes/liter in a compromised condition or patients with less than 0.5×10^9 granulocytes/liter in good condition, whom we treat with i.v. third generation cephalosporins alone; and finally patients with less than 0.5×10^9 granulocytes/liter in poor condition, who receive "triple" therapy (e.g., amikacin, ceftazidime, and flucloxacillin). If there is no improvement within 4 days, we give triple therapy if only one antibiotic was used previously, or else consider antifungal therapy.

In the patients with septicemia, *Escherichia coli, Klebsiella pneumoniae* and *Pseudomonas aeruginosa* are the most frequently observed gram-negative bacilli, and *Staphylococcus aureus* and streptococci the most frequently observed gram-positive bacteria. Among the fungi *Candida, Aspergillus,* and *Mucor* species predominate.

While *Pneumocystis carinii* pneumonia characteristically occurs after recovery from severe myelosuppression, *Clostridium perfringens* peritonitis, perianal and skin infections, meningitis, brain abscess and encephalitis more often occur when myelosuppression is most severe.

Other infections such as herpes zoster, cryptococcal meningitis, and *postsplenectomy septicemia* are related to specific host susceptibility, as in CMV interstitial pneumonia observed after total body irradiation given in the context of bone marrow transplantation. Other iatrogenic septicemias, such as *Staphylococcus epidermidis* and *Corynebacterium* species, are related to the increasing use of indwelling catheters.

Besides specific antibiotic treatment, high dose i.v. immunoglobulin, 0.4 g/kg daily for 1-4 days has been helpful in all of these infections.

Blood Component Replacement and Bone Marrow Transplantation [1, 4]

Prevention and treatment of anemia (<90 g hemoglobin/liter) and bleeding (< 10×10^9 platelets/liter) are generally accepted indications for red cell or platelet replacement, and hypertransfusion or coagulation disorders for administration of fresh frozen plasma. The indications for granulocyte replacement are less clear. We use granulocyte replacement (5×10^9/kg daily $\times$ 3-5) mainly for granulocytopenic patients with bacterial septicemia who do not respond to adequate antibiotic and high dose i.v. immunoglobulin.

Indications for allogeneic bone marrow transplantation are patients with acute nonlymphoblastic leukemia in first remission, patients with acute lymphoblastic leukemia relapsing while on therapy in second remission, and patients with juvenile and adult-type chronic myeloid leukemia (CML) in the chronic phase. If no compatible bone marrow donor is available, we recommend autologous bone marrow transplantation with or without purging in the situations enumerated above except CML. Autologous bone marrow transplantation is also recommended for patients over 2 years with stage IV neuroblastoma in first remission or Murphy stage IV Non-Hodgkin lymphoma with CNS infiltration or certain types of large (> 8 cm) Ewing's sarcoma in first complete remission.

Psychosocial Concomitants of Cancer in Children and Adolescents [5, 6]

The psychosocial concomitants of cancer in the young cannot be adequately assessed without knowing the specificities of human psychomotor development and psychosocial integration, nor can they be assessed without considering the personalities of the parents, siblings, other relatives, friends, teachers, etc.

One way to discuss psychosocial concomitants of cancer is to follow a patient through his illness and to describe the impact of the different phases on him. Another approach is to study the reactions of the parents and other family members to investigation, diagnosis, hospitalization, treatment, side-effects, relapse, death, and time after death. The most critical phases are probably the first information, relapse, death, and time after death.

It takes time and experience to inform the parents on the true nature of the disease, on treatment and prognosis, on how to guarantee optimum therapy, on the philosophy one has if there is little or no hope, on how to inform the child and siblings, etc. It takes time and experience to inform and guide parents and the patient if a relapse occurs and if the child deteriorates and dies slowly, in the course of weeks or even months. It might be of great importance to prevent suicides or the destruction of a family after a child or an adolescent with cancer has died. It might also take time to reintegrate a child or adolescent after he/she has had to struggle for life and has not received school or professional training and is not well integrated or accepted by peers.

Final Remarks

As demonstrated above, supportive care in pediatric oncology is a very vast and complex field which becomes even more complex with increasing numbers of survivors. Perhaps the most important aspect is that supportive care should always be part of a general concept of treatment and should never be considered alone. Of those with cancer who survive there will always be a fraction with no sequelae, a fraction with acceptable side-effects, and a fraction with unacceptable long-term side-effects. Although the latter becomes gradually smaller, it becomes harder to accept and live with irreparable damage and to be or to become totally dependent. In no age group is supportive care as efficient but also as dangerous as in the young with cancer because those who will survive do so for a long time, a whole life.

References

1. Altmann AJ, Schwartz AD (1983) Oncologic emergencies. In: Altmann AJ, Schwartz AD (eds) Malignant diseases of infancy, childhood and adolescence. Saunders, Philadelphia, pp 136-176
2. Bodey GP (1986) Infection in cancer patients. A continuing association. Am J Med [Suppl 1A] 81: 11-26
3. Brown AE (1985) Management in the febrile, neutropenic patient with cancer: therapeutic considerations. J Pediatr 106: 1035-1042
4. Deisseroth AB, Abrams R, Holohan T, Bode U, Fontana J, Colvert D, Wright D (1982) Blood component replacement, applications of the continuous flow centrifuge, and bone marrow transplantation. In: Levine AS (ed) Cancer in the Young. Masson, New York, pp 285-298
5. Lansky SB (1985) Management of stressful periods in childhood cancer. Pediatr Clin North Am 32: 625-632
6. Levine AS, Hersh SP (1982) The psychosocial concomitants of cancer in young patients. In: Levine AS (ed) Cancer in the Young. Masson, New York, pp 367-387
7. Pizzo PA (1982) Infectious complications in the young patient with cancer: etiology, pathogenesis, diagnosis, management and prevention. In: Levine AS (ed) Cancer in the Young. Masson, New York, pp 299-337
8. Pizzo PA, Hathorn JW, Hiemenz J, Browne M, Commers J, Cotton D, Gress J, Longo D, Marshall D, McKnight J, Rubin M, Shelton J, Thaler M, Wesley R (1986) A randomized trial comparing ceftazidime alone with combination antibiotic therapy in cancer patients with fever and neutropenia. N Engl J Med 315: 552-558
9. Spiegel RJ, Pizzo PA (1982) Symptomatic and supportive care of the cancer patient. In: Levine AS (ed) Cancer in the Young. Masson, New York, pp 339-365

Cancer: A Family Disruption

J. Johnson

North Cancer Center, 3300 Oakland Avenue, Robbinsdale, MN 55422, USA

Cancer is a potent agent of change. Regardless of the magnitude or direction of change, cancer consistently disrupts a family's established patterns of daily living. The availability and complexity of today's medical treatments extends life and heightens the unknown for people with cancer. As patients find themselves facing a life defined by uncertainties, remissions, exacerbations, and changes in treatments; the family, likewise, is confronted with continual change. Each member of the family, patient included, must deal with the ramifications of the cancer diagnosis for themselves as individuals while attempting to cope as a family with the disease and its treatment.

Cohen and Wellisch [1] proposes using a "dual-analysis" approach to examining the impact cancer has on a family system. The family must deal simultaneously with the sudden impact of the news of cancer, as well as the slow motion movement of the disease itself. Crisis theory and intervention is helpful at the time of diagnosis when people suddenly find themselves in an acute crisis situation. The nature and resolution of this acute crisis is dependent on factors identified in crisis theory. The long-term effects of cancer on family structure and development makes it necessary to also view cancer as creating a crisis that is ongoing and chronic in nature. This chronic type of crisis presents a different type of challenge for families. Cancer patienthood draws the entire family into new modes of interaction, interdependence and concern - all of which are mandated by the disease and its treatment. For this reason it is appropriate to call cancer a family disease.

The family as a whole is a living system that is distinct from, yet connected to, the life of its individual members. It is a complex, dynamic network of interconnected and interactive relationships. As a system, every family adopts its own unique way for structuring roles, relationships and responsibilities that direct their family life. They each also have their own system for handling life's differing crises, emotional upheavals, conflicts and demands. Families affirm, protect, and define standards of acceptable behavior, values and beliefs. The ways in which they have historically functioned provides the basis for how they approach their present situation. It is helpful to recognize this aspect of family system theory when assisting a family through the crises surrounding the cancer diagnosis.

Recent Results in Cancer Research, Vol. 108

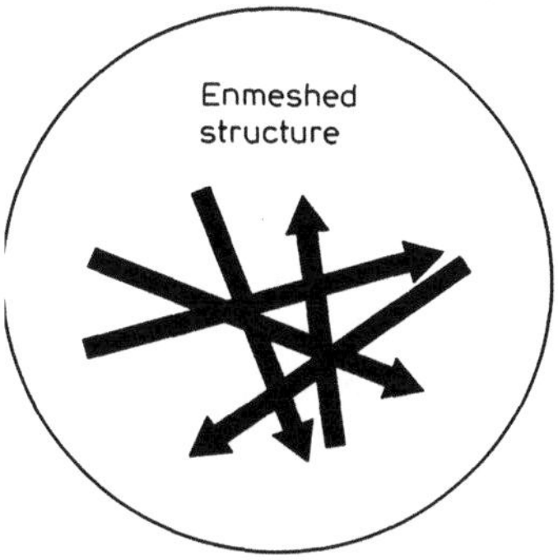

Fig. 1. Enmeshed family system

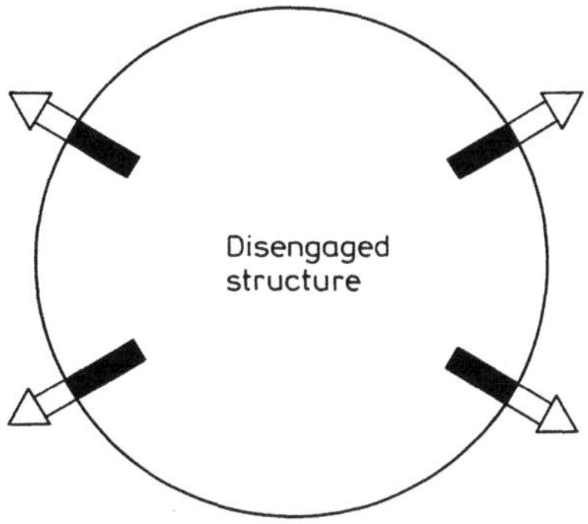

Fig. 2. Disengaged family system

Insight into another aspect of family systems theory provides the basis for understanding why families react differently at times of crisis. Two contrasting family systems that occur with some frequency are referred to as *enmeshed and disengaged* [2]. An enmeshed family (Fig. 1) is characterized by lack of individual differentiation of its members, dependent and "parasitic" type relationships, restrictions against outside support, resistance to change, discipline by disapproval, unspoken expectations, emphasis on "conditional love" and a tone of heaviness and protectiveness. In a severely enmeshed system seeking outside help is not acceptable. Regardless ofthe magnitude of the problem an enmeshed family will hold to the view that they can manage the situation themselves. A disengaged family system (Fig. 2) operates in the opposite mode from an enmeshed system. It is characterized by weak or nonexistent internal bonds, low family structure, the tendency of members to do their own thing independent of the others, relationships which are fragmented, conflicting, and isolating, lack of commitment and involvement with each other, minimal touching, and a tone of alienations and emptiness. Information exchange, and communication at times of crisis is not apt to occur. Nor will emotions be shared or support offered among the family members. Most families can be described as being on a continuum between these two extreme systems. Olsen [3] stresses that families who make a good adjustment to illness have a clear separation of generations; flexibility within and between roles; direct and consistent communication; and above all, tolerance for individuation. When a family member becomes ill, it is essential to view the family as a whole rather than think in terms of interactions between two or more members. It is also helpful to examine the family dynamics and appreciate the manner in which they operate as a system.

Cassileth [4] has identified some specific ways in which cancer imposes on families. They include:

1. *Threaten or disruptive patterns of interaction.* Roles and relationships of family members can either intensify or disintegrate. Some families have clearly defined roles for their members whereas others have a free-for-all type of structure. One frequent role change that occurs following a cancer diagnosis is that duties and responsibilities are taken away from the sick family member and assumed by

another. The result often is that one person feels a sense of loss while the other person feels burdened by the added responsibilities.

Communications is a key factor in a family's adaptation to cancer. Who tells who "the news"? The pattern of how families have previously shared sorrow, fear, and anger will be consistent with how they share their feelings about the cancer diagnosis. Frequently people want to protect their children from these anxiety producing feelings and will chose not to tell them, at least at first. Many families are good at communicating informational facts to one another but need encouragement to express their emotional needs. This is understandable given the intense and fragile nature of these emotions. When the patient is the one who directs the flow of family communication an even bigger change is created in how a family talks to each other.

2. *Disturbance of future plans*. The roller-coaster effect of cancer makes it difficult for families to be futuristic. It creates an environment of uncertainty. Setting goals and having dreams for the future gives families a sense of specific purpose, direction and uniqueness. These goals may be temporarily or permanently disrupted when a member has cancer. Displacement of family plans causes frustration, anger and grief.
3. *Alteration of external reference groups*. The work setting provides people with an important identity outside the family. Cancer frequently impinges on a person's capacity to work which in turn alters their working relationships with fellow employees. There are reports of family members being treated with overconcern from co-workers to that of total lack of acknowledgment that they are experiencing a family crisis. Families along with the patient experience the social stigma of cancer. Extended family members are another reference group that changes. They may become a vital part in the daily lives of the nuclear family unit where as prior to the illness their involvement as a relative was the occasional family gathering. When families live at a distance it becomes necessary for decision making to be done by phone which gives little opportunity for family discussion.

New reference groups are also created by a cancer diagnosis. Doctors, nurses, social workers and other patients on the same treatment schedules become familiar names and faces. These new people assume great importance for cancer families. Trips to the doctor and clinic are frequent events that are time consuming. These visits dominate family life and conversation.

The value of a family assessment is apparent when one recognizes the wide variation among individuals, families, and cultures. There is no one right way how a family should act or respond in time of crisis. More emphasis needs to be placed on assessing the family as a system. This data will provide the health care team with valuable information on family structure, expectations and previous crisis experience. Because medical treatment of cancer patients continues over months and years a plan for helping families can be established and reassessed on a regular basis. Hill and Hansen from the University of Minnesota [5] have developed a framework for family assessment in chronic illness that is an excellent reference point. This framework explores four factors that influence a family's ability to cope. It may take more than one interview to complete the form but the format will provide a consistency in the data gathering process which is directed at the family as a unit of care.

1. *Characteristics of the Illness*
   a) What is the family's understanding of the diagnosis?
   b) What is the perceived degree of pain, disability, threat to life?
   c) What is understood about treatment and related side effects?
   d) What belief is held as to prognosis and potential for regaining health?
2. *Perceived Threat to Family Relationships, Status and Goals*
   a) How does the family define roles, relations, and communication patterns?
   b) What are the decision-making patterns before and after the illness?
   c) What are the family goals and how are they affected by the illness?
   d) How do individual member's feel about changes created by the illness?
3. *Available Resources*
   a) What financial resources are available if income is threatened?
   b) What are the family's support resources: relatives, friends, community support groups, etc.?
4. *Past Experiences with Similar Situations*
   a) What coping strategies has the family used in past crises?
   b) What is the cancer history of the family and what were those experiences like for the family?

Having this information will enable the health care team to assist the family more fully. They can determine what information the family needs in order to maximize their coping skills and anticipate the types of resources and support needed in the future.

It is the challenge of the oncology team members to find ways and means for addressing the needs of cancer families throughout the continuum of care. This means providing services that extend from simply being available for understanding, support, and affirmation to providing programs specifically designed to incorporate the cancer family in its entirety. Three goals have been identified that encourage families to utilize positive coping skills. These should be incorporated into the design for family centered programs. They are:

1. Improve problem-solving techniques used by families.
2. Strengthen families' sense of self-esteem.
3. Increase families' interactional skills.

Examples of programs that are currently being used to help families in adapting to the cancer diagnosis are:

1. Family conferences at various times in the course of illness conducted by the doctor and other health care team members.
2. Audiotapes of family conferences for families to replay at their chosing.
3. Groups for patients and family members that provide information and support.
4. One to one visitation programs utilizing ex-patients and their family members.

A program, with which I have been closely associated, addresses family concerns in a retereat type setting [6]. Named the "We Can Week-end", this program is based on the simple premise that every cancer family can actively participate in the restoration process. Participants are encouraged to see that in striving to regain a balance in family life it is helpful to learn about the facts and feelings surrounding cancer. The commitment of our oncology team has been to design a program that is flexible to include all ages of children, is directive in discussing cancer and its ramification, provides a broad selection of educational activities and promotes communication within the family about their feelings concerning cancer. The longe range goal of the "We Can Week-end" is to help families utilize positive skills for coping with the cancer in their family.

Sixteen to eighteen families spend two days and an overnight together along with a staff of twenty health professionals. The selected site offers classrooms, sleeping and eating facilities, gymnasium, swimming pool, and a large outdoor recreation area. Art, movement, and music activities are integrated throughout the 2-days to create group togetherness and sensitivity. This program, offered two times a year at our hospital, has received positive response from families. It is being replicated in a number of other places in the United States.

The concept of cancer care needs to be expanded to include all family members. As health care professionals we have the skills to assess and plan ways to address family needs. We are key people in guiding cancer families toward the establishment of healthy patterns of coping during the crisis and recurrent times of stress brought on by cancer. There is strong justification for health care facilities to provide family centered programs throughout the continuum of cancer care.

References

1. Cohen M, Wellisch D (1978) Living in limbo: psychosocial interventions in families with a cancer patient. Am J Psychother 32 (4): 561
2. Brenner P (1985) Hospice applications of family systems theory. Am J Hospice Care 2 (6): 13-16
3. Olsen EH (1970) The impact of serious illness on the family system. Postgrad Med: 169-174
4. Cassileth BR (1979) The cancer patient, social and medical aspects of care. Lea and Febiger, Philadelphia
5. Hill R, Hansen DA (1964) Families under stress. In: Christensen HT (ed) Handbook of marriage and the family. Rand McNally, Chicago
6. Johnson J, Norby P (1981) We can weekend: a program for cancer families. Cancer Nurs 4 (1): 23-28

Quality of Life/Education About Cancer

Psychological and Social Support of Cancer Patients: Report on a Program of the Radiotherapy Department, Erlangen

R. Sauer[1] and M. Seitz[2]

[1] Strahlentherapeutische Klinik, Universität Erlangen-Nürnberg, Universitätsstraße 27, 8520 Erlangen, FRG
[2] Institut für Pastoraltheologie, Universität Erlangen-Nürnberg, Kochstraße 6, 8520 Erlangen, FRG

The term radiation therapy is all too readily associated with the idea of "technical medicine" and the dictates of technology, with the general human needs of the patient simply being overwhelmed. But in Erlangen, in particular, we are of the opinion that the task of the physician is not merely to provide the patient with the highest level of medical care, but also to support him as a complete and individual fellow human being. We would therefore like to report on a combined medical and pastoral training program which is probably unique in nature and which, to our minds, might serve as a model to be copied.

The program is a training project comprising both an initial theoretical part and a subsequent practical part in which theory is put into practice. Our project has three main aspects:

1. In a series of lectures we demonstrate, on the basis of talks with seriously ill patients, how a physician and a priest or social worker can communicate with patients with cancer. Between 50 and 60 students attend these interviews during which they are free to put their own questions to the patient. These students are studying medicine, theology, or psychology, or are social workers.
2. During the semester, the theologist accompanies the physician on ward rounds. There are two reasons for this: firstly, we wish to demonstrate that spiritual counselling forms part of our clinical supportive care; secondly, we wish to familiarize the priest with the medical problems of the cancer patients.
3. The students gain practice in communicating with the cancer patients in the ward. They form a visiting service, and also participate in the work of the ward, e.g., by making beds, handing out meals, distributing the necessary drugs to patients, or helping on the way to the therapeutic unit.

Here, we would like to report briefly on five aspects of our experience:

1. Our idea of what man is
2. Our attitude toward disease
3. Communication with the patient - information and honesty
4. The hopes of the cancer patient
5. The cooperation among all those involved in providing supportive care to cancer patients

Recent Results in Cancer Research, Vol. 108

Our Idea of Man and Human Dignity

In this connection, there are three basic things of which we have to be aware:

The Uniqueness (Individuality) of the Patient. Although about 200000–250000 people develop cancer every year in Germany, for each of the victims it is a unique, quite personal, event. It is never always the same disease, and is certainly never experienced by two patients in quite the same way. For every disease strikes the patient in his quite specific life situation, which itself is embedded in his own particular life history.

The Solitude (Isolation) of the Patient. Solitude is a result of our individuality or uniqueness. In the first instance, this does not necessarily have to do with the absence of other people. Solitude (isolation) is not eliminated by living together with one's family, by visits, or by telphone calls. Even when participating in a conversation, or as a member of a group, a person can be fully aware of his loneliness. And each and every one of us experiences and lives his illness alone.

The limitations of Understanding and Communication of the Patient. We all find it extremely difficult to talk about the things that really move and concern us. We lack the words and the ability to express our thoughts. The sick person signals his needs in more or less clearly understandable remarks about his state of health and often projects his fears and anxieties onto his environment. In the final resort, however, we always find the following four questions arising:

- What have I got?
- Why me?
- Why right now?
- What is the point of it all? That is, the question as to the meaning, if any, of the illness.

Unfortunately, physicians in particular often seem to have little awareness of this problem of understanding and communication.

Our Attitude Toward Disease

More and more people seem, as it were, to be losing sight of severe illness. More than 50% of the seriously ill now die in hospital, and this seems to be generally regretted. For, although illness is an inseparable part of life, it is more or less seen as a sort of mechanical failure, and the hospital nothing more than a repair shop. And this is the reason why so much is expected of us physicians. So many people appear to believe that by paying their health insurance contributions they have done the best they can to ensure that, in the event of their falling ill, they will be made well again. This principle might be compared with an automatic vending machine in which a coin is inserted ast the top and the desired item taken out at the bottom.

In reality, disease may be considered a warning sign (comparable with a road sign). At the same time, however, it may trigger a process that can result in the patient's reaching completely new shores. Of course, in the first instance, it means a loss. It means a restriction on the possibilities previously available to him. At the same time, however, it may also represent an increase in reality - that is, an enhancement of the intensity of life. Many patients have reported to us that their attitude to life underwent a change. They may express this by saying something like: Having cancer has been a help to me. The stability and depth of friendships, for example, may suddenly be revealed. Only recently, a patient told us how she and her husband now read to each other. This is a sign of the intensification of a relationship.

Communication with the Cancer Patient - Information and Honesty

The general problem of patient information is wide-ranging, and one that is constantly cropping up. In the situation under consideration here, of course, it is not simply a question of providing information about the diagnosis, but also about the prognosis, which is of primary importance throughout the whole course of the illness. This is not the place to go into detail on the pros and cons of honesty vis-à-vis the patient: however, it does seem unbelievable to the authors that so many lies are still being told to cancer patients. And it is those in particular who scarcely ever have any lengthy talks with a cancer patient who are against providing him with accurate information which, they maintain, would be cruel. They introduce such vague terms as hope and belief, and warn against the possibility of suicide, which, it is claimed, is so widespread in particular among young cancer patients. We cannot go into too much detail here, and shall cotent ourselves with a guidelines, all of which have been tested in talks with many patients:

- Our aim is to have open, honest talks with the patient, and we never resort to lying. It is nevertheless important to distinguish between what is correct and what is true. Correctness (or accuracy) represents the facts of the actual situation as, to the best of our knowledge, they are. Truth is an absolute term that represents a dynamic process, a complete understanding of which we humans do not as a rule possess.
- We say what we know and also, if asked, what we hope. In certain circumstances we adhere to the motto of the German Army Command in the First World War, namely: we do not tell everything we know, but what we tell is correct.
- We never talk to the patient's relatives behind his back. Anything we can legally and humanely say to relatives, we can also say in the presence of the patient.
- We adhere to the principle of not destroying hope, but strengthening it. In this connection, for example, we explain the facts of the illness and what treatment can be expected to achieve. In a moment I shall return to this point.

This approach is, of course, easy enough when we have something to offer, i.e., when surgery, radiotherapy, or chemotherapy is possible. The situation becomes more difficult when there is nothing more we can actively do, that is, when all that is left to us is to provide nursing care. At such a point, most of those who are in favor of telling the truth "at any price" actually fail, and begin to resort to lying.

Even here, however, we adhere to the principle of openness in our communication with the patient. We believe that Dietrich Ritschel accurately summarized the problems and anxieties that move the physician, family members, and spiritual counsellors, when he said:

It is not enough simply to condemn the physicians in our society for continuing regularly to lie to the seriously ill and dying patient. Rather, we should consider what freedom they themselves enjoy, and what hopes they cherish. For here is where the problem lies, and not in the question as to how much truth a patient can tolerate and how much his reserves of strength may be reduced by letting him know the truth too soon. And, anyway, truth is not simply a matter of information. It is a process that needs to develop over a lengthy period of time. This can be observed in patients who have been supported in their illness over a number of years.

The Hopes of the Cancer Patient

Giving hope, holding out hope, not taking hope away - these expressions are used by many who in fact often have only a vague idea of what they really mean. The little word hope is very frequently received with a bending of the knee and a respectful silence. Holding out hope to a patient does not mean simply saying to him: Chin up, everything will turn out all right. Rather it means going into details. It is as if an assistant comes to us with the remark that a patient is unwell. Our response must be to ask why is he not well, and what is his present need? Only then can I be of help to him. Here, too, we must ask, in what can hope be found; what is there? We shall see that hope, too, is a dynamic process.

The content of hope changes not only with age, but also in the course of cancer.

- Initially, the patient hopes that he can be helped.
- Then, he hopes that he will become well again. In many cases, we are justified in holding out this hope. But if this is not possible, what then?
- The patient asks who will help me in this or the other situation? He might ask: How are things to go on at home, who will help my wife run the farm? What can I still expect to do for my children? What can I do with the rest of the time left to me?
- The patient hopes - within the limitations imposed upon him by his illness - to lead a normal life. It goes without saying that normal means something quite different for the patient than for a healthy person. In the Hebrew, normality is expressed by the word shalom, which means something like well-being, a state in which something, like a relationship, can grow. And this is why some patients are of the opinion that they have changed their lives, that they can differentiate between important and unimportant, and that they can derive pleasure from the little things of daily life, etc.
- In the case of the very severely ill patient, talk of hope has something of the ambiguity of harvesting and leave-taking. Here, we are referring to death without specifically mentioning it by name. For example: I am worried about leaving my husband on his own. The reason I am still fighting is to be here for his sake for as long as possible.

- Finally, even talks with the dying are frequently more realistically oriented to the actual situation, and easier to hold than many physicians believe. Such questions are asked as: What happens when one dies? What must I expect? A possible answer might, for example, be: we shall be with you; we shall take away your pain.

On the question of hope, a patient once wrote to one of us:

> Only what belongs to the same category as the evil that makes comfort necessary in the first place, can be truly comforting. Hope belongs to a quite different category - it is not to be defined as some sort of specific expectation, but, rather, as a principle that touches the question of the meaning of existence. Thus, in common with fear, transitoriness, and disease, it represents a major element of basic human existence. It is like the tree that we plant although we know that the world will be destroyed on the following day. The inexorable destruction of the world robs the act of planting the tree, and the deep wonder that this act symbolizes, of nothing of its meaning or value.

Cooperation Among Those Providing Care to the Cancer Patient

Today, the patient is in the care, not of one, but of several physicians. Further care providers are members of the family, spiritual counsellors, psychologists, and social workers. This fact requires not merely good cooperation, but also appropriate knowledge on the part of the carers. It is this knowledge we are trying to impart with our training project.

Helmuth Thielicke once said: "No-one can give what he does not own." It is to be hoped that we might all feel something of the needs of our patients, and of the soil on which these needs have grown. Perhaps we have succeeded in some small way in showing what holding out hope might mean. In this area we can all be physician and spiritual counsellor. We should not avoid painful talks, but rather try to make the fears involved, concrete and thus be of some help, even in situations that might be medically hopeless.

Quality of Life for Patients Receiving Chemotherapy and Hormonal Therapy

R. Tiffany

Royal Marsden Hospital, Fulham Road, London SW3 6JJ, Great Britain

This chapter will examine some of the issues relevant to chemotherapy and hormonal therapy, and the challenges that they present particularly, but not exclusively, to the nursing profession. One cannot, of course, separate treatment of the disease from the disease process itself and its impact on the patient and family. Patients' attitudes to cancer vary considerably depending upon cultural, ethnic, social, economic, and educational factors, but probably the most important and prominent attitude is fear – fear of having cancer, fear of it being fatal, fear of disfiguration, fear that it will cause severe pain, fear of treatment and its side-effects. Such fears will vary in intensity and frequency, as will the patient's reaction to them.

For the majority of patients undergoing treatment by chemotherapy or hormonal therapy, cure is not the expected outcome; rather they enter the "snakes and ladders" domain of treastment, remission, relapse, and perhaps further treatment that will characterise the rest of their illness career. And the minority who are cured have to learn to live for the rest of their lives with the threat of a malignant diagnosis hanging over their heads like a medical sword of Damocles; they never truly free themselves from the yoke of their diagnosis as they are called back into the system for their progress tobe monitored.

Other contributions to this book have emphasised the importance of communication and information as means of assisting the patient to cope with his or her fears and anxiety, and I would like to add a few comments myself on these two points.

On Communication

Sometimes listening to health care professionals talk about communication one could be fooled into believing that we have a choice: that is, whether or not we wish to communicate. However, most communication in hospital happens accidentally and is quite outside the control of staff. This is because communication is not limited to those moments when a member of staff makes a conscious decision to tell a patient or relative something, but is going on all the time at a nonverbal

Recent Results in Cancer Research, Vol. 108

level. The atmosphere created on a hospital ward, the attitudes and expressions of staff as they go about their work, and the way other patients and relatives seem to be reacting to the situation are all aspects of communication. Therefore we are not in a position to decide whether or not there should be communication between staff, patients, and relatives; rather it is a given fact of hospital life. Indeed, it may be that patients will learn more of their illnesses if they have been *told* nothing, since they will constantly be on the lookout for any clues to clear the fog of mystification. However, in such a situation we cannot be sure of the accuracy of the perceptions of the patient. The only decision we can make is whether or not we wish to be *consciously* involved and to understand what is happening, and to convey information positively to support him or her and the family.

On Information

Perhaps one of the most sensitive issues in oncology is who can and who cannot give information to patients and their families and whose role it is to counsel patients concerning their disease and treatment. Perhaps in the not too distant future we will reach a stage of maturity when jockeying for position between doctor, social worker, nurse, and psychologist will cease and when we will allow the patients to have a greater choice as to with whom they wish to communicate. Some might argue that planned sessions of information giving are the appropriate mechanism to use. I have no doubt as to the value of such sessions. However, I am reminded of the patient who during the long hours of darkness eventually has the courage to ask of the night nurse "Have I got cancer?". To have this, or some other important question, met by a wall of silence can be devastating for the patient and emotionally draining for the nurse. "I knew the situation was bad when the nurse could not tell me anything" was one comment recently expressed by a patient. A team approach utilising the appropriate person giving appropriate information at the appropriate time should offer a solution to this dilemma. However, whoever provides information requires knowledge and skill in this area to be really effective, and the lack of such skills among health care professionals gives cause for concern.

The evidence is now overwhelming that truth and openness with patients enhances the relationship between them and their care givers, recognising, of course, that we must allow patients the choice of denial if this is the strategy that they choose as a coping mechanism. Also in giving information we must ensure that we do not assault patients with the violence of our words and that truth is conveyed with a sensitivity that engenders hope rather than despair.

Coping Strategies

Other contributors to this book have highlighted the spiritual dimensions of care and the role of music and other arts in assisting patients to cope with cancer and its treatment and in improving the quality of their lives. The use of beauticians and other nontraditional health care workers can also greatly enhance tolerance to treatment and help patients and their families face an uncertain future positively. Nutritional aspects of support receive considerable attention, and rightly so. Weight loss is not an obligatory accompaniment of cancer and chemotherapy. For many patients, even those having to tolerate nausea and vomiting, weight can be maintained and improved. Individually tailored, nutritionally sound dietary programmes can offer the patient significant support and by involving the patient and family in planning may prevent them from seeking alternative and often inappropriate and harmful diets.

Maintaining family integrity during illness is a challenge to us all. Judy Johnson has reminded us that "cancer is a potent agent of change that disrupts the pattern of daily living." She also outlined some of the strategies which could be employed to unite families in the acute crisis of diagnosis and the chronic crisis of disease progression. In addition, the valuable role that social workers can play in regard to family financial structures and employment-related issues should be emphasised.

So far I have discussed psychosocial skills needed to support patients. For nurses the development of practical skills is equally important. For, unless the nurse is confident of his or her abilities to perform often complex clinical procedures he or she will not have the freedom of mind to concentrate on the individual's other needs. Over the past few years many nursing strategies have been developed to improve the quality of care given to patients receiving chemotherapy. These developments fall into three main categories:

1. Techniques related to the administration of cytotoxic drugs that improve the comfort and safety of the procedure
2. Interventions to reduce the side-effects of treatment, e.g., relaxation and other techniques to reduce anticipatory vomiting and scalp cooling to reduce the incidence of alopecia
3. Manipulation of the environment to assist the patient in coping with the negative aspects of treatment.

We have at our disposal new tools that can help patients and families cope with cancer and chemotherapy or hormonal therapy and that enhance the quality of their lives. Unfortunately, too often they are not utilised to bring about what we know is possible.

Additionally, nursing and medical research is exploring new methods of care and support. The same commitment and enthusiasm is required for these studies as for studies into treatment protocols if we are justly to earn the title given to us collectively as caring professionals.

Public Information and Professional Education About Cancer

F. van der Linde

Gesundheitsdepartement des Kantons St. Gallen, Moosbruggstraße 11,
9001 St. Gallen, Switzerland

As the term "public information" in the title implies, the scope of this presentation goes beyond the topic of supportive care and will cover some problems of cancer information and education which concern the public, that is the entire population at risk of cancer. Many of the principles and rules discussed will, however, be applicable to the situation of the cancer patient and his environment as well. "Professional education," which is to be discussed in the second part, has two different aspects which will have to be dealt with separately: the information which has to be provided to the health professional on the one hand and the messages and educational efforts which are delivered by physicians, nurses, and other health professionals to the patients and the public on the other. The focus of this presentation will be on the arguments for the need for good public information on such a difficult and multidimensional problem as "cancer" and on some methodological aspects which often pose problems especially for the medical profession. Often it can even be observed that the role of the physician in cancer information and education is being underestimated and viewed by doctors as a subject of minor importance. Some special attention will therefore be given to the role of physicians in professional and public education; but the issues discussed here are of course of importance for all health professionals in the field of cancer.

Why Do We Need Public Information About Cancer?

The question of why we need public information about cancer is not just of theoretical relevance when we consider what people actually *do* with information given to them. Cancer as a substantial contributor to morbidity and mortality in the population is frequently not just perceived as one among other diseases, but is - more often than in the case of other diagnoses with comparable or worse prognoses - associated with fear and irrational behavior. This fact is well known to the mass media, which find in the cancer field an almost inexhaustible source of news and stories. I am not saying that all this information is bad, but we have to be well aware of the fact that the media in the first place have to sell news to the public and are not primarily concerned with the potentially deleterious effects of their

Recent Results in Cancer Research, Vol. 108

messages. From our professional point of view, information is not an end in itself, but should be in one way or another a help for the public or the patient. To put it in simple terms: the aim of any cancer information from the standpoint of health professionals should be to enable the public or the patient to cope better with the problem of cancer. This is true regardless of the target population of our information. The key question with any kind of information is which psychological effects it will arouse in the recipient, be it in the context of prevention, early detection, diagnosis, treatment, rehabilitation, or permanent care.

Information coming from health professionals is often linked with specific intentions on our part: we want the patient or the public to do or to abstain from something (to seek medical advice in the presence of certain symptoms, not to smoke, etc.). Thus we find ourselves in some kind of educational setting. Using the term "education" we go beyond the transmission of knowledge. What we really do in addition to this is to try to bring about *changes in attitudes* and ultimately *behavior modification*. Usually the methods used by health professionals to motivate people to adopt a specific behavior are basically informational. It is presupposed that people will respond "rationally" to protect themselves against cancer or to stick to a recommended treatment, once the steps they should take have been explained. However, behavior that is "rational" from a professional point of view is not necessarily compelling from an individual's. Irrational psychological forces often compete to divert people away from the recommendations made in cancer education. Taking as an example the early detection of breast cancer, it is obvious that a women needs some knowledge of the disease and - in the case of a healthy person even more important - of the technique of self-examination. She will, however, hardly put to use this knowledge unless she perceives breast cancer personally as a relevant problem and in addition is convinced that self-examination can be a useful tool for early detection and better prognosis. To create this attitude is not just a matter of giving information but is dependent on many accompanying psychosocial factors, and not least on the amount of confidence someone has in the person transmitting the relevant information.

Other attitudes, such as those toward medical treatment of cancer in general, are also important determinants which may interact with a person's attitude toward our professional view of the problem. But even in the case of a generally positive attitude there is no guarantee as to the actual *behavior* of a person (does the woman in our example really practice breast self-examination?). It seems, however, that attitudes play a more important role in explaining and predicting behavior than does factual knowledge, although the latter is generally an indispensable part of cancer education.

Attitudes to cancer arise in part and in varying degrees from fear. Cancer is a significant, objective threat in everyone's life. Fear of it is in no way abnormal. In fact, fear (like pain) is important in producing adaptive responses. However, psychological defence mechanisms are sometimes used maladaptively to reduce the anxieties aroused by the threat of cancer. Such defence mechanisms are maladaptive because they may lead people to bypass the medical pathways for dealing effectively with the organic disease. A person who discovers a symptom which he knows could signify cancer will not necessarily seek medical attention. He might deny the relevance of the symptom or repress awareness of it. This use of the defence mechanisms of denial and/or repression is likely to be at least partially successful in relieving initial anxieties about cancer. For the time being, anxiety can be reduced to a tolerable level and the unconsciously employed psychological strategy is thus rewarded and therefore is likely to be used again in similar circumstances.

In designing public information and education programs, greater account should undoubtedly be taken of the irrational side of human nature, provided this does not lead to manipulative techniques of persuasion such as additional fear arousal, alarmism, or, at the other extreme, deceitful optimism. Even apart from ethical considerations, such techniques might well in the long run be self-defeating.

Public information is, as has been mentioned before, an indispensable part of cancer education, be it as a prerequisite for inducing changes of attitudes or to counterbalance inappropriate messages given by some mass media. Information is useful as long as we recognize its inherent limitations in directly influencing individual behavior. Transmission of information has therefore to be planned carefully. Two guiding questions stand at the beginning of any planning process:

1. What do I want the public (patient) to learn?
2. What does the public (patient) already know or perceive about this topic?

They seem trivial at first sight but prove on second thoughts to be of utmost importance. I will not elaborate on the first question, although we have to realize that particularly in the field of cancer information it may be rather difficult to determine the precise content of our message, be it in the context of prevention or, for instance, of supportive care. The second question may pose even more problems. People have an enormous amount of knowledge, pseudoknowledge, or superstitions about cancer. This puts the cancer educator in the uncomfortable situation that his message has to compete with preexisting beliefs and attitudes and that perhaps his ideas are even unwelcome. Finding out what our patients or the public already know about the topic we want to discuss may provide us with leads for setting priorities in preparing and transmitting adequate information. If, for example, we want the population to acquire a differentiated view about the seriousness of the different kinds of cancer it will be useful to collect data about this question at regular intervals. As an example, in Fig. 1 the results from a recent Swiss representative population survey are shown [1]. It seems surprising that leukemia is associated with such an ominous prognosis and it must be assumed that the therapeutic progress of the past decades has not been taken notice of by a considerable part of the population. Data of this kind cannot, of course, be extrapolated to other countries, but must be interpreted in the context of the particular local situation.

Information can be distributed by different kinds of channels, and again, before we plan any activities as health professionals, it may prove useful to know where people acquire their knowledge about cancer. Figure 2 shows, based on the same Swiss survey, some sources of information for the population as a whole [1]. The more detailed results not shown here naturally disclose some variance between specific subgroups, e.g., according to age or socioeconomic status, but the overwhelming importance of the mass media is obvious in all subgroups. What this picture shows is the preferred source of information for general knowledge

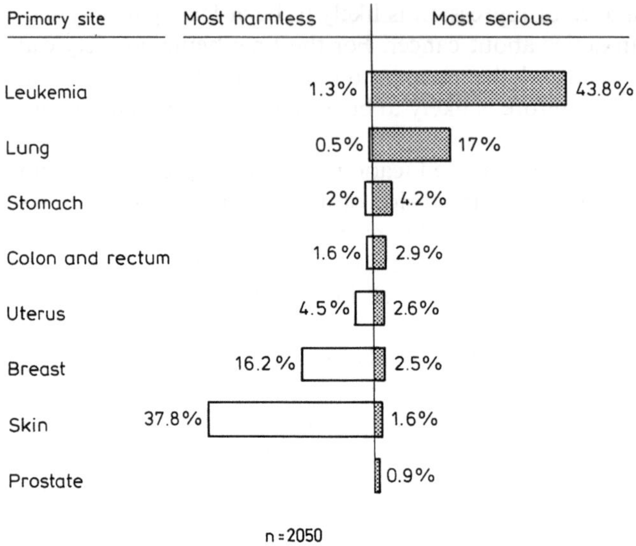

Fig. 1. Perception of the seriousness of cancer (Swiss Population, 1982). (Hornung [1])

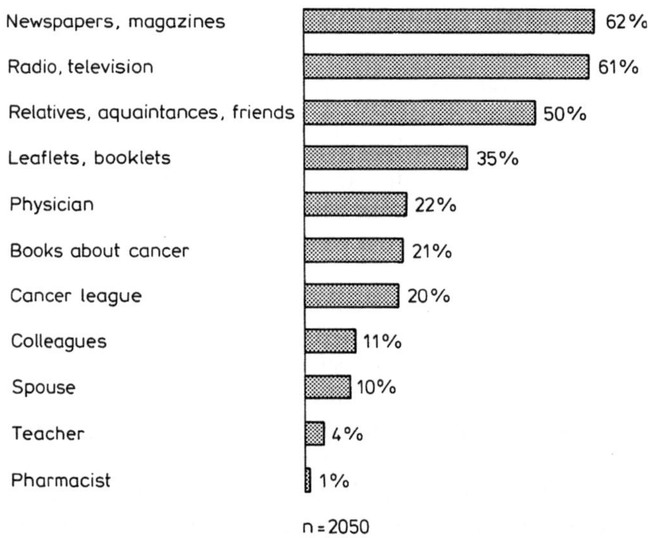

Fig. 2. Sources of information about cancer (Swiss Population, 1982). (Hornung [1])

about the problem. When people were asked where they would actively seek information in the context of a specific cancer-related problem, 75% answered they would consult a physician. This result is important when we plan any professional activity which goes beyond the mere transmission of knowledge and thus provides the link between the topics of public and of professional education. The mass media are certainly the most effective way of informing people about something.

They are important sources of impersonal knowledge and as such act as triggers for the first steps in the process of influencing attitudes. However, as soon as adoption of attitudes and behavioral changes are the scope of our efforts - not only in a therapeutic but also in a preventive setting - face-to-face methods are more effective. Since public education about cancer from the professional viewpoint is ultimately aimed at behavior change and not merely the creation of awareness, the interpersonal persuasive efforts of all health professionals are of vital importance.

Why Professional Education About Cancer?

The problems discussed above have pointed to the need for a person-to-person relationship in cancer information and education. The results of the mentioned survey data leave no doubt about the eminent role of the physician in this communication process as a source of information. In the last decade, a group of experts have, in collaboration with the International Union Against Cancer (UICC), made considerable efforts to analyze this role of the physician and to stress the need to involve doctors to a greater degree in public education about cancer [2, 3]. The following summary of their conclusions points specifically to the role of the physician, but there is no reason to exclude other health professionals from these arguments, provided they act as credible and competent persons in the field of cancer care. The main conclusions can be summarized as follows [3]:

1. *Doctors have direct continuing access to the public.* No central public health agency or cancer society has regular access in a private consulting relationship with so many people as does (collectively) the medical profession. Moreover, primary care physicians often have extended contact with patients that may last many years.
2. *Doctors have captive audiences.* Unlike a TV set, a doctor giving a health message cannot easily be "turned off." His audience usually hears him out, so that at least the first step in the process of effective communication is guaranteed.
3. *Doctors are credible authorities.* Because of their training and experience, doctors are considered the most knowledgeable group on matters of health. Communication research has shown repeatedly that the credibility of the communicator is an important factor determining whether advice contained in messages is adopted.
4. *Doctors are trusted.* Doctors may be criticized in the media; orthodox medical ideas may be attacked; we hear of epidemics of iatrogenic disease. Yet in spite of this development, most people trust the advice of their *own* doctor.
5. *The medical consultation is a powerful educational context.* Health education is a field where success stories are rare, yet within this field *patient* education programs are one of the most promising areas [4]. Education by doctors focused upon the patient's complaint has the advantage of enhanced motivation in the patient. Although such strong motivation is absent when a doctor attempts to educate a healthy person, even among the not sick the medical consultation may nevertheless engender a higher-than-usual motivation to comply with advice.

These general rules apply also and in some respects even more to the hospital situation, where the interaction between physician (or any other health personnel) and patient can be especially effective. A hospitalized patient will be particularly receptive to instructions from the doctor, and likely to follow them. On account of the frequency of situations involving personal interaction and because of a great deal of individualized information about the patient collected from observations and examinations, the hospital can be a particularly effective setting for patient information and education.

Considering these favorable conditions for a physician to act as a source of information and as an educator for patients and for the public, it may at first sight seem surprising that in the view of other health professionals many doctors meet these demands rather poorly. Frequently complaints are heard about the difficulties in involving physicians in this special kind of cancer care which seems to be quite remote from their professional background. In one of the UICC workshops on the topic of involving doctors in public education about cancer a list of problems and possible reasons for this discrepancy was elaborated by the participants, who included health professionals in the cancer field from different countries (physicians, nurses, social workers, health educators, etc.). The top ten problems that emerged from this survey were [5]:

Rank	Problem
1	Doctors lack appropriate communication skills
2	Doctors do not have time to educate patients about cancer
3	Doctors do not see themselves in an educator role
4	Doctors have negative attitudes to cancer education
5	Doctors do not believe that their involvement would produce the desired results
6	Doctors are fatalistic about cancer
7	Postqualification training does not include public education about cancer
8	Doctors lack educational skills
9	Doctors lack up-to-date knowledge about cancer
10	Undergraduate medical training does not include public education about cancer

Of course, these spontaneous statements by a group of some 30 health professionals interested in problems of cancer education are not of scientific value and may not reflect the situation as perceived by the majority of physicians. But at least they point to a field where many doctors may not be performing too well. If we accept the general trend of these statements, they reveal deficiencies mostly at the levels of attitudes and behavior, but in addition clearly rank the lack of skills in communication techniques as problem number one. Without going into a deeper analysis of these statements one conclusion which has to be drawn seems obvious: there must be a deficiency in professional information not only in the sense of physicians being the source of information, but also in the education of doctors regarding communication techniques. Why some physicians - according to this limited survey - seem to have pessimistic views about cancer and about the effectiveness of their own interventions cannot be further investigated here, but is certainly an observation which has to be taken very seriously.

To conclude, it has become clear that cancer information and education is a task connected with many more problems and difficulties than are usually anticipated. It most certainly needs a multidisciplinary approach, especially in the planning process, and it has to be realized by all professionals involved that the physician carries a great responsibility. His behavior can be a crucial factor in the acceptance or rejection of information or recommendations by the patient or the public. It seems therefore to be of substantial importance that doctors as well as other health professionals become familiar with the mechanisms involved in a process of planning and communicating cancer information, even if one particular doctor or nurse or social worker plays only a limited role in the sequence of this process.

Figure 3 summarizes the steps that are basic to planning cancer education - or any kind of education - in the form of six questions, including the problem of

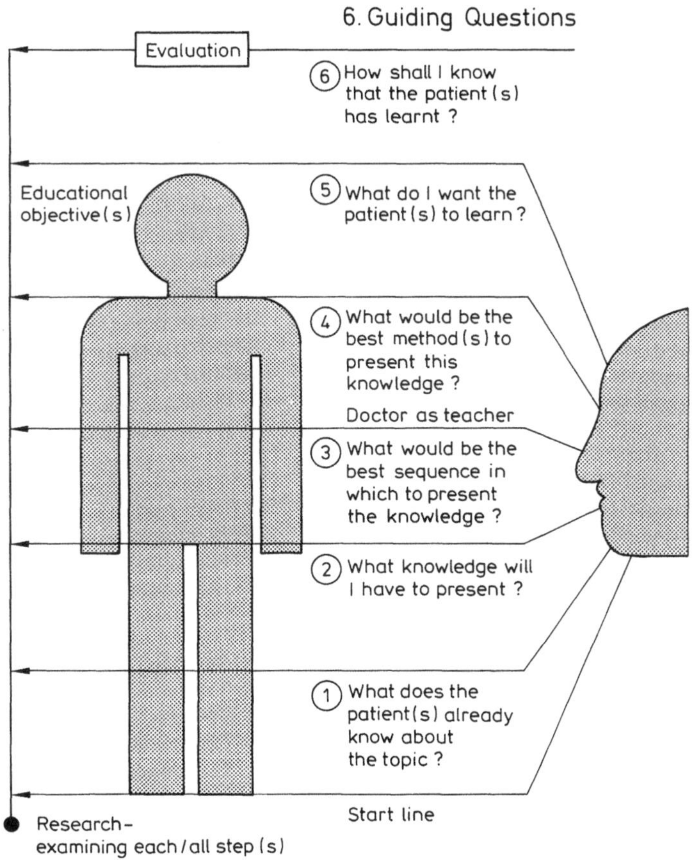

Fig. 3. Guiding questions for planning cancer education. (Hill et al. [3])

evaluating the communication process [3]. For a professional health educator this implies the use of the traditional methods of scientific research, but in addition the physician in his daily practice is able to make observations on an individual basis to ascertain whether his message has been understood and put into practice by the patient.

With regard to cancer information which should help the patient and the public to cope better with the cancer problem, it is appropriate for this presentation to end not with theoretical models but with an appeal to all professionals in the field of cancer to be fully aware of the paramount importance of the personal element of the communication process. Any media, from T.V. to printed leaflets, can be helpful, especially in public education, but should never be taken as a substitute for the personal interaction between the doctor, the nurse, or any other health professional and the cancer patient.

References

1. Hornung R (1986) Krebs: Wissen, Einstellungen und präventives Verhalten der Bevölkerung. Huber, Bern
2. Wakefield J (ed) (1978) Public education about cancer. Recent research and current programmes. UICC Technical Report Series 31:
3. Hill DJ, Heffernan MW, Rice DI (1979) Involving doctors in health education about cancer. UICC Technical Report Series 44:
4. Haggerty RJ (1977) Changing lifestyles to improve health. Prev Med 6: 276–289
5. UICC Workshop on Doctor Involvement in Public Education about Cancer, Manchester, England, 1981

The Role of Traditional Chinese Medicine in Supportive Care of Cancer Patients

Y. Sun

Department of Medical Oncology, Cancer Institute (Hospital), Chinese Academy of Medical Sciences, P. O. Box 2258, 100021 Beijing, People's Republic of China

Traditional Chinese medicine (TCM), with a history of several thousand years, represents an ancient cultural legacy accumulated by the Chinese people in the treatment and prevention of various diseases. A number of Chinese herbs may augment the host defense mechanisms, and others are effective in helping patients to recover from acute infection as well as in treating some chronic diseases. During the past two decades, experimental studies on the use of TCM in cancer patients have been carried out. This communication briefly reports the results in the supportive care of cancer patients.

Promotion of the Immune System

According to the basic theory of TCM, there is always some kind of deficiency before and during the course of diseases, including cancer. Fu-zheng therapy is one of the main principles in TCM; it literally means "promoting or enhancing the natural host defense mechanism" in various diseases. In TCM, the strategy in the management of diseases usually consists of two arms - to support the host and to attack the pathogenic factors.

Beginning in 1974, we started clinical trials and laboratory research to study the effect of several TCM herbs as biological response modifiers (BRMs) in cancer patients [1-6]. In a collaborative study of over 500 patients with different types of cancer at various stages, the preliminary results suggested some modulation of nonspecific cell-mediated immunity. This was also the case in a clinical trial using *Astragalus membranaceus* and *radix ginseng* in colon and stomach cancer patients (Tables 1, 2). Other herbs known to have an immunomodulating effect are shown in Table 3. Some set prescriptions also showed the same efficacy in cancer patients as well as in laboratory studies. Traditionally we usually use these kinds of herb in combination according to the dialectical approach, but they are also effective when used as single drugs.

The isolation and identification of effective components are underway in several laboratories. Components E from *Ligustrum lucidum* and F3 from *Astragalus membranceus* are highly effective both in vitro and in vivo. LL-E is now undergoing clinical trials in cancer and hepatitis patients.

Table 1. Changes in percentage phagocytosis of macrophages with Fu-zheng therapy in patients with malignant diseases (mean values)

Groups	No. of pts.	Observation period (months)						*P* value	
		Pre-treatment	-6	7-12	13-24	24+	Post-treatment	Against-pre-treatment levels	Against controls
Control	21	55.0	44.4	54.0	43.3		48.0	<0.001	
F-Z therapy	50	44.9	57.6	56.0	65.7	65.2	59.2	<0.001	<0.01
Lymphomas	26	43.4	56.8	57.3	65.7	65.2	60.3	<0.001	<0.01
Others	24	46.5	58.4	54.4	65.7	65.2	57.7	<0.01	<0.01

Table 2. Function of macrophages in colon and stomach cancer patients after *Astragalus membranaceus* and *ginseng extracts*

Parameters	No. of pts.	Before treatment	After treatment	*P*
Percentage of phagocytosis	15	32 ±2.3	44 ±3.9	<0.01
Index of phagocytosis	15	0.36±0.03	0.51±0.05	<0.05

Table 3. Medicinal herbs and animal known to have an immunomodulating effect

Astragalus membranaceus	*Ligustrum lucidum*
Radix anconiti praeparata	*Poris cocos*
Coriolus versicolor	*Tris pallasii* Fischer
Polysticus versicolor (Laoshan)	*Lentimus edoesa*
Polyporus versicolor	*Herba cistanches*
Herba epimedii	*Polyporum umbellatus*
Polygopyrum cymosum (Trer)	*Stichopus japanicus* Selenka

The polysaccharide of *Polyporum umbellatus* is also used in lung cancer patients with favorable results. A polysaccharide preparation was isolated from the artificial culture of *Polysticus versicolor* grown in the suburbs of Ningjing, in the Lao-shen forest. It is similar to the Japanese product PSK. The in vivo inhibitory effect on transplantable animal tumors was tested, and confirmed as not cytotoxic but host mediated. A preliminary clinical trial is also underway, and enhancement of cell-mediated immunity and protection of bone marrow function have been observed. Acid mucopolysaccharide from *Stichopus japanicus* Selenka is also tested in animals. After injection of the acid mucopolysaccharide 30 mg/kg per day intraperitoneally for a week, the phagocytosis of macrophages in nude mice was enhanced significantly ($P < 0.001$); such injection for 3-5 days also increased the delayed hypersensitivity response ($P < 0.05$-0.01) and returned to a normal level the cell-mediated immunity of immunosuppressed mice.

Some kinds of TCM herb may improve long-term results in cancer patients, as will be discussed later.

Table 4. Combination of TCM and irradiation *(IR)* in the treatment of nasopharyngeal carcinoma (randomized clinical trial)

Treatment	No. of pts.	Survival rate (%)		
		1-yr	3-yr	5-yr
IR	105	80	32	24
IR+TCM	92	91	67	53
		$P=0.05$	$P<0.01$	$P<0.05$

Use of Medicinal Herbs as Radio- and Chemosensitizers

Some medicinal herbs known as ABC (activate blood circulation) drugs may have a radiosensitizing effect, as proved both in experimental animals and clinically. According to the theory of TCM, blood stasis is a major factor in several diseases. Studies by several Chinese scientists have demonstrated that the majority of ABC drugs can promote circulation, in part by decreasing arterial resistance. In addition, some of the herbs also exhibit heparin-like activity, inhibiting platelet aggregation, preventing the formation of fibrin, acclerating the degradation of fibrin or fibrinogen, inhibiting fibrin stabilizing factor, and possibly activating the plasminogen-plasmin system. All these findings may explain the effectiveness of ABC drugs in the treatment of various vascular diseases, including coronary heart disease, thromboangiitis, thrombic obstruction of the retinal veins, occlusive cerebrovascular disease, and ischemic stroke.

In our hospital, when this kind of herb was used as an adjuvant to irradiation in patients with nasopharyngeal cancer, the 5-year survival rate was twice as high among those who received ABC drugs plus standard radiotherapy as among those who received radiotherapy alone (53% vs. 24%) (Table 4) [7].

Irisqunone was isolated from the seeds of *Iris pallasii* Fischer [*Iris lactes pall.* ssp. *Chinensis* (Fisch) Koidz]. Using Ma 737 breast cancer on mice, the radiosensitizing enhancement ratio was 1.3 in a hypoxic condition, and 1.68 on Hela cells. Randomized clinical trials were carried out in lung cancer patients. The complete remission rate and the response rate (complete plus partial remission) of patients who received Irisqunone 60 mg three times a day orally combined with radiation were 37% and 87% respectively, while those of patients who received conventional fractional radiation were 13% and 47% respectively. The 2-year survival rate was 21% in the combined modality group as compared to 14% in the control group ($P<0.05$) (Table 5). Radiosensitizing enhancement against esophageal and other malignancies was also evident. The clinical toxicity of Irisqunone was very low, with anorexia or nausea occurring in only a few patients. Furthermore, Irisqunone reduced the side-effects of radiotherapy, the bone marrow function was protected, and the immunity of patients was enhanced significantly. Thus, the quality of survival among patients so treated was improved.

The plant *Rabdosia subesceus* (Donglingcao), which is a perennial herb that grows in the mountain areas of Henan province, has been studied during the past 10 years for its ability in esophageal cancer patients to potentiate the therapeutic

Table 5. Clinical results in lung cancer patients treated with irradiation and Irisqunone

Treatment	No. of pts.	Response rate	CR	2-year-Survival
Irradiatior	32	47%	13%	14%
Irradiation + Irisqunone	30	87%	37%	21%

effect of bleomycin A_5 (pingyangmycin) and nitrocarphane (AT-1258). In a study of 80 patients, the response rate was 31% in the combined group, and only 7% in the pingyangmycin-nitrocarphane group ($P < 0.05$). The active component, named Oridonin, which is a diterpene and cyclopentanone, was isolated and tested. Its cytotoxic effect in vitro against esophageal cell lines EA-109 and CaEs-17 was comparable to that of 5-fluorouracil. It also prolonged life span or inhibited tumor growth in experimental tumor-bearing animals. Oridonin can synergistically inhibit the DNA synthesis of tumor cells induced by pingyangmycin, and the content of P-450 in the microsomes of the rat liver could be induced by a combination of Oridonin and pingyangmycin although there was no effect on the content of P-450 when each drug was used alone.

Protection of Bone Marrow, Adrenal Cortex, and Liver Function

In patients undergoing irradiation and/or chemotherapy, TCM herbs such as *Astragalus membranaceus* and *Ligustrum lucidum,* Oridonin, Irisqunone, and some set prescriptions have been observed to protect bone marrow, adrenal cortical function, and liver function. Laboratory studies showed that some herbs potentially may protect the peripheral white blood cells after administration of cytotoxic agents such as cyclophosphamide (Table 6). Further, some herbs are able to stimulate colony-forming units of bone marrow in tumor-bearing animals (Table 7). The active component F3, isolated from *Astragalus membranaceus,* is also capable of improving the rat's peripheral white blood cell counts.

In a randomized clinical trial, we measured the plasma hydrocortisone level in patients with stage II carcinoma of the cervix. The average level before and after irradiation was 8.0 and 6.1 μg/100 ml in 18 patients, but 9.5 and 9.1 μg/100 ml in patients who received irradiation and Fu-zheng herbs for 2 months.

Protection against hepatitis due to chemotherapeutic agents was also observed. A drug developed from the medicinal herb *Fructus schisandrae* [*Schisandra chinensis* (Turcz.) Baill.] is called diphenyl dimethyl dicarboxylate (DDB). A randomized clinical trial showed that in 19 of 23 patients (83%) who received intensive chemotherapy and DDB daily, the serum SGPT level returned to normal within 10 days; by contrast it did so in only 13% (3/23) of the control group. Among the patients in the control group, there were two deaths from hepatic coma, while in the treated group all recovered within 20 days. DDB thus shortens the time intervals between courses of chemotherapy, which are often prolonged owing to chemical hepatitis. An active component of *Ligustrum lucidum,* known to have antihepatitis virus activity, has also been found to have a protective effect on hepatic function during chemotherapy.

Table 6. Changes in peripheral WBC count after using medicinal herbs in mice

Drugs	Peripheral WBC (per mm³) 4 days after cyclophosphamide 100 mg/kg	*P*
Control	3499 ± 133	<0.001
Fructus ligustri lucidi	6183 ± 548	<0.001
Purrosia lingua (Thumb.) Farw.	5840 ± 920	<0.001
Psoralea corylifolia L.	5594 ± 721	<0.001
Cornus officinalis Sieb. et zucc.	5663 ± 1434	<0.05
Radix scrophulariae	5430 ± 1539	<0.05

Table 7. Effect of Fu-zheng therapy on colony-forming units - spleen of mice

	CFUs (No./femur)	
	C57-BL mice	LACA mice
Fu-zheng therapy	4867 ± 819** (9)	3085 ± 1068.94* (15)
Control	2137 ± 318 (4)	1857 ± 523.86 (7)

* $P<0.05$.
** $P<0.001$.

Table 8. Long-term results in patients with carcinoma of the cervix and breast cancer treated by irradiation alone and irradiation plus FZ therapy (randomized clinical trial)

Groups	Number of patients	Long-term results		*P*
		Surviving NED	Dead	
Carcinoma of cervix[a]				
Irradiation	15	6 (40%)	9 (60%)	NS
Irradiation + FZ therapy	16	9 (56%)	7[c] (44%)	
Carcinoma of cervix[b]				
Irradiation	19	13 (68%)	6 (32%)	NS
Irradiation + FZ therapy	17	15 (88%)	2 (12%)	
Carcinoma of breast				
Irradiation	12	6 (50%)	6 (50%)	<0.05
Irradiation + FZ therapy	10	9 (90%)	1 (10%)	

NED, no evidence of disease.
[a] Patients treated in 1974, mostly stage-III patients.
[b] Patients treated in 1975, mostly stage-II patients.
[c] Two patients died from other reasons, 5 died from cancer.

Improvement of Long-term Results

In a randomized prospective clinical trial of cervical and breast cancer patients who received irradiation or irradiation plus Fu-zheng herbs, the 10-year survival rates suggested some advantage for the combined modality (Table 8).

Table 9. Survival rate of lung cancer patients treated with chemotherapy and TCM

Type of lung cancer and treatment	No. of pts.	Survival rate		Median survival time (days)
		1-yr	2-yr	
Squamous carcinoma				
Chemotherapy	30	33%	3%	204
Chemotherapy + TCM	30	67%	13%	465
Adenocarcinoma				
Chemotherapy	32	24%		192
Chemotherapy + TCM	30	54%		324

The results from the Shanghai Cancer Hospital show that, among 31 patients with stage II hepatomas receiving radiotherapy and Fu-zheng therapy, the mean survival time was 20 months compared to 9 months for 18 patients receiving radiotherapy only. In a second group of hepatoma patients treated with chemotherapy, the survival time nearly doubled among the patients given Fu-zheng therapy (12.5 vs. 6.4 months).

In Shanghai College of Traditional Medicine, a prospective randomized clinical trial was carried out in advanced non-small cell lung cancer patients treated with chemotherapy (cyclophosphamide, vincristine, and fluorouracil for squamous carcinoma, and mitomycin C, vincristine, and fluorouracil for adenocarcinoma) alone or combined with TCM (Table 9). Again, an advantage was found for the combined modality.

A nationwide collaborative study is under way to confirm the above results, so that we may provide some drugs that are useful adjuvants to irradiation and chemotherapy in the treatment of cancer.

Study of Mechanisms

It is still too early to discuss the mechanisms involved in the efficacy of most traditional Chinese medicinal herbs. Some recent data show that several mechanisms might play an important role in their biological activities.

Using the coculture system in cancer patients, we showed that the extracts of *Astragalus membranaceus* and *Ligustrum lucidum* may suppress the activity of excess Ts cells. MNC of cancer patients depressed the mitogen responses of normal cells in a coculture system. This was partially abrogated in most situations by preincubating the patients' cells in the herb extract for 45 min or by irradiation of the patients' cells. There was a significant correlation between the presence of immunodeficiency and the presence of suppressor cell activity. It was also demonstrated that the reduction of Ts cells was correlated with the clinical response to anticancer drug treatment. Thus, the reduction of suppressor cell activity may restore immunocompetence and inhibit tumor growth, and potentially improve the prognosis of the patients.

Astragalus membranaceus may augment the interferon response in mice to virus, and is able to prevent infection by the common cold virus. It potentially has antiviral activity, since it prevented influenza and upper respiratory tract infections in a field study. *Astragalus membranaceus* may affect the content of 3′5′-cyclic adenosine monophosphate in patients' plasma. Because similar changes in cyclin nucleotides occur during stimulation of lymphocytes, the effects of these herbal extracts might be mediated through some changes in cyclic nucleotides in various cellular components of the immune system. In a recent study by our group, a synergistic effect of F3 from *Astragalus membranaceus* and rIL-2 on the induction of lymphokine-activated killer (LAK) cell activity was observed, and an antioxygenation effect of LL-E is also apparent. This may further explain the efficacy of these TCM herbs. The content of some trace elements, such as zinc and magnesium, which are important in the immunity of normal subjects and patients showed some differences.

Future Perspectives

Traditional Chinese medicine can play an important role in the management of cancer patients, especially when used as an adjuvant to other modalities and in supportive care. More than 20 herbs are under investigation, and more than ten have been proved to have an immunomodulating or blood circulation accerating effect. But, in general, many important questions remain to be answered concerning the binding activity of the active components to lymphocytes or monocytes, the target cell, and the molecular mechanisms of action. The following studies are currently underway:

1. Studies to isolate and identify effective components
2. The screening of useful medicinal herbs, either traditional or new
3. Studies of the mechanism of Fu-zheng herbs, including suppression of T cell activity, a synergistic effect with rIL-2 on LAK cells, an effect on interferon production, antiviral activity, etc.
4. Pharmacological study
5. Clinical trials and collaborative studies, including use of herbs as adjuvants and radio- and chemosensitizers, and to combat carcinogenesis in some precancerous diseases, especially in certain high risk groups

References

1. Sun Y et al. (1981) Effect of Fu-zheng therapy in the management of malignant diseases. Chin Med J [Engl] 61: 97-101
2. Sun Y et al. (1983) Preliminary observations on the effects of Chinese medicinal herbs *Astragalus membranaceus* and *Ligustrum lucidum* on lymphocytes' blastogenic responses. J Biol Response Mod 2: 227-237
3. Sun Y et al. (1983) Immune restoration and/or augmentation of local graft versus host reaction by traditional Chinese medicinal herbs. Cancer 52: 70-73
4. Sun Y (1984) Immunomodulating effect of Fu-zheng medicinal herbs. Zhong Xi Yi Tie He Za zhi Ho Tsa Chih 4: 368-370
5. Sun Y et al. (1983) Laboratory studies on the immuno-promoting effect of *Astragalus membranaceus* and *Ligustrum lucidum*. Zhonghua Weishengwuxue He Mianyixue zazhi 3: 211-221

6. Sun Y (1986) Chinese medicinal herbs as biological response modifiers. In: Lotzova E, Herberman RB (eds) Natural immunity against cancer and biological response modification. Karger, Basel, pp 206-211
7. Cai WM et al. (1982) Combination of Chinese herbal medicine and radiotherapy in the treatment of nasopharyngeal carcinoma. J Amer College Trad Chin Med 2: 1-8
8. Li WM et al. (1985) The effects of acid mucopolysaccharide from *Stichopus japanicus* Selenka (SJAMP) on the immune function of mouse. Zhong Guo Zhong Liu Lin Chnang 12: 118-121

Subject Index

MIX
Papier aus verantwortungsvollen Quellen
Paper from responsible sources
FSC® C105338

If you have any concerns about our products,
you can contact us on
ProductSafety@springernature.com

In case Publisher is established outside the EU,
the EU authorized representative is:
Springer Nature Customer Service Center GmbH
Europaplatz 3, 69115 Heidelberg, Germany

Printed by Libri Plureos GmbH
in Hamburg, Germany